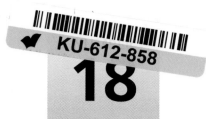

Recent Advances in

Histopathology

Edited by

David G. Lowe MD FRCS FRCPath FIBiol

Professor of Surgical Pathology, St Bartholomew's and The Royal London
School of Medicine and Dentistry, Queen Mary and Westfield College,
University of London, London, UK

James C. E. Underwood MD FRCPath

Joseph Hunter Professor of Pathology and Head of Department, Department
of Pathology, University of Sheffield, Sheffield, UK

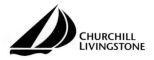

CHURCHILL
LIVINGSTONE

EDINBURGH LONDON NEW YORK PHILADELPHIA SYDNEY TORONTO 1999

CHURCHILL LIVINGSTONE
An imprint of Harcourt Brace & Company Limited

© Harcourt Brace & Company Limited 1999

First published 1999

ISBN 0-443-060363

ISSN 0-0143 6953

British Library Cataloguing in Publication Data
A catalogue record for this book is available from the British Library

Library of Congress Cataloging in Publication Data
A catalog record for this book is available from the Library of Congress

Medical knowledge is constantly changing. As new information becomes available, changes in treatment, procedures, equipment and the use of drugs become necessary. The editors and the publishers have, as far as possible, taken care to ensure that the information given in this text is accurate and up to date. However, readers are strongly advised to confirm that the information, especially with regard to drug usage, complies with current legislation and standards of practice.

Commissioning Editor – Laurence Hunter
Project Controller – Frances Affleck
Designer – Sarah Cape

Typeset by B.A. & G.M. Haddock
Printed in China
NPCC/01

Recent Advances in

Histopathology

DATE DUE		
GAYLORD		PP

Recent Advances in Histopathology 17

Edited by Peter P. Anthony, Roderick N. M. MacSween & David G. Lowe

ISBN 0-443-05766-4
ISSN 0143 6953

You can place your order by contacting your local medical bookseller or Customer Service Department, Harcourt Brace and Company Ltd, Foots Cray High Street, Sidcup, Kent DA14 5AP, UK

Tel: +44 (0)181 308 5710
Fax +44 (0)181 309 0807

Contents

Preface

As the incoming Editors of *Recent Advances in Histopathology* we owe a great deal to Peter Anthony and Roddy MacSween, our predecessors for the last 20 years. Under their guidance *Recent Advances* became established as essential reading for all histopathologists. By their thoughtful choice of topics and authors they succeeded admirably in including in each edition a balanced mixture of scientific principles and practice, taking readers to the leading edge of advancing knowledge and aiming to reconcile controversy. Trainees firmly (but mistakenly) believed that with each edition Peter and Roddy set the syllabus for the examinations of the Royal College of Pathologists and similar professional bodies outside the UK; consultants and senior specialists recognised this book as the principal source of guidance on good professional practice. The success of their mission is evident from the sales of the books in the series, from the well-thumbed copies of previous editions, and from the numerous citations of articles from *Recent Advances* in the reference lists of scientific papers.

We now have the challenge and the advantage of inheriting this successful venture that reflects so well the sterling work of Peter and Roddy.

1999

D.G.Lowe
J. C. E. Underwood

Contributors

Peter H. Bartels PhD
Professor of Pathology, Optical Sciences Center, University of Arizona, Tucson, Arizona, USA

Ian D. Buley MA BM BCh FRCPath
Consultant Pathologist, Department of Cellular Pathology, John Radcliffe Hospital, Headington, Oxford, UK

Simon S. Cross BSc MD MRCPath
Senior Lecturer and Honorary Consultant Histopathologist, Department of Pathology, University of Sheffield Medical School, Sheffield, UK

Paola Domizio BSc MBBS, FRCPath
Senior Lecturer in Histopathology, St Bartholomew's and The Royal London School of Medicine and Dentistry, Queen Mary and Westfield College, University of London, London, UK

Richard G. A. Faragher BSc DPhil
Senior Fellow, Ocular Research Group, Department of Pharmacy and Biomolecular Studies, University of Brighton, Brighton, UK

Thomas Gahm PhD
Vice President Computer Science, Autocyte Inc., Burlington, North Carolina, USA

Andrew K. Graham PhD
Telepathology Coordinator, Nuffield Department of Pathology and Bacteriology, University of Oxford, John Radcliffe Hospital, Oxford, UK

Robert P. Hasserjian MD
Senior Lecturer, Department of Histopathology, Imperial College School of Medicine, Hammersmith Hospital, London, UK

Amanda Herbert MB BS FRCPath
Consultant Cyto/Histopathologist, Histopathology Department, St Thomas' Hospital, London, UK

James W. Ironside BMSc MBChB FRCPath
Reader in Pathology, University of Edinburgh and Honorary Consultant Neuropathologist, Western General Hospitals Trust, Edinburgh, UK

Sezgin M. Ismail MRCP FRCPath
Senior Lecturer in Pathology, University of Wales College of Medicine, Cardiff, UK

Stephen R.D. Johnston MA MRCP PhD
Senior Lecturer and Honorary Consultant in Medical Oncologist, Department of Medicine, The Royal Marsden NHS Trust, London, UK

David Kipling BA(Hons) DPhil
Senior Lecturer in Cancer Biology, Fellow of the Lister Institute for Preventive Medicine, Department of Pathology, University of Wales College of Medicine, Cardiff, UK

Thomas Krausz MD FRCPath
Professor of Surgical Pathology, Department of Histopathology, Imperial College School of Medicine, Hammersmith Hospital, London, UK

F. Joel W-M. Leong MB BS
Clinical Lecturer, Nuffield Department of Pathology and Bacteriology, University of Oxford, John Radcliffe Hospital, Oxford, UK

David G. Lowe MD FRCS FRCPath FIBiol
Professor of Surgical Pathology, St Bartholomew's and The Royal London School of Medicine and Dentistry, Queen Mary and Westfield College, University of London, London, UK

Sebastian B. Lucas FRCP FRCPath
Professor of Clinical Histopathology, UMDS Department of Histopathology, St Thomas' Hospital Medical School, London, UK

David MacVicar MRCP FRCR
Consultant Radiologist, Academic Department of Diagnostic Radiology, Royal Marsden NHS Trust, Sutton, UK

Jo E. Martin MA MBBS PhD MRCPath
Professor of Neuropathology, St Bartholomew's and The Royal London School of Medicine and Dentistry, Queen Mary and Westfield College, University of London, London, UK

James O'D. McGee MD PhD FRCPath FRCP MA
Professor and Head of Department, Nuffield Department of Pathology and Bacteriology, University of Oxford, John Radcliffe Hospital, Oxford, UK

Rodolfo Montironi MD FRCPath
Associate Professor of Pathology, Institute of Pathological Anatomy and

Contributors

Histopathology, School of Medicine, University of Ancona, Azienda Sanitaria 'Umberto 1°', Torrette di Ancona, Italy

Jem Rashbass BSc MBBS PhD MRCPath
Clinical Director of Biomedical Computing and Honorary Consultant Haematopathologist, Cambridge University, Addenbrooke's Hospital, Cambridge, UK

Neil A. Shepherd MBBS FRCPath
Consultant Pathologist and Visiting Professor at Cranfield University, Department of Histopathology, Gloucestershire Royal Hospital, Gloucester, UK

Virpi V. Smith PhD
Clinical Scientist and Honorary Lecturer, Institute of Child Health and Camelia Botnar Labs, Great Ormond Street Hospital for Children NHS Trust, London, UK

Deborah Thompson MSc
Principal Systems Programmer, Optical Sciences Center, University of Arizona, Tucson, Arizona, USA

Wiebren A. A. Tjalma MD
Department of Obstetrics and Gynaecology, Division of Gynaecological Oncology, Antwerp University Hospital (UZA), Edegem, Belgium

James C. E. Underwood MD FRCPath
Joseph Hunter Professor of Pathology and Head of Department, Department of Pathology, University of Sheffield, Sheffield, UK

Peter A. van Dam MD PhD
Consultant Gynaecological Oncologist, Department of Obstetrics and Gynaecology, Sint Augustinus Hospital, Wilrijk, Belgium

Bryan F. Warren MBBS MRCPath
Consultant Gastrointestinal Pathologist, Department of Cellular Pathology, John Radcliffe Hospital, Oxford, UK

James W. Ironside

CHAPTER 1

New variant Creutzfeldt-Jakob disease

Creutzfeldt-Jakob disease (CJD) is one of a group of disorders known as transmissible spongiform encephalopathies (TSE; Bastian 1991; Brown & Bradley 1998). These rare fatal neurodegenerative disorders, which occur in man and animals, have attracted considerable scientific, public and political interest in recent years after advances in scientific understanding of the unconventional agents associated with these diseases, and in light of the large epidemic of bovine spongiform encephalopathy (BSE) in the UK. The first TSE to be recognised was scrapie, a naturally occurring disorder affecting sheep and goats, which is endemic in the UK (Kimberlin 1981). Most of the scientific studies on the nature of the transmissible agents in TSE have been undertaken in scrapie, using experimental transmission to mouse or hamster (Kimberlin 1981, Prusiner 1993, 1998). Although the precise nature of the transmissible agents in TSE remains uncertain, there is increasing evidence to support the prion hypothesis, which states that the transmissible agent is composed entirely of a protein, the prion protein (PrP), which is a modified form of a normal cell surface glycoprotein that is highly conserved in mammals (Prusiner 1982). It is distributed in a wide range of tissues and expressed at highest levels in neurones in the central nervous system (CNS; Prusiner 1993). Earlier studies on the TSE agents indicated that they were remarkably small, resistant to physical and chemical agents which inactivate the conventional viruses and bacteria, and transmissible both within and among animal species (Pattison 1965, Adams et al 1969, Kimberlin 1981). Transmission from one species to another is usually hindered by the species barrier, where the initial transmission is often characterised by a prolonged incubation period and changes in the distribution of pathological changes in the brain (Kimberlin & Walker 1988, Prusiner 1993, 1994). Subsequent passage in the recipient species, however, is usually characterised by adaptation to the new host, with a shortened incubation period and a more reproducible pattern of brain pathology (Kimberlin & Walker 1988).

Dr James W. Ironside, CJD Surveillance Unit, Western General Hospital, Edinburgh EH4 2XU, UK

Table 1.1 Human TSE

Idiopathic	Sporadic CJD
Acquired	Iatrogenic CJD New variant CJD Kuru
Genetic	Familial CJD GSS (classical and variants) Fatal familial insomnia

Prion protein (PrP) is encoded by a gene on the short arm of chromosome 20 in human beings and the entire open reading frame is contained in a single exon (Prusiner 1993). Studies of the PrP gene in human beings have identified a number of pathogenic mutations and insertions that are associated with familial CJD and other inherited forms of human TSE (Baker & Ridley 1992, Goldfarb et al 1994). At codon 129 in the PrP gene, there is a naturally occurring polymorphism (of either methionine or valine) which is of major importance as it affects both clinical and pathological disease phenotypes (de Silva et al 1994, Parchi et al 1996, MacDonald et al 1996), and influences disease susceptibility in human beings (Collinge et al 1991, Palmer 1991).

HUMAN TSE

CJD was the first human TSE to be described, in the third decade of this century (Creutzfeldt 1920, Jakob 1921). However, review of Creutzfeldt's original case has indicated that it is probably not an example of a human TSE but may represent a metabolic encephalopathy. Jakob's original descriptions included a family with CJD: subsequent analysis of material from one of the family members revealed a pathogenic mutation in the PrP gene (Brown et al 1994a). Human TSE can occur as a sporadic, familial or acquired disorder (Table 1.1; Bastian 1991, Prusiner 1994). The commonest human TSE is sporadic CJD, which occurs with a world-wide incidence of about 1 case per million population per year, occurring most frequently in individuals aged 60–69 years (Brown et al 1986, Will et al 1998). A wide age range may be involved, however, from very occasional cases occurring in teenagers (Brown et al 1985, Berman et al 1988) to patients in the tenth decade of life (Brown et al 1986, Will 1993).

Most cases of sporadic CJD present as a rapidly progressive dementia associated with movement disorders including myoclonus, pyramidal and extra-pyramidal rigidity, cerebellar ataxia and visual abnormalities (Brown et al 1986, Brown et al 1987, Will 1993). Human TSE is invariably fatal, and most patients in the UK with sporadic CJD are dead within 5 months of disease onset (Will 1991, Will 1996). There is a wide range of clinical phenotypic variation, including groups of patients who present with particular clinical features, such as cerebellar signs and symptoms or prominent visual symptoms (Brown et al 1986, Bastian 1991, Richardson & Masters 1995). About two-thirds of patients with sporadic CJD have a characteristic abnormality in the electroencephalogram (EEG), with a prominent triphasic complex occurring with a periodicity of 1 Hz (Bortone et al 1994, Will 1996). Epidemiological studies have not established the cause of sporadic CJD (Brown et al 1987, Will 1993, Will 1996) and there is no evidence to suggest that this disorder results from exposure to animal TSE, particularly scrapie in sheep. Homozygosity at codon 129 in the PrP gene is a relative risk factor for both sporadic and acquired forms of CJD (Collinge et al 1991, Palmer et al 1991), though the disease mechanism behind this observation is uncertain.

Familial forms of human TSE may account for up to 15% of all cases; most of the patients have a family history of a neurological disorder (Baker & Ridley 1992, Goldfarb et al 1994). The first PrP genetic mutation associated with a human disease was a proline–leucine mutation at codon 102 (Hsiao et al 1989), which is associated with the Gerstmann-Straussler-Scheinker syndrome (GSS), a rare familial disorder characterised by progressive ataxia (Gerstman et al 1936). Since then, an increasing number of genetic abnormalities have been identified in the PrP gene, most of which are pathogenic (Baker & Ridley 1992, Goldfarb et al 1994). In addition to point mutations, a number of pathogenic insertions have been identified in the octapeptide repeat region (Owen et al 1989, Goldfarb et al 1994). Phenotypic variation in clinical and pathological terms also occurs in the genetic forms of human TSE, a particularly striking example of which is found at codon 178, where an aspartic acid–asparagine mutation can occur in an allele that encodes either methionine or valine at codon 129. If methionine is encoded, the patients usually have the clinical features of fatal familial insomnia, with prominent sleep disturbances, hypo-thalamic and endocrine abnormalities and an absence of dementia (Medori et al 1992). If a valine allele is present at codon 129 in addition to the codon 178 mutation, the affected patient exhibits clinical features characteristic of CJD (Goldfarb et al 1991).

Human TSE were also recognised to occur as acquired disorders in two main groups of patients: those with iatrogenic CJD (Brown et al 1992, Brown et al 1994b) and with kuru (Klatzo 1959, Alpers et al 1987). CJD has been accidentally transmitted from one patient to another during invasive surgical and medical procedures, including the use of neurosurgical instruments and stereotactic EEG electrodes that had been inadequately decontaminated, by corneal and dura mater grafts and, most frequently, by human pituitary hormone replacement with either growth hormone or gonadotrophins extracted from cadaveric pituitary glands. As might be expected with such a wide range of exposure routes, the clinical and pathological features of these iatrogenic CJD cases are variable. However, it has been observed that most cases with 'central' inoculation (corneal and dura mater grafts and contaminated neurosurgical instruments) have clinical and pathological features similar to those of sporadic CJD, while the pituitary hormone recipients with a 'peripheral' route of exposure (such as intravenous or intramuscular injection) have a more prolonged illness with prominent cerebellar signs and symptoms and a neuropathological profile that is centred on severe cerebellar degeneration (Brown et al 1992)

Kuru was an unusual example of human TSE that was transmitted through practices associated with ritualistic cannibalism. It occurred predominantly in the Fore tribe in Papua New Guinea and, in the 1950s, was a major cause of death in the tribe, affecting mostly women and children who were exposed to brain tissue at the funeral ritual (Alpers 1987). Kuru was also characterised by predominant cerebellar signs and symptoms, but with other features including emotional lability and changes in personality and intellectual function. The neuropathology of kuru is also concentrated in the cerebellum, which often contains amyloid plaques composed of prion protein – the so-called 'kuru plaques' (Klatzo et al 1959).

Studies on kuru and iatrogenic CJD have provided some interesting data on incubation periods for human TSE. In 'central' inoculation of the CJD agent, incubation periods are shortest, usually about 18 months (Brown et al 1994b). With 'peripheral' routes of exposure in cases associated with pituitary hormone therapy the incubation period is longer, at about 12 years (Brown et al 1992, Brown et al 1994b). Similar findings have been reported in kuru, which is presumably due to gastro-intestinal exposure to the transmissible agent (Alpers 1987). The youngest case of kuru occurred in a child of about 5 years, which gives a minimum incubation period for the disease. Although the ritualistic practices associated with the transmission of kuru have been abandoned, occasional cases still occur representing the end point of incubation, which may be well over 30 years (Alpers 1987).

DIAGNOSIS OF HUMAN TSE

Clinical criteria have been formulated for the diagnosis of CJD and related human TSE. For sporadic CJD, cases can be classified on clinical grounds as probable or possible depending on the clinical features and EEG findings (Will 1996). Confirmation of the clinical diagnosis can be made only after examination of brain tissue by biopsy or necropsy. This places a high priority on securing necropsy on patients with these disorders, and for the development of sensitive and specific techniques for neuropathological diagnosis (Budka et al 1995, Kretzschmar et al 1996). Although CJD is transmissible, there is no apparent occupational risk in healthcare professionals, including mortuary technicians, neuropathologists and laboratory technical staff (Brown et al 1986, Will 1991, Will 1993). The main risk of accidental transmission of CJD is inoculation of brain tissue into the body, which can be avoided during the course of necropsy by the use of appropriate instruments and protective clothing, including cut-resistant or chain mail gloves (Ironside & Bell 1996). Because of the limited number of strategies available for decontamination of the CJD agent (Table 1.2), the main aim at necropsy is to minimise contamination to the environment. It has, therefore, been suggested that autopsy can be performed in a body bag on such cases, using absorbent material to contain spillages and leaks. Disposable instruments should be used wherever possible, and non-disposable items, such as handsaws, should be cleaned, decontaminated (Table 1.2) and autoclaved. Operating policies for autopsy procedures and tissue handling in human TSE have been recently published (Ironside & Bell 1996, Bell & Ironside 1993, Budka 1995).

The neuropathological diagnosis of human TSE depends upon the autopsy, followed by brain fixation and selection of a suitable number of CNS blocks in order to reveal the full spectrum of pathology in each case (Budka et al 1995,

Table 1.2 Decontamination procedures for human TSE agents

Autoclaving (porous load)	A single cycle 134°C, 30 lb psi, 18 min holding time at temperature
	Six separate cycles 134°C, 30 lb psi, 18 min holding time at temperature
Chemicals	Exposure (1 h) to sodium hypochlorite containing 20 000 ppm available chlorine
	Exposure (1 h) to 2 M sodium hydroxide with constant rewetting of surfaces

Kretzschmar et al 1996). Ideally this should include several areas of cerebral cortex including all the main lobes, hippocampus, basal ganglia and thalamus, hypothalamus, cerebellum, brainstem and spinal cord. Histological diagnosis has for many years depended on the identification of the characteristic spongiform change in the neuropil (Fig. 1.1; Masters & Richardson 1981), which affects the grey matter and may begin as small irregular rounded lesions, 2–10 µm in diameter, with neuronal loss and reactive gliosis as secondary, but non-specific, features. Occasional patients with human TSE have amyloid plaques: these occur particularly in patients with sporadic CJD in those who are either valine homozygotes or heterozygotes at codon 129 in the PrP gene (de Silva et al 1994, Parchi et al 1996); with kuru (Klatzo et al 1959); with familial TSE (including GSS; Bastian 1991, Bell & Ironside 1993); and with iatrogenic CJD, particularly following inoculation with human growth hormone (Bell & Ironside 1993, Billette de Villemeur et al 1994). These small amyloid plaques can occasionally be hard to detect on conventional microscopy but their presence is beautifully revealed by immunocytochemical techniques for PrP (Kitamoto & Tateishi 1988, Hayward et al 1994, Bell et al

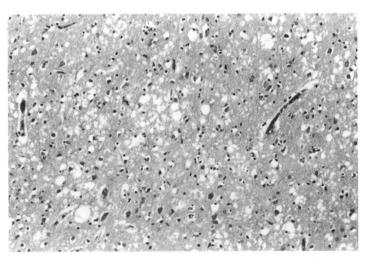

Fig. 1.1 The cerebral cortex in sporadic CJD shows widespread spongiform change, with confluent vacuolation in several cortical regions. No amyloid plaques are present. Haematoxylin and eosin × 180.

1997). There are no sequence differences between the normal and disease-associated forms of PrP (Prusiner 1994) and, consequently, most PrP antibodies cannot distinguish between these isoforms (Kitamoto & Tateishi 1988, Bell et al 1997). In order to overcome this potential difficulty, proteinase K is used in Western blots to permit distinction between normal and disease-associated PrP isoforms (Parchi et al 1996). This enzyme degrades the normal PrP isoform leaving a partially degraded disease-associated isoform that has differential proteinase K sensitivity, which may relate to conformational changes that, in turn, are influenced by codon 129 genotype and protein glycosylation (Prusiner 1998). Prion protein has two potential glycosylation sites which permit detection of differential glycosylation in the disease-associated PrP isoform (Parchi et al 1996).

Table 1.3 Tissue pretreatments for PrP immunocytochemistry

Float 5 μm sections on to Vectabond-coated slides
Sections to water
Picric acid 15 mM (to remove formalin pigment)
Water
Autoclave in distilled water at 121°C for 10 min, or microwave at full power for 3 × 5 min
Water
96% formic acid, 10 min
4 M guanidine thiocyanate 2 h at 4°C
Water, then Tris buffer
Blocking serum 10 min
Primary PrP antibody (Bell et al 1997, Kitamoto & Tateishi 1988)
Wash in Tris buffer
Secondary antibody
Wash in Tris buffer, then visualise, counterstain, dehydrate and mount

Immunocytochemistry can be performed for PrP on paraffin wax embedded and formalin fixed tissues, though this requires pretreatment steps to minimise staining of any residual normal PrP and enhance the immunostaining of disease-associated PrP (*see* Table 1.3; Bell et al 1997). The development of reliable techniques for PrP immunocytochemistry has greatly facilitated diagnosis and research in human TSE. In paraffin wax sections, there is a remarkable variation in the distribution and nature of the PrP accumulation in CJD which is partly influenced by the codon 129 genotype in the PrP gene (see above; Parchi 1996, MacDonald et al 1996). Likewise, there is a wide spectrum in the morphology of PrP deposits and plaques occurring in familial and iatrogenic diseases and in kuru. In the acquired forms of human TSE, it is not certain whether this availability reflects strain differences in the transmissible agent responsible for these disorders or whether host factors are involved.

BSE was first reported in the UK in 1986 (Wells et al 1987), since when the disease reached epidemic proportions, with around 1200 cattle per week dying of the disease in 1992–1993 (Anderson et al 1996, Ministry of Agriculture 1996). Early epidemiological studies identified that meat and bonemeal animal feed was the source of the epidemic and a ban on the use of this animal feed for cattle in 1988 undoubtedly limited the peak incidence of BSE in subsequent years (Wilesmith et al 1991, Anderson et al 1996). The source of the contamination of meat and bonemeal feed is unknown; it has been suggested that sheep scrapie may have initially caused a disease in cattle that was then subsequently passaged into other cattle (Wilesmith et al 1991), or possibly that BSE was a rare sporadic disease in cattle which then spread rapidly throughout the cattle population through contaminated meat and bonemeal. BSE affected predominantly dairy herds, most of whom are in the south and south-west of England. Its incidence is now declining greatly in the UK after the implementation of measures to control the use of meat and bone meal in feedstuffs for farm animals (Anderson et al 1996, Ministry of Agriculture 1996). BSE is a stereotyped disease in terms of both clinical and pathological features. Confirmation of the diagnosis of BSE depends on neuropathological examination of the brain, which in most cases shows spongiform change that is most severe in the brain stem, where neuronal vacuolation is prominent (Wells et al 1987). Analysis of the clinical and pathological features of BSE suggested a single agent 'strain' and this was subsequently confirmed by strain typing studies in inbred mice, which showed that all the cases of BSE studied had a similar strain of TSE agent in terms of the uniform incubation period in the mice and the characteristic neuropathological changes occurring in the mouse brains (Bruce et al 1994, 1996).

The incidence of BSE has greatly declined in the UK – recent estimates indicate that at least 700,000 cattle died with the disease during the period 1986–1996 (Anderson et al 1996). BSE has been transmitted to other species, including domestic and wild cats (Wyatt et al 1991, Willoughby et al 1992), and exotic antelopes and other ungulates in zoos (Kirkwood & Cunningham 1994). For the domestic cats and zoo ungulates, the exposure to BSE was thought to be through animal meat and bone meal. In the wild cats in zoos, it is presumed that these ate cattle carcasses that were contaminated with BSE. It, therefore, appears that the enteral route of infection with BSE is most likely for these other animals, despite the 'species barrier'. Although there is no history to suggest that the pre-existing animal TSE, scrapie, was a risk to human health, the identification of the new disease, BSE, in cattle in the UK in the late 1980s prompted additional consideration of whether the BSE agent could cause disease in humans. This resulted in the establishment of the National CJD Surveillance Project in 1990.

CJD SURVEILLANCE

Surveillance of CJD in the UK was re-instituted in May 1990 to detect any changes in the incidence or disease phenotype of CJD (in terms of clinical and pathological features) that might represent the effects of the BSE agent in man. Case notification occurs from healthcare professionals (mainly neurologists and neuropathologists) throughout the UK to the CJD Surveillance Unit in Edinburgh (Will 1996). Detailed epidemiological and clinical data are obtained within the framework of a case control study, which uses identical methodology to other parallel studies in European countries with a much lower incidence of BSE (Delasnerie-Laupretre et al 1995). The epidemiological data are largely obtained by a questionnaire that is administered to the relatives of the patient. Blood is taken with informed consent from suspected patients for PrP genetic studies. Additional clinical data, including EEG and neuroradiological imaging studies, are also reviewed and the cases classified on clinical grounds as probable or possible CJD (Will 1996). Necropsy is performed in about 70% of all suspected cases, though in younger patients the autopsy rate is over 90%. Autopsies are generally performed by neuropathologists operating in regional centres throughout the UK, though many general pathologists are also able to undertake autopsies in cases of suspected CJD and occasional cases are referred directly to the Surveillance Unit in Edinburgh.

The results of the autopsies are studied and most cases reviewed in the CJD Surveillance Unit laboratory, where PrP immunocytochemistry is performed on fixed tissues. All pathologists undertaking a necropsy in a case of suspected CJD are encouraged to freeze a portion of tissue from the brain for further studies, including Western blot analysis of PrP and for potential transmission studies (Table 1.4). The CJD Surveillance Unit runs a brain bank for fixed and frozen tissues from cases of CJD and controls (including age-matched non-demented individuals and individuals dying with other forms of dementia) and for non-CNS tissues (Bell & Ironside 1997). This invaluable resource of material is extensively used for research purposes both within the UK and overseas.

Table 1.4 What to take in a CJD autopsy

Essential	Frozen brain tissue (frontal lobe and cerebellum minimum, a half frozen brain may be easier)
	Fixed brain and pituitary gland
	Other organs relevant to the immediate cause of death or medical history
Desirable	Spinal cord
	Lymphoid tissue (tonsil, lymph nodes and spleen) fixed and frozen
	Frozen blood for DNA analysis

A similar prospective surveillance project for CJD was carried out in the UK in 1980–1984, based in Oxford. Retrospective data have been studied (including all death certificates in which CJD and related diseases were mentioned), enabling figures for the incidence of CJD to be collected and analysed retrospectively since 1970 (Cousens et al 1997). The CJD Surveillance Unit produces an annual report which contains the results of clinical, pathological and epidemiological data, including findings from the case-control studies.

NEW VARIANT CJD

In 1996, the CJD Surveillance Unit published details of a series of 10 patients with a TSE which represented an apparently new variant of CJD (Will et al 1996). The clinical features in these patients were relatively uniform and characterised by an early age at disease onset (16–39 years, mean 26 years) in contrast to sporadic CJD in the UK (mean age at onset 65 years). The clinical presenting features were also unusual, and comprised psychiatric features in about two-thirds of patients (including personality change, depression and behavioural alterations) (Zeidler et al 1997a), with sensory abnormalities in the remaining patients (including paraesthesiae and dysaesthesiae affecting the face, hands, legs and feet) (Zeidler et al 1997b). The initial referral was variable, often to a psychiatrist or general physician, but patients were referred to neurologists once neurological symptoms had been identified. The first neurological symptom to appear in most cases was cerebellar ataxia, which was later accompanied by other movement disorders including myoclonus, chorea and pyramidal and extrapyramidal signs and symptoms (Will et al 1996). Dementia was present in most cases, though most patients died without severe intellectual impairment, and was often accompanied by visual abnormalities and akinetic mutism in the final stages of the illness. The duration of this illness was unusually lengthy for CJD, on average around 14 months (range 9–30 months) in contrast to sporadic CJD with which patients survive for about 5 months. None of the patients exhibited the characteristic EEG changes associated with sporadic CJD. Genetic analysis showed that all cases were methionine homozygotes at codon 129 in the

Table 1.5 Comparison between new variant and sporadic CJD

	New variant CJD	Sporadic CJD
Incidence and distribution	37 cases in UK, 1 in France	Worldwide incidence of 1/million/annum
Mean age at onset (years)	26	65
Mean duration of illness (months)	14	5
Clinical presentation	Psychiatric features, sensory symptoms	Rapidly progressive dementia
PrP codon 129 genotype	MM 100%	MM 80%, VV 10%, MV 10%
EEG	No specific abnormality	Periodic sharp wave complexes
Experimental transmission to mice	Transmissible agent is identical BSE	Transmissible agents are distinct from BSE

PrP gene, with no pathogenic insertions or mutations detected (Will et al 1996). The major clinical differences between sporadic and new variant CJD are summarised in Table 1.5.

Since the initial report, one similar case has been identified in France (Chazot et al 1996) and 27 others in the UK. The subsequent patients have shown a relatively uniform clinical phenotype (Zeidler et al 1997b), and though the mean age is about 26 years, the oldest patient was 52 years old at disease onset. The additional cases show a similar PrP genotype to the first 10 patients. There is no evidence of clustering of cases in terms of their place of residence in the UK and no common occupational exposure to BSE has been identified (Cousens et al 1999). Detailed clinical and epidemiological studies have not so far identified any other specific risk factors for this new disease and, in particular, no source of possible iatrogenic infection has been identified. All patients have eaten meat or meat products for at least part of the 1980s and, therefore, could have been exposed to the BSE agent at that time.

Table 1.6 Characteristic neuropathological features of new variant CJD

- Multiple florid plaques in cerebral and cerebellar cortex on haematoxylin and eosin, periodic acid/Schiff, Alcian blue and Gallyas stains
- Spongiform change most marked in basal ganglia
- Severe posterior thalamic gliosis
- Multiple small cluster PrP plaques on immunocytochemistry in most brain regions
- Amorphous PrP deposits around neurones and capillaries on immunocytochemistry in cerebral and cerebellar cortex
- Perineuronal and periaxonal PrP accumulation in the basal ganglia on immunocytochemistry
- PrP glycosylation pattern after proteinase K digestion on Western blots is identical to BSE and distinct from sporadic CJD

NEUROPATHOLOGY OF NEW VARIANT CJD

All cases of new variant CJD exhibit a characteristic spectrum of neuropathology (Will et al 1996, Ironside 1996) which comprises the four characteristic features of other TSEs – spongiform change, neuronal loss, reactive gliosis and amyloid plaque formation – but is clearly separable on morphological and immunocytochemical grounds from other forms of CJD (Table 1.6). The most striking neuropathological abnormality is in the grey matter of the cerebral cortex and cerebellum, where spongiform change is accompanied by numerous amyloid plaques with a fibrillary structure surrounded by a halo or rim of spongiform change (Figs 1.2–1.4; Ironside et al 1996). This type of plaque resembles the so-called 'florid' plaque which was first described in experimental mice following transmission of Icelandic scrapie (Fraser 1979). The amyloid component of the plaques varies in size from around 5–50 µm. The plaques are scattered throughout the cerebral and cerebellar cortex and are occasionally present in the subpial space. Spongiform

Fig. 1.2
The cerebral cortex in new variant CJD also shows spongiform change, but contains amyloid plaques surrounded by a peripheral rim of vacuolation (centre). Haematoxylin and eosin × 240.

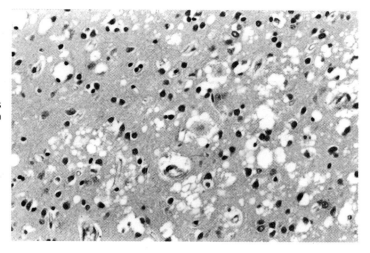

Fig. 1.3
A high power view of the characteristic plaques in new variant CJD shows a central dense eosinophilic core with a fibrillary periphery, surrounded by an irregular rim of vacuolation. Haematoxylin and eosin × 360.

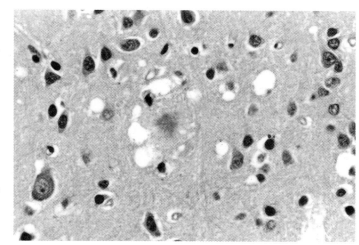

Fig. 1.4
The cerebellar cortex in new variant CJD shows spongiform change and gliosis, particularly in the molecular layer, which also contains a fibrillary plaque with surrounding spongiform change (centre). Haematoxylin and eosin × 240.

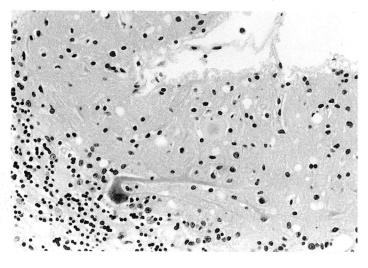

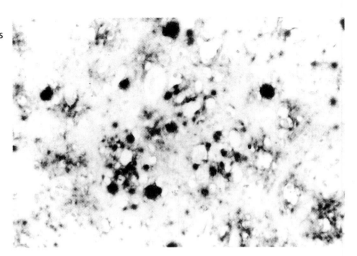

Fig. 1.5
Immunocytochemistry for PrP in the cerebral cortex in new variant CJD shows several large densely-staining plaques, multiple smaller plaques which tend to occur in clusters, and amorphous PrP deposits around small neurones. KG9 monoclonal antibody × 240.

change and plaque formation is most conspicuous in the occipital cortex and, elsewhere, the spongiform change is often patchy, occurring at any layer within the cerebral cortex. Severe spongiform change is accompanied by astrocytosis and neuronal loss which is most evident in the occipital cortex. The amyloid plaques stain strongly with periodic acid–Schiff, Alcian blue and the Gallyas technique, which also stains smaller plaques which are not evident on routine stained sections. These plaques also stain strongly by immunocyto-chemistry for PrP, which demonstrates the large florid plaques, smaller plaques frequently occurring in clusters within the intact neuropil, and accumulation of PrP around the capillaries and cells within the cortex (including small neurones and occasional glial cells) (Fig. 1.5). These diffuse deposits of PrP are particularly characteristic for new variant CJD and are not encountered in sporadic, iatrogenic or familial CJD (Bastian 1991, Bell & Ironside 1993, Budka et al 1995, Kretzschmar et al 1996, Parchi 1996, Ironside 1998).

Hippocampal involvement is characterised by patchy spongiform change involving the CA1 region, parasubiculum, subiculum and temporal cortex. Occasional plaques are identified within the areas of spongiform change and immunocytochemistry for PrP shows strong staining of these plaques with a more diffuse or synaptic pattern of positivity in the grey matter. Spongiform change is particularly prominent in the basal ganglia, especially in the caudate nucleus (Fig. 1.6). Amyloid plaques are occasionally present in this region, and immunocytochemistry for PrP shows a pattern of PrP accumulation different from that in the cerebral and cerebellar cortex, which may reflect the different synaptic organisation in this region of the brain. Perineuronal and peri-axonal deposits of PrP are particularly common, with numerous linear deposits occasionally forming small plaque-like structures or nodular aggregates around neurones (Fig. 1.7). In the thalamus and hypothalamus, a more synaptic pattern of PrP accumulation is noted with occasional plaques, but the most striking abnormality in these regions is severe gliosis and neuronal loss in the dorsomedial nucleus, posterior thalamic nuclei and pulvinar (Fig. 1.8). The severity of the thalamic pathology may reflect the sensory abnormalities experienced by some patients as thalamic pain (Zeidler et al 1997b). In the

Fig. 1.6
The caudate nucleus in new variant CJD shows severe spongiform change with accompanying gliosis, but few amyloid plaques are present. Haematoxylin and eosin × 180.

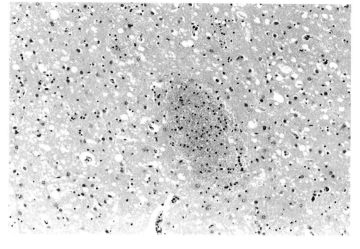

Fig. 1.7
Immunocyto chemistry for PrP in the caudate nucleus in new variant CJD shows strong staining of neurones and linear PrP accumulation around axons (centre) in contrast to the patterns of accumulation in the cerebral cortex (Fig. 1.5). KG9 monoclonal antibody × 360.

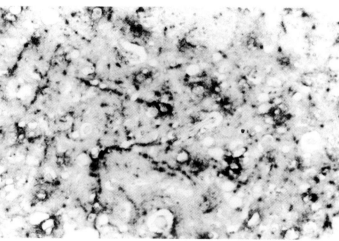

Fig. 1.8
The posterior thalamus in new variant CJD shows severe neuronal loss with extensive and severe gliosis, but relatively little spongiform change and very few amyloid plaques. Haematoxylin and eosin × 240.

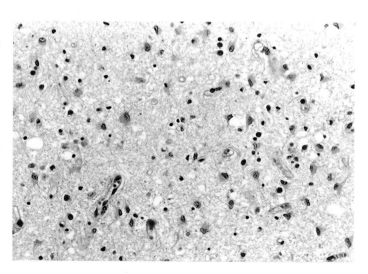

Fig. 1.9
The pontine nuclei in new variant CJD show punctate positivity for PrP in an irregular distribution, apparently within the cytoplasm and also at the cell boundary, suggesting synaptic accumulation. KG9 monoclonal antibody × 360.

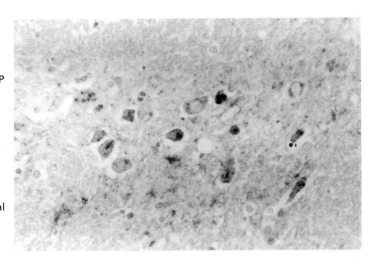

brain stem, spongiform change and amyloid plaques are not prominent features though there is widespread accumulation of PrP in the diffuse or synaptic pattern, particularly in the peri-aqueductal grey matter and colliculi, and in the pontine nuclei. Many of the neurones in the pontine nuclei show punctate positivity for PrP partly in the cytoplasm (Fig. 1.9). In the cerebellum, the patterns of PrP accumulation are similar to those in the cerebral cortex with numerous plaques also present in the granular layer and occasionally in the white matter (Fig. 1.10). Neuronal loss is variable in the cerebellum and usually involves the granular layer, with accompanying gliosis in a patchy distribution. This is reflected in the cerebellar atrophy which has been identified on naked eye examination of the brain in occasional patients. Quantitative studies of the neuropathology in new variant CJD confirms the severe involvement of the occipital lobe and cerebellar cortex in terms of PrP accumulation, while astrocytosis is more pronounced in the thalamus than in other brain regions (Ironside et al 1996).

Comparison of the neuropathology of new variant CJD with sporadic CJD in older patients who are methionine homozygotes shows an entirely different pattern of pathology, with the sporadic CJD patients showing spongiform change particularly involving the cerebral cortex in the absence of amyloid plaques (de Silva et al 1994, Parchi et al 1996). PrP accumulation in these cases is usually perivacuolar or synaptic with none of the complicated plaque structures or the perivascular or pericellular deposits seen in new variant CJD (MacDonald et al 1998, Ironside 1998). Likewise, new variant CJD is distinguishable from iatrogenic CJD after peripheral inoculation of human growth hormone (Bell & Ironside 1993, Billette de Villemeur et al 1994), particularly in terms of the widespread cortical pathology, numerous florid plaques and high levels of PrP accumulation. Comparison with kuru shows a much more widespread accumulation of PrP in new variant CJD with florid plaques not being a prominent feature of the pathology in kuru, and plaque-like deposits being relatively small and less widespread in terms of distribution and numbers than in new variant CJD (McLean et al 1997). None of the inherited forms of human prion diseases shows a similar neuropathology to new variant CJD (Ironside 1998).

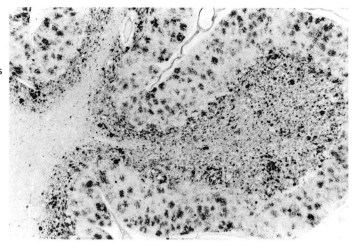

Fig. 1.10
The cerebellum in new variant CJD shows extensive PrP accumulation with large plaques in the molecular and granular layers, occasional small plaques in the white matter (left) and numerous amorphous deposits of PrP around small blood vessels and neurones in the molecular layer. KG9 monoclonal antibody × 100.

SIGNIFICANCE OF THE FLORID PLAQUE IN CJD

Florid plaques are a major feature of the neuropathology in new variant CJD, but are not specific for this disorder and were first described in experimental transmissions of Icelandic scrapie into mice (Fraser 1979). The focal spongiform change around these plaques may possibly represent dilated neuritic processes. Florid plaques occur in other TSE and are a prominent feature of the neuropathology in chronic wasting disease in deer (Williams & Young 1993). Occasional florid plaques have been identified in iatrogenic CJD after dura mater transplantation in Japan (Takashima et al 1997), and detailed examination of the brain in sporadic CJD may demonstrate occasional florid plaques, though these are usually confined to single lesions in individual cases. Although florid plaques are, therefore, not specific for new variant CJD, their number, size and extent of distribution are highly characteristic. However, diagnosis of new variant CJD can be made on brain biopsies in the absence of florid plaques if the other characteristic neuropathological features are present on PrP immunocytochemistry, where small clusters of PrP plaques, perivascular and pericellular deposits are present (Table 1.6).

LYMPHORETICULAR INVOLVEMENT IN NEW VARIANT CJD

Earlier studies of lymphoid tissue in both natural and experimental scrapie indicated that infectivity may be present in both the clinical and, in some cases, the preclinical phases of the illness (Kimberlin & Walker 1988), accompanied by positive staining for PrP on immunocytochemistry (van Keulen et al 1996). Tonsillar tissue in an autopsy case of new variant CJD was found to contain disease-associated PrP on both immunocytochemistry (with labelling of follicular dendritic cells within germinal centres) and by Western blotting (Hill et al 1997). Since this initial report, this finding has been confirmed in other cases of new variant CJD (Hill et al 1999). Similar investigations on sporadic CJD have yielded negative results (Kawashima et al 1997). Involvement of lymphoid tissue in new variant CJD raises the possibility of using tonsillar biopsy as a diagnostic investigation, and this is currently under evaluation(Hill et al 1999). The involvement of lymphoid tissue in new variant CJD also raises the possibility that circulating lymphoid cells might also be associated with infectivity, which has, in turn, raised questions concerning infectivity in blood and blood products (Ludlam 1997, Will & Kimberlin 1998). This concern has been reinforced by recent experimental data which indicate that functional B lymphocytes are required for the transmission of scrapie by a peripheral route (Klein et al 1997). There is no evidence that sporadic CJD is transmitted by either whole blood or blood products (Esmonde et al 1993), but the evidence of involvement of the lymphoid system in new variant CJD indicates that this situation should be reconsidered for the new disease, and scientific investigations are currently under way to assess this possibility.

RELATIONSHIP BETWEEN NEW VARIANT CJD AND BSE

The initial description of new variant CJD suggested that the emergence of this new disorder in the UK was a consequence of exposure of the population to the BSE agent (Will et al 1996). This suggestion was based on the association of new variant CJD with the BSE epidemic, whereas similar epidemiological studies in other European countries with very small numbers of BSE have not revealed any new variant CJD cases. Although one case of new variant CJD has been reported in France (Chazot et al 1996), this does not invalidate the suggestion, as British food exports are eaten in France. Furthermore, the time interval between the first identification of BSE and new variant CJD (about 10 years) is consistent with known incubation periods for human prion diseases. The association between BSE and new variant CJD was reinforced by neuropathological and clinical studies on three macaque monkeys which had been intracerebrally inoculated with BSE (Lasmezas et al 1996). Neuropathological studies of these animals showed florid plaques and other neuropathological features which were very similar to new variant CJD, and the documented clinical features of the illness in the animals were also comparable with those in new variant CJD. Biochemical studies of the prion protein in Western blots from new variant CJD showed a predominance of highly glycosylated PrP, a feature shared with PrP extracted from cases of BSE and from experimental BSE and BSE which had occurred in other species, including antelopes and domestic cats (Collinge et al 1996). Transmission of BSE and new variant CJD into transgenic mice, in which the mouse PrP gene had been disrupted and a human PrP gene inserted, have also shown a similar biochemical profile (Hill et al 1997).

Unlike scrapie, in which numerous strains of the transmissible agent have been identified on transmission to groups of inbred mice, studies on BSE have revealed only a single strain of transmissible agent (Bruce et al 1994, Bruce 1996). A similar strain of agent has been identified from cases of TSE occurring in antelopes and domestic cats, indicating that BSE is responsible for these novel TSE (Bruce et al 1994, Bruce 1996). Recent experiments in new variant and sporadic CJD have now shown that the transmissible agent in new variant CJD shows strain characteristics identical to BSE in terms of the incubation period in mice and the neuropathological lesion profile in the mouse brains (Bruce et al 1997). However, sporadic cases of CJD show entirely different findings in terms of incubation period and lesion profile, including cases of sporadic CJD occurring in two dairy farmers in the UK. These findings provide strong evidence to support the initial suggestion that exposure to BSE has resulted in transmission of the BSE agent to humans, causing new variant CJD (Pattison & Almond 1997).

FUTURE STUDIES IN NEW VARIANT CJD

New variant CJD may now be considered as 'human BSE' (Pattison & Almond 1997), but much additional information is required to understand the mode of transmission which (in the absence of any other evidence) appears to be dietary. The infective dose required to cause new variant CJD in humans is also unknown, and it is not certain whether a single relatively large dose is essential or whether cumulative low doses may also result in disease transmission. The incubation period is also uncertain and the significance of the uniform host PrP genotype remains to be determined. Cattle and most other animal species encode methionine at the equivalent position in their PrP gene and this perhaps indicates that methionine homozygotes in human are most susceptible to BSE, or that this genotype may result in a shorter incubation period than for individuals with other PrP genotypes. Other host susceptibility factors are uncertain, though it is clearly conceivable that other genes may be involved in determining susceptibility. The spread of the BSE agent in humans and the peripheral pathogenesis of new variant CJD are also poorly understood, though the evidence for the involvement of the lymphoid system supports the suggestion that a 'neuro-immune' connection is important in establishing disease, perhaps involving interaction between lymphoid cells and the peripheral nervous system, i.e. in the spleen, which then allows spread of the transmissible agent to the spinal cord and thence to the brain (Aguzzi 1997).

In the light of the considerable uncertainties in our knowledge of this disease, few attempts have been made to predict the likely future numbers of new variant CJD in the UK; it is, therefore, difficult to state with accuracy whether an epidemic may occur and if so, its likely magnitude (Cousens et al 1997). At present, the rate of increase in new variant CJD in the UK is relatively constant and, given that the incubation period for this new disease is likely to be lengthy, continuing surveillance will be required over the next few years to monitor disease trends and predict more accurately the likely numbers of future cases. The possibility of an epidemic of new variant CJD has focussed attention on the possibilities for treatment of TSE. At present, there are no known drugs which will protect against TSE and, though a number of compounds have been found to prolong experimental disease incubation periods, these are often associated with other toxic side effects (Tagliavini et al 1997) or effective only before neurological involvement occurs. Manipulation of the 'neuro-immune connection' (Aguzzi 1997) might provide a possible avenue for new therapeutic approaches; the possibility also exists of finding compounds which might inhibit or delay the conversion of PrP from the normal to the disease-associated isoform.

CONCLUSIONS

Surveillance of CJD in the UK has identified a new variant of this disease which represents the effect of the BSE agent in humans. At present, it is not possible to predict with certainty the likely numbers of future cases and continuing surveillance is required to provide additional data for more accurate future disease modelling. Much remains unknown concerning the pathogenesis of new variant CJD, including the various agent and host factors which determine disease phenotype and susceptibility. Although it is possible to use tonsillar biopsy for early diagnosis, neuropathology remains the only way to confirm a diagnosis of new variant CJD. This places a high priority on necropsy in patients with suspected new variant CJD, with histological, immunocyto-chemical and biochemical studies in all cases. Finally, the prospect of identification of other 'new variant' forms of CJD must still be faced, as BSE in individuals of different PrP genotypes (other than methionine homozygotes at codon 129) might result in a different clinical and pathological phenotype. Continuing surveillance of CJD will also help answer this intriguing possibility.

ACKNOWLEDGEMENTS

I am most grateful to my colleagues Dr J E Bell, Professor R G Will and Dr R Knight for helpful discussion and to Ms B A Mackenzie for help in preparation of the manuscript. Mrs L McCardle, Miss S Lowrie and Mrs M LeGrice are thanked for their technical expertise in the CJD Surveillance Unit Laboratory. The CJD Surveillance Unit is supported by the Department of Health and the Scottish Home and Health Department, with additional research funding by BBSRC and MRC. The CJD Surveillance Project is critically dependent on the co-operation of neurologists, neuropathologists and histopathologists across the UK, whose invaluable contribution to this project is gratefully acknowledged.

References

Adams DH, Caspary EA, Field EJ 1969 Susceptibility of scrapie agent to ionising radiation. Nature 221: 90–91

Advisory Committee on Dangerous Pathogens Spongiform Encephalopathy Advisory Committee 1998 Transmissible spongiform encephalopathy agents: safe working and the prevention of infection. London:The Stationary Office

Aguzzi A 1997 Neuro-immune connection in spread of prions in the body? Lancet 349: 742–743

Alpers M P 1987 Epidemiology and clinical aspects of kuru. In: Prusiner S B, McKinley M P (eds) Prions: novel infectious pathogens causing scrapie and Creutzfeldt-Jakob disease. San Diego: Academic Press, pp 451–465

Anderson R M, Donnelly C A, Ferguson N M et al 1996 Transmission dynamics and epidemiology of BSE in British cattle. Nature 382: 779–788

Baker H F, Ridley R M 1992 The genetics and transmissibility of human spongiform encephalopathy. Neurodegeneration 1: 3–16

Bastian FO (ed) 1991 Creutzfeldt-Jakob disease and other transmissible human spongiform encephalopathies. St Louis: Mosby Year Book

Bell J E, Ironside J W 1993 How to tackle a possible Creutzfeldt-Jakob disease necropsy. J Clin Pathol 46: 193–197

Bell J E, Ironside J W 1993 Neuropathology of spongiform encephalopathies in humans. Br Med Bull 49: 738–777

Bell J E, Gentleman S M, Ironside J W et al 1997 Prion protein immunocytochemistry – UK five centre consensus report. Neuropathol Appl Neurobiol 23: 26–35

Bell J E, Ironside J W 1997 Principles and practice of 'high-risk' brain banking. Neuropathol Appl Neurobiol; 23: 281–288

Berman P, Davidson G S, Becker L E 1988 Progressive neurological deterioration in a 14-year-old girl. Pediatr Neurosci 14: 42–49

Points of best practice

- Autopsy in suspected cases of CJD can be safely performed in most routine mortuaries, following published guidelines.

- Autopsy procedures in CJD should include the collection of frozen brain tissue whenever possible.

- There is no evidence for an increased incidence of CJD in mortuary technicians, pathologists or laboratory staff, but care should be taken when handling suspected CJD tissues to avoid accidental inoculation and minimise contamination of the surrounding workspace.

- Details of all recommended procedures for handling tissues, blood and other specimens from suspected CJD patients are available in: Transmissible Spongiform Encephalopathy Agents: Safe Working and Prevention of Infection. London, The Stationary Office 1998.

- Neuropathological studies are required to investigate all cases with a clinical diagnosis of suspected CJD and are the only means at present of confirming a diagnosis of new variant CJD.

- Immunocytochemistry for PrP is essential for CJD diagnosis and research; detailed protocols are now available which can be used in most neuropathology laboratories.

- All diagnosed or suspected cases of CJD in the UK should be referred to the CJD Surveillance Unit (Tel: 0131 537 1980; Fax: 0131 343 1404).

- The CJD Surveillance Unit will be pleased to assist in any aspect of CJD diagnosis, including autopsy procedures and PrP immunocytochemistry, upon request.

Billette de Villemeur T, Gellott A, Deslys J P et al 1994 Iatrogenic Creutzfeldt-Jakob disease in three growth hormone recipients: a neuropathological study. Neuropathol Appl Neurobiol 20: 111–117

Bortone E, Bettoni L, Giorgi C, Terzano M G, Trabattoni G R, Mancia D 1994 Reliability of EEG in the diagnosis of Creutzfeldt-Jakob disease. Electroenceph Clin Neurophysiol 90: 323–330

Brown P, Bradley R 1998 1755 and all that: a historical primer of transmissible spongiform encephalopathy. BMJ 317: 19–26

Brown P, Cathala F, Labauge R, Pages M, Alary J C, Baron H 1985 Epidemiologic implications of Creutzfeldt-Jakob disease in a 19-year old girl. Eur J Epidemiol 1: 42–47

Brown P, Cathala F, Castaigne P, Gajdusek D C 1986 Creutzfeldt-Jakob disease: clinical analysis of a consecutive series of 230 neuropathologically verified cases. Ann Neurol 20: 597–602

Brown P, Cathala F, Roberts R F, Gajdusek D C, Cataigne P 1987 The epidemiology of Creutzfeldt-Jakob disease: conclusion of a 15-year investigation in France and review of the world literature. Neurology 37: 895–904

Brown P, Preece M A, Will R G 1992 Friendly fire in medicine: hormones, homografts and Creutzfeldt-Jakob disease. Lancet 340: 24–27

Brown P, Crevenakova L, Boellaard J W, Stavrou D, Goldfarb L G, Gajdusek D C 1994a Identification of a PRNP gene mutation in Jakob's original Creutzfeldt-Jakob disease family. Lancet 344: 130–131

Brown P, Cervanakova L, Goldfarb L G et al 1994b Iatrogenic Creutzfeldt-Jakob disease: an example of the interplay between ancient genes and modern medicine. Neurology 44: 291–293

Bruce M E 1996 Strain typing studies of scrapie and BSE. In: Baker H F, Ridley R M (eds) Prion diseases. New Jersey: Humana, pp 223–236

Bruce M E, Chree A, McConnell I, Foster J, Pearson G, Fraser H 1994 Transmission of bovine spongiform encephalopathy and scrapie to mice. Strain variation and the species barrier. Philos Trans R Soc Lond B Biol Sci 343: 405–411

Bruce M E, Will R G, Ironside J W et al 1997 Transmissions to mice indicate that 'new variant' CJD is caused by the BSE agent. Nature 389: 498–501

Budka H, Aguzzi A, Brown P et al 1995 Neuropathological diagnostic criteria for Creutzfeldt-Jakob disease (CJD) and other human spongiform encephalopathies (prion diseases). Brain Pathol 5: 459–466

Budka H, Aguzzi A, Brown P et al 1995 Tissue handling in suspected Creutzfeldt-Jakob disease (CJD) and other human spongiform encephalopathies (prion diseases). Brain Pathol 5: 319–322

Chazot G, Broussolle E, Lapras C L, Kopp N 1996 New variant of Creutzfeldt-Jakob disease in a 26-year-old French man. Lancet 347: 1181–1182

Collinge J, Palmer M S, Dryden A J 1991 Genetic predisposition to iatrogenic Creutzfeldt-Jakob disease. Lancet 337: 1441–1442

Collinge J, Sidle K C L, Meads J, Ironside J W, Hill A F 1996 Molecular analysis of prion strain variation and the aetiology of 'new variant' CJD. Nature 383: 685–690

Cousens S N, Linsell L, Smith PG et al 1999 Geographical distribution of variant CJD in the UK (excluding Northern Ireland). Lancet 353: 18–21

Cousens S N, Vynnyncky E, Zeidler M, Will R G, Smith P G 1997 Predicting the CJD epidemic in humans. Nature 385: 197–198

Cousens S N, Zeidler M, Esmonde T F et al 1997 Sporadic Creutzfeldt-Jakob disease in the United Kingdom: analysis of epidemiological surveillance data for 1970–96. BMJ 315: 389–396

Creutzfeldt H G 1920 Uber eine eigenartige herdformige Erkrankung des Zentralnervensystems. Z ges Neurol Psychiatr 57: 1–18

de Silva R, Ironside J W, McCardle I, Esmonde T F G, Bell J E, Will R G 1994 Neuropathological phenotype and 'prion protein' genotype correlation in sporadic Creutzfeldt-Jakob disease. Neurosci Lett 179: 50–52

Delasnerie-Laupretre N, Poser S, Pocchiari M, Wientjens D P W M, Will R G 1995 Creutzfeldt-Jakob disease in Europe. Lancet 346: 898

Esmonde T F G, Will R G, Slattery J M et al 1993 Creutzfeldt-Jakob disease and blood transfusion. Lancet 341: 205–206

Farquhar C, Dickinson A, Bruce M 1999 Prophylactic potential of pentosan polysulphate in transmissible spongiform encephalopathies. Lancet 353: 117

Fraser H 1979 The pathogenesis and pathology of scrapie. In: Tyrell D A J (ed) Aspects of slow and persistent virus infections. The Hague: Martinus Nijhoff, pp 30–58

Gerstmann J, Straussler E, Scheinker I 1936 Uber eine eigengartige hereditarfamiliare Erkrankung des Zentralnervensystems. Z ges Neurol Psychiatr 154: 736–762

Goldfarb L G, Haltia M, Brown P et al 1991 New mutation in scrapie amyloid precursor gene (at codon 178) in Finnish Creutzfeldt-Jakob disease kindred. Lancet 327: 445

Goldfarb L G, Brown P, Cervenakova L, Gajdusek D C 1994 Molecular genetic studies of Creutzfeldt-Jakob disease. Mol Neurobiol 8: 89–97

Hayward P A R, Bell J E, Ironside J W 1994 Prion protein immunocytochemistry: the development of reliable protocols for the investigation of Creutzfeldt-Jakob disease. Neuropathol Appl Neurobiol 20: 375–383

Hill A F, Butterworth RJ, Joiner S et al 1999 Investigation of variant Creutzfeldt-Jakob disease and other human prion diseases with tonsil biopsy samples. Lancet 353: 183–189

Hill A F, Desbruslais M C, Joiner S et al 1997 The same prion strain causes nvCJD and BSE. Nature 389: 448–450

Hill A F, Zeidler M, Ironside J W, Collinge J 1997 Diagnosis of new variant Creutzfeldt-Jakob disease by tonsil biopsy. Lancet 349: 99–100

Hsiao K, Baker H F, Crow T J et al 1989 Linkage of a prion protein missense variant to Gerstmann-Straussler syndrome. Nature 338: 342–345

Ironside J W 1996 Creutzfeldt-Jakob disease. Brain Pathol 6: 379–388

Ironside J W 1998 Prion diseases in man. J Pathol 186: 227–234

Ironside J W, Bell J E 1996 The 'high-risk' neuropathological autopsy in AIDS and Creutzfeldt-Jakob disease: principles and practice. Neuropathol Appl Neurobiol 22: 388–393

Ironside J W, Sutherland K, Bell J E et al 1996 A new variant of Creutzfeldt-Jakob disease: neuropathological and clinical features. Cold Spring Harbor Symp Quant Biol 61: 523–530

Jakob A 1921 Uber eigenartige Erkrankungen des Zentralnervensystems mit bemerkenswertem anatomichen Befunde (Spastische Pseudosklerose-Encephalomyelopathie mit disseminierten Degenerations-herden). Z ges Neurol Psychiatr 64: 147–228

Kawashima T, Furukawa H, Doh-ura K, Iwaki T 1997 Diagnosis of new variant Creutzfeldt-Jakob disease by tonsil biopsy. Lancet 350: 68–69

Kimberlin R H 1981 Scrapie. Br Vet J 137: 105–112

Kimberlin R H, Walker C A 1988 Pathogenesis of experimental scrapie. In: Bock G, Marsh R J (eds) Novel infectious agents and the central nervous system. Ciba Foundation Symposium 135. Chichester: Wiley, pp 37–62

Kirkwood J K, Cunningham A A 1994 Epidemiological observations on spongiform encephalopathies in captive wild animals in the British Isles. Vet Rec 135: 296–303

Kitamoto T, Tateishi J 1988 Immunohistochemical confirmation of Creutzfeldt-Jakob disease with a long clinical course with amyloid plaque core antibodies. Am J Pathol 131: 435–443

Klatzo I, Gajdusek D C, Vigas V 1959 Pathology of kuru. Lab Invest 8: 799–847

Klein M A, Frigg R, Flechsig E et al 1997 A crucial role for B cells in neuroinvasive scrapie. Nature 390: 687–690

Kretzschmar H A, Ironside J W, DeArmond S J, Tateishi J 1996 Diagnostic criteria for sporadic Creutzfeldt-Jakob disease. Arch Neurol 53: 913–920

Lasmezas C I, Deslys J-P P, Demalmay R et al 1996 BSE transmission to macaques. Nature 381: 743–744

Ludlam C 1997 New variant Creutzfeldt-Jakob disease and treatment of haemophilia. Lancet 350: 1704

MacDonald S T, Sutherland K, Ironside J W 1996 Prion protein genotype and pathological phenotype studies in sporadic Creutzfeldt-Jakob disease. Neuropathol Appl Neurobiol 22: 285–292

Master CL, Gajdusek DC 1982 The spectrum of Creutzfeldt-Jakob disease and the virus-induced subacute spongiform encepahlopathies. In: Smith WT, Cavamagh JB, eds. Recent Advances in Neuropathology, 2nd edn. Edinburgh:Churchill Livingstone, pp137–163

Masters C L, Richardson E P 1981 Subacute spongiform encephalopathy (Creutzfeldt-Jakob disease). The nature and progression of spongiform change. Brain 104: 559–588

McLean C A, Ironside J W, Masters C L 1997 Comparative neuropathology of kuru and new variant CJD. Brain Pathol 7: 1247

Medori R, Tritschler H J, Leblanc A C et al 1992 Fatal familial insomnia is a prion disease with a mutation at codon 178 of the prion protein gene. N Engl J Med 326: 444–449

Ministry of Agriculture, Fisheries and Food 1996 Bovine spongiform encephalopathy in Great Britain. A progress report. London: MAFF

Owen F, Poulter M, Lofthouse R et al 1989 Insertion in prion protein gene in familial Creutzfeldt-Jakob disease. Lancet i: 51

Palmer M S, Dryden A J, Hughes J T, Collinge J 1991 Homozygous prion protein genotype predisposes to sporadic Creutzfeldt-Jakob disease. Nature 352: 340–342

Parchi P, Castellani R, Capellari S et al 1996 Molecular basis of phenotypic variability in sporadic Creutzfeldt-Jakob disease. Ann Neurol 39: 669–680

Pattison I 1965 Resistance of the scrapie agent to formalin. J Comp Pathol 75: 159-164

Pattison J, Almond J 1997 Human BSE. Nature 389: 437–438

Prusiner S B 1982 Novel proteinaceous infectious particles cause scrapie. Science 216: 136–144

Prusiner S B 1993 Genetic and infectious prion diseases. Arch Neurol 50: 1129–1153

Prusiner S B 1994 Biology and genetics of prion disease. Annu Rev Microbiol 48: 655–686

Prusiner S B 1998 The prion diseases. Brain Pathol 8: 499-513

Richardson E P, Masters C L 1995 The nosology of Creutzfeldt-Jakob disease and conditions related to the accumulation of PrP^{CJD} in the nervous system. Brain Pathol 5: 33–41

Tagliavini F, McArthur R A, Canciani B 1997 Effectiveness of anthracycline against experimental prion disease in Syrian hamsters. Science 276: 1119–1122

Takashima S, Tateishi J, Taguchi Y, Inoue H 1997 Creutzfeldt-Jakob disease with florid plaques after cadaveric dural graft in a Japanese woman. Lancet 350: 865–866

van Keulen L J M, Schreuder B E C, Meloen R H, Mooij-Harkes G, Vromans M E W, Langeveld J P M 1996 Immunohistochemical detection of prion protein in lymphoid tissues of sheep with natural scrapie. J Clin Microbiol 34: 1228–1231

Wells G A H, Scott A C, Johnson C Y et al 1987 A novel progressive spongiform encephalopathy in cattle. Vet Rec 121: 419–420

Wilesmith J W, Ryan J B M, Atkinson M J 1991 Bovine spongiform encephalopathy: epidemiological studies on the origin. Vet Rec 128: 199–203

Will R G 1991 Epidemiological surveillance of Creutzfeldt-Jakob disease in the United Kingdom. Eur J Epidemiol 7: 460–465

Will R G 1993 Epidemiology of Creutzfeldt-Jakob disease. Br Med Bull 49: 960–970

Will R G 1996 Surveillance of prion diseases in humans. In: Baker H F, Ridley R M (eds) Prion diseases. New Jersey: Humana, pp 119–137

Will R G, Alperovitch A, Poser S et al 1998 Descriptive epidemiology of Creutzfeldt-Jakob disease in six European countries, 1993–1995. Ann Neurol 43: 763–767

Will R G, Ironside J W, Zeidler M et al 1996 A new variant of Creutzfeldt-Jakob disease in the UK. Lancet 347: 921–925

Will R G, Kimberlin R H 1998 Creutzfeldt-Jakob disease and the risk from blood or blood products. Vox Sang 75: 178–180

Williams E S, Young S 1993 Neuropathology of chronic wasting disease of mule deer (Odocoileus hemionus) and elk (Cervus elaphus nelsoni). Vet Pathol 30: 36–45

Willoughby K, Kelly D F, Lyon D G, Wells G A H 1992 Spongiform encephalopathy in captive puma (Felis concolor). Vet Rec 131: 431–434

Wyatt J M, Pearson G R, Smerdon T N, Gruffydd-Jones T J, Wells G A H, Wilesmith J W 1991 Naturally occurring scrapie-like spongiform encephalopathy in five domestic cats. Vet Rec 129: 233–236

Zeidler M, Bamber R W K, Dickens C M et al 1997a New variant Creutzfeldt-Jakob disease: psychiatric features. Lancet 350: 908–910

Zeidler M, Stewart G E, Barraclough C R et al 1997b New variant Creutzfeldt-Jakob disease: neurological features and diagnostic tests. Lancet 350: 903–907

Sebastian B. Lucas

Imported infectious diseases

In *Recent Advances in Histopathology* a decade ago, *Aspects of infectious disease* (Lucas 1989) considered the diagnosis and differential diagnoses of some of the commoner non-standard infectious diseases that histopathologists in the UK encounter. These included leprosy, leishmaniasis, amoebiasis, the coccidioses and microsporidiosis, anisakiasis, strongyloidiasis, the filariases, and schistosomiasis. The effect of the global pandemic of HIV/AIDS on prevalent infections in hospitalized patients and cadavers was emerging, with pathologists confidently diagnosing infections such as intestinal *Cryptosporidium* and disseminated *Mycobacterium avium* complex and the fungus *Pneumocystis carinii* – hitherto rare entities.

Since then, infectious disease in the UK and globally has changed in several respects:

1. HIV has become yet more prevalent globally with more than 30 million adults and children living with HIV/AIDS (UNAIDS 1997); in the UK, 31,000 HIV-infected persons have been diagnosed since reporting started in 1984 (PHLS CDSC 1998). The range of opportunistic infections and tumours (Schultz et al 1996, Waddell et al 1996) that such patients acquire continues to widen, and the pathology the agents induce is often novel. Conversely, several infections that were predicted to be more severe in numbers and morbidity because of HIV turned out to be relatively unaffected by HIV: these include falciparum malaria, leprosy, strongyloidiasis (Fig. 2.1) and amoebiasis (*Entamoeba histolytica*; Lucas 1990, 1993).

2. Recent highly active anti-retroviral therapy (HAART) has dramatically altered the clinical pathology of HIV/AIDS (British HIV Association 1997), with moribund patients rapidly improving, their CD4+ve T-cell counts rising, and several opportunistic infections, such as cryptosporidiosis, and

Prof. Sebastian B. Lucas, UMDS Department of Histopathology, St Thomas' Hospital, Lambeth Palace Road, London SE1 7EH, UK

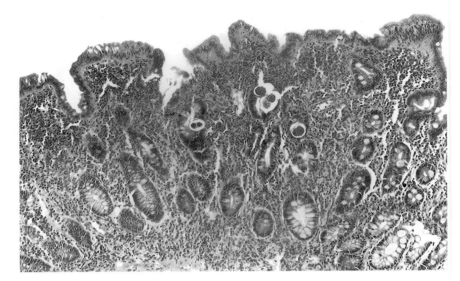

Fig. 2.1 Strongyloidiasis. Duodenal biopsy from a British traveller in Africa with diarrhoea. There is villous blunting and, in several crypts, cross-sections of female nematode worms. This is virtually diagnostic of *Strongyloides stercoralis* infection (the differential is *Capillaria philippinensis*, which is rare and geographically restricted). H&E.

tumours, such as Kaposi's sarcoma, resolving without specific therapy (Carr et al 1998, Sepkowitz 1998).

3. The incidence of tuberculosis in UK declined until the early 1990s and has risen again (Ormerod 1996) this is due to particularly high rates among Indian subcontinent immigrants and ethnic Africans and, in part, to HIV co-infection. Multi-drug resistant forms are also increasing (though they are no more infectious than drug-sensitive *Mycobacterium tuberculosis*). Hepatitis C virus (HCV) infection is more common than previously appreciated (Di Bisceglie 1998). Like tuberculosis and HIV, HCV poses infectious hazards in the laboratory and mortuary to which many pathologists and technical staff are reluctant to expose themselves, and which may necessitate upgrading of facilities. The general appreciation of infectious hazard and risk reduction is undoubtedly rising as hospitals tighten up on standards, and laboratory accreditation emphasizes health and safety.

4. UK inhabitants travel abroad in ever greater numbers returning with non-endemic infections such as leishmaniasis, malaria and schistosomiasis.

5. As a result of well-publicized recent overseas' epidemics, of contagious and morbid infections such as Ebola virus in Zaire and Gabon (Rollin & Ksiazek 1998), and unusual leptospirosis in Nicaragua (Zaki & Shieh 1995), there has been a greater awareness among medical practitioners of the possibilities of such hazardous infections in returning nationals and visitors.

6. Certain new infections have been identified (Schwartz et al 1995), mainly overseas, such as Cyclospora (Bendall et al 1993); further microsporidial

species (Yachnis et al 1996, Cowley et al 1997), and bacillary angiomatosis in HIV-infected patients; Hantavirus pulmonary syndrome (Nolte et al 1995), and the tick-born bacterial infection erlichiosis (a cause of ring-granulomas in the liver; Walker & Dumler 1997).

7. Polymerase chain reaction (PCR) technology has enabled identification of many infections in tissues, even when formalin-fixed and paraffin wax-embedded, with greater sensitivity than the classical staining methods.

If referral patterns are an indicator, the significant imported diseases that cause problems for UK pathologists are leishmaniasis, tuberculosis, schisto-somiasis, strongyloidiasis, mycetoma and malaria. Tuberculosis and its differential diagnosis, when unfixed material for culture is not available, remains a problem which PCR has not yet resolved. The histological nuances of leprosy are not generally appreciated and, like uncommon cancers, should be managed in a few specialist centres.

Tables 2.1 and 2.2 indicate many of the infectious disease problems for pathologists, according to whether they can be acquired only abroad or perhaps more commonly acquired outside the UK. In this chapter, several problematic infections will be reviewed, concentrating on diagnosis and pathogenesis.

BACTERIAL INFECTIONS

LEPROSY

Leprosy is declining in incidence and prevalence in many countries (World Health Organization 1997) as a result of the introduction of systematic multidrug anti-leprosy therapy (MDT) in the 1980s and the prophylactic effect of mass BCG vaccination against tuberculosis (though, unfortunately, in the most tuberculosis-endemic areas of the world, BCG has no impact on tuberculosis incidence; Pönnighaus et al 1992). Each year, 15–30 new patients are diagnosed with leprosy in the UK, all imported infections, and virtually all are biopsied. As described previously (Lucas 1989), the major problems in histopathological diagnosis have not changed. Paucibacillary leprosy, i.e. with no detectable acid-fast bacilli, is the main challenge. With the decline in incidence, diagnoses are being sought earlier in the course of the disease and diagnostic tests, such as skin biopsy, become more difficult to interpret. A comparability study of early leprosy lesions involving three experienced leprosy histopathologists and repeated evaluations of the biopsies found a high discordant rate in diagnostic certainty between them, with different patterns of interpretive behaviour over the two rounds of the study (Fine et al 1993). Much depended on how hard bacilli were searched for.

Early leprosy, with a small number of pale macules on the skin, is always difficult to diagnose unless there is definite granulomatous disruption of a dermal nerve (i.e. early tuberculoid leprosy) or a non-artefactual acid-fast bacillus is identified in a critical site such nerve, subepidermal location, or arrector pili muscle. A recent study of 5 such patients in India involved the study of an average of 145 modified Ziehl-Neelsen stained sections per case.

Table 2.1 Infections only acquired outside UK (with the name of the disease caused if not evident)

Virus	Rabies Yellow fever Dengue Ebola/Lassa/Marburg Sin Nombre virus (Hantavirus pulmonary syndrome)
Bacteria	*Rickettsia* spp. (non-Q fever) *Yersinia pestis* (plague) *Klebsiella rhinoscleromatis* (scleroma) *Pseudomonas pseudomallei* (melioidosis)
Mycobacteria	*Mycobacterium leprae* *Mycobacterium ulcerans* (Buruli ulcer)
Fungi	*Histoplasma capsulatum* *Coccidioides immitis* *Paracoccidioides brasiliensis* *Blastomyces dermatiditis* *Penicillium marneffei* (penicilliosis)
Protozoa	*Plasmodium falciparum* (malaria) *Pl. vivax, Pl. malariae, Pl. ovale* *Trypanosoma brucei, T. cruzi* *Leishmania* spp. *Isospora belli* *Sarcocystis* spp. *Cyclospora cayetanensis*
Nematodes	Hookworms & ascarids *Strongyloides stercoralis* *Trichuris trichuria* (whipworm) *Onchocerca volvulus* (onchocerciasis) *Wuchereria bancrofti* (lymphatic filariasis) *Loa loa* (loiasis) *Dirofilaria* spp. (dirofilariasis)
Trematodes	*Schistosoma mansoni* *S. japonicum, S. haematobium* *Paragonimus* spp. *Clonorchis* spp.
Cestodes	*Spirometra* spp. (sparganosis) *Echinococcus multilocularis* (alveolar hydatid cyst)

Sub-epidermal AFB were found in all five but only two had AFB in the dermal nerve (Job et al 1997a). Apart from showing how difficult it may be to discover AFB, the findings also challenge the accepted notion that leprosy is acquired via the respiratory tract with haematogenous dissemination to nerves and then skin; perhaps some skin lesions are genuine primary infection sites.

PCR has shown that detectable DNA declines rapidly in multibacillary leprosy lesions after effective chemotherapy (Jamil et al 1993), faster than the bacilli fragment and become morphologically non-viable. Can PCR assist in diagnosing paucibacillary leprosy? There is no doubt that epidemiological surveys of nasal carriage of bacilli using PCR on swabs provides information

Table 2.2 Infections acquired in UK but also commonly imported

Virus	Hepatitis A, B, C, D, E, F, G HTLV-1 HIV-1 (HIV-2 is rare in UK but could be transmitted)
Bacteria	Q-fever *Chlamydia trachomatis* *Corynebacterium diphtheriae* *Vibrio cholerae* *Salmonella* spp. *Shigella* spp. *Brucella* spp. *Treponema pallidum* *Borrelia* (relapsing fever) *Calymmatobacterium granulomatis* (donovanosis, granuloma inguinale) *Haemophilus ducreyi* (chancroid)
Mycobacteria	*Mycobacterium tuberculosis*
Fungi	Mycetoma Chromomycoses
Protozoa	*Entamoeba histolytica* *Acanthamoeba*. spp
Nematodes	Trichinella
Cestodes	*Echinococcus granulosus* (classical hydatid cyst) Taenia adult worms *Taenia solium* (cysticercosis)

on infection rates in populations (Klatser et al 1993), but the quest for 100% sensitivity and specificity in detecting *Mycobacterium leprae* DNA in fixed skin biopsies has not yet been successful. While PCR does have a higher sensitivity rate than histological detection of AFB in skin biopsies, in most studies there is a persistent problem of false positives (De Wit et al 1991, Job et al 1997b). This approach continues, but one practical solution appears to be coming from changes in policy in managing patients with definite and suspect leprosy. Recent trials of patients with multibacillary leprosy show that MDT can be shortened to one year at most without significant increase in rate of relapse. Further, an apparently successful trial of single-dose MDT in patients with single lesion leprosy in India (McDougall 1997) heralds the likelihood of more empirical anti-leprosy therapy in suspect cases without requiring definite proof of diagnosis.

TUBERCULOSIS

Many parts of the UK have experienced a marked increase in tuberculosis, in part because of HIV infection, but mainly because of immigration of ethnic subgroups from the Indian sub-continent and sub-Saharan Africa with high rates of indigenous tuberculosis (Ormerod 1996). Because tuberculosis can

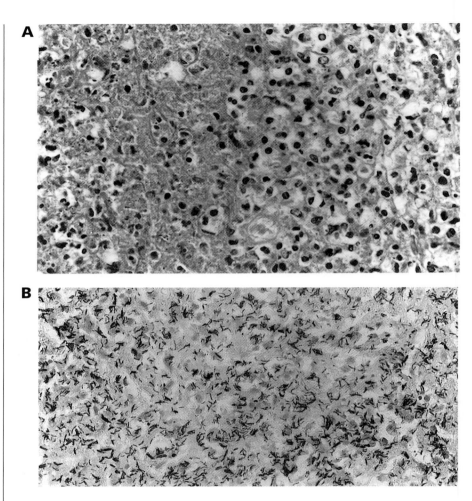

Fig. 2.2 Non-reactive tuberculosis. (**A**) Lymph node from a patient with advanced AIDS and tuberculosis. There is a dirty necrosis with apoptoses and hydropic macrophages. H&E. (**B**) The Ziehl-Neelsen stain shows very numerous acid-fast bacilli.

present in any organ, pathologists need an even higher index of suspicion than clinicians for the disease. Epithelioid cell and Langhans' giant cell granulomas with caseation necrosis are the prototypical histopathology of tuberculosis, but almost any pattern of inflammation can be seen, including acute inflammation (Santa Cruz & Strayer 1982, Lucas 1998).

One form that may not automatically raise the possibility of tuberculosis is anergic or non-reactive tuberculosis, where there are no granulomas or epithelioid cells or giant cells, just necrosis with much cellular debris; ZN stains shows enormous numbers of bacilli (Fig. 2.2; Nambuya et al 1988). This is seen in patients with advanced cellular immunodeficiency; HIV infection is the commonest underlying mechanism now, but leukaemia, malnutrition, advanced age, cytotoxic drugs and steroids can all predispose to this pattern.

Because AFB detection in histological sections requires a minimum density of 1000 bacilli per cubic centimetre of tissue, it was hoped that PCR analysis would provide an optimal means of proving or excluding suspected tuberculosis. There is, however, a significant lack of consistency in sensitivity and specificity among microbiology laboratories in detecting *M. tuberculosis* in standardised samples (Noordhoek et al 1996). Using formalin-fixed and paraffin wax-embedded tissues, PCR has proved sensitive, and has identified *M. tuberculosis* DNA in tuberculid skin lesions, where culture is regularly negative (and has even, thereby, identified a putative fourth type of tuberculid; Baselga et al 1997, Hara et al 1997). However, in trying to distinguish tuberculosis from sarcoidosis, PCR using various primers has yielded positive signals from sarcoid tissues (Saboor et al 1992, Richter et al 1996). While this informs the controversy over the aetiology of sarcoidosis, it does not help in case management. Another promising potential use for PCR is for determining the species of mycobacteria in fixed tissues (Richter et al 1995).

BRUCELLOSIS

Brucellosis, usually imported, is another granulomatous disease to consider. As a lymphoreticular infection, it presents with fever, lymphadenopathy, hepatosplenomegaly, and sometimes ascites (Lucas 1994, Christou et al 1997). A biopsy of these organs or the bone marrow reveals granulomas, sometimes with necrosis. One does not see the Gram-negative *Brucella* spp. bacilli but, like tuberculosis, a high index of suspicion has rewards: brucellosis is readily diagnosable by serology and blood culture, and responds to antibiotic therapy.

VIRAL INFECTIONS

VIRAL HAEMORRHAGIC FEVERS (VHF)

In the 1970s, there was a scare in the UK about imported VHF: two patients from West Africa presented in London hospitals with Lassa fever, but no secondary infections occurred among health care workers. In 1997, a patient from Zimbabwe died in the UK of an undiagnosed haemorrhagic illness that on serological tests may have been Crimean-Congo haemorrhagic fever (CCHF; Dr G. Lloyd, CAMR, personal communication). There was no autopsy.

The viral haemorrhagic fevers are placed in hazard group 4 by the Advisory Committee on Dangerous Pathogens (ACDP 1995). They include Lassa fever, Marburg and Ebola virus infection. With modern air transportation, further patients with VHF may arrive in the UK and present with a non-specific fever, asthenia and headache before the more indicative conjunctival and cutaneous haemorrhagic rash and bleeding from the gastro-intestinal tract develop. As these viruses are inactivated by formalin, there is no hazard in a fixed biopsy. In Ebola, the histopathology of the illness is better studied experimentally than in human beings (Zaki et al 1996, Davis et al 1997). The Ebola filovirus is present in large quantities free in the blood, throughout the mononuclear phagocyte system, in endothelial cells, in hepatocytes and adrenal cells and in gastro-intestinal epithelia. The fibroblastic reticular cell network of lymph nodes is particularly heavily infected and damaged, perhaps a mechanism of reducing the immune response to the infection. The lungs in fatal cases show features of shock. The liver has focal necrosis. Immunostaining with monoclonal antibodies to Ebola shows intense staining in the sinusoids.

The human pathology of CCHF in South Africa has been recently reviewed (Burt et al 1997). The liver and lung histopathology is similar to that in Ebola, with the liver showing a range from numerous apoptotic Councilman bodies to large foci of necrosis: the virus is distributed similarly.

The ACDP guidelines (ACDP 1995) state that autopsies should not be performed in cases of known or suspected VHF, as being too hazardous. Should such cases occur, then careful post-mortem needle biopsy of liver tissue and aspiration of blood for virus culture, electron microscopy and serology will provide, in consultation with microbiological experts, a confirmatory diagnosis.

RABIES

Because of quarantine restrictions, rabies is not endemic in the UK and imported infections are rare. The last two instances were in 1996 and 1987, both in African patients (Raman et al 1988, personal observations). Histopathologists are most likely to encounter rabies at autopsy, though it has been established for years that a nuchal skin biopsy can be immunostained with a monoclonal antibody against rabies antigen to demonstrate positive nerve staining (Blenden et al 1984). This can be used as a diagnostic test in a suspect patient with abnormal cerebration. After the ascent of the virus via the peripheral nerves to the brain, there is the phase of centrifugal spread of infection via cerebrospinal and autonomic nerves; hence, the infectiousness of saliva and the diagnostic skin features.

The pathology of the brain in rabies is variable. Macroscopically it may be swollen or normal. Microscopically there may be encephalitis or no inflammation. The typical viral inclusions – Negri bodies and the less rounded and discrete lyssa bodies – are not always found in the cytoplasm of neurones, being identified in up 71% of cases. The most likely sites to detect inclusions are the Purkinje cells, hippocampal and brain stem neurones, ahead of cerebral cortex neurones (Mrak & Young 1994). Fresh brain tissue from these sites may be collected and examined rapidly by immunostaining under safe conditions.

In addition to encephalitis, rabies causes a myocarditis which may be the predominant clinical feature at some stage. There is chronic lymphohistiocytic inflammation with focal muscle fibre necrosis and, in some cases, acute inflammation. Negri bodies have been found in cardiac neurones and, by immunocytochemistry, rabies antigen can be demonstrated in the cytoplasm of degenerate muscle fibres (Metze et al 1991).

The practical problem for pathologists is that of health and safety in the mortuary. Rabies is in hazard group 3 and, in the 1996, case the relevant authorities in the UK strongly recommended that the autopsy be done by a pathologist and mortuary technical officer with previous rabies vaccination. In addition, neoprene gloves that prevent cuts should be worn under the outer rubber gloves.

HANTAVIRUS PULMONARY SYNDROME (HPS)

In 1993, a new respiratory disease with a high mortality was identified in the southwest USA; the cause was previously undescribed rodent-born hantavirus

(Sin Nombre virus, SNV; Zaki et al 1997). Retrospectively, further cases were diagnosed with confirmation by immunocytochemistry. The disease is so far restricted to the north and south Americas, but hantaviruses are carried by rodents throughout the world (Schmalijohn et al 1997) and are causes of nephropathies.

The lung is the main target in HPS. There is an interstitial pneumonia, with oedema, fibrin exudate, and focal hyaline membranes. Characteristically, there are large immunoblasts in the lung tissues and the peri-arteriolar lymphoid tissue in the spleen (Nolte et al 1995, Zaki et al 1997). Immunostaining shows SNV antigen in endothelial cells and follicle dendritic cells. As with Legionnaires' disease in the 1970s, in HPS the autopsy was the means of identifying a new disease, and of pursuing its epidemiology prospectively and retrospectively.

FUNGAL INFECTIONS

HISTOPLASMOSIS

Apart from tuberculosis, the differential diagnoses of nodules of caseous and other patterns of granulomatous necrosis in the lung include Wegener's granulomatosis and *Histoplasma capsulatum* infection. In histoplasmosis, there are often tiny deposits of calcification throughout the necrosis. Histoplasmas are not readily seen on H&E stain but do stain with Grocott, this stain revealing live and dead yeast forms (Fig. 2.3). The presentation of this infection is often a chance radiological finding with subsequent biopsy at thoracotomy, and it usually represents an old healed primary infection that is unlikely to recrudesce. However, in a patient co-infected with HIV or with other risk

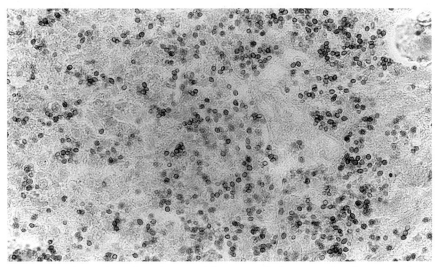

Fig. 2.3 Histoplasmosis. Solitary lung nodule removed after a routine chest X-ray from a British traveller. There was uniform caseous necrosis with a granulomatous cuff. No yeasts were evident with H&E stained sections. The Grocott silver stain shows numerous round yeasts of *H. capsulatum*.

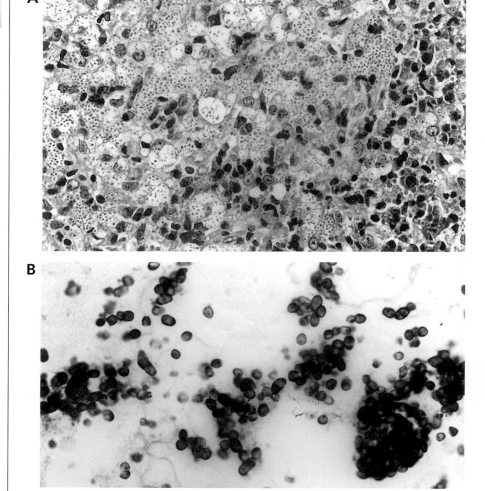

Fig. 2.4 Penicilliosis. (**A**) Lymph node from an HIV-infected patient. Abundant small yeasts are seen in the macrophages; no granuloma formation is evident. H&E. (**B**) The Grocott silver stain shows round and ovoid yeasts. Several are splitting (as opposed to budding), characteristic of *P. marneffei*.

factors for immunosuppression, there is a risk of disseminated infection (Wheat et al 1982, Miller et al 1994).

PENICILLIOSIS

Penicillium marneffei is a saprophytic fungus infection that parasitises the macrophages of man as small yeasts that resemble *Histoplasma capsulatum* in size (DiSalvo et al 1973). It occurs only in the Far East, and the cases of infection encountered in the UK have been among HIV-infected travellers. The fungus is inhaled, establishing the primary infection (as with tuberculosis, histoplasmosis and many systemic mycoses), and disease is probably a reactivation of latent infection. Immunocompetent persons occasionally develop disease. Those with non-HIV-related immunosuppressive conditions are more susceptible, but the major increase in penicilliosis now seen is due to HIV co-infection (Cooper & McGinnis 1997). In some hospitals in Thailand, HIV-associated penicilliosis parallels the importance of HIV-associated tuberculosis in Africa (Duong 1996).

Clinical presentation is with fever, cough, hepatosplenomegaly, anaemia, lymphadenopathy and often with skin nodules or ulcers. The bone marrow is also involved. The pathology – as with many mycoses – includes tuberculoid granulomas, suppuration and necrosis. In immunosuppressed patients, there is diffuse proliferation of yeasts in macrophages usually without granuloma formation (Fig. 2.4). The yeasts are oval and elongated up to 5 μm; they do not bud, but split with the formation of a central septum, and can thus be distinguished from *H. capsulatum* (Tsui et al 1992, Hilmarsdottir et al 1993, Cooper & McGinnis 1997).

PROTOZOAL INFECTIONS

CYCLOSPORIASIS

Cyclospora cayetanensis is a coccidian protozoan infection of the gut (it was once thought to be a cyanobacterium blue-green alga) that was first identified in stool samples of patients with diarrhoea in Papua New Guinea about 20 years ago (Eberhard et al 1997). Water- and food-borne, it causes diarrhoea and may be associated with HIV infection. Most cases are reported from southern USA, the Caribbean and Central America; occasionally, it is encountered as an imported disease in the UK and Europe (Bendall et al 1993, van Nhieu et al 1996). The readiest diagnostic technique is parasitological examination of stool and identification of oocysts; but schizonts (2–3 μm) and elongated merozoites (5 μm long) are identifiable with some difficulty in the enterocytes of the small bowel. Duodenal biopsy shows moderate inflammation and some villous blunting (Fig. 2.5). The parasites are better seen in 5 μm H&E sections than in thinner ones (van Nhieu et al 1996); though similar to the life cycle stages of *Isospora belli*, they are smaller and are not PAS positive. They are less refractile than the rounded spores of microsporidia.

LEISHMANIASIS

Leishmania spp. are acquired from sand-fly bites in many parts of South America, the Middle East, the Indian subcontinent, Africa and, notably, in the countries that line the Mediterranean Sea. Many tourists become infected. Some present with cutaneous or visceral leishmaniasis as the disease develops (Lucas 1989), but many acquire a latent infection that can emerge many years or even decades later, often under circumstances of decreasing cellular immunity. In Europe, there is an epidemic of HIV-associated visceral leishmaniasis (Albrecht et al 1997, Alvar et al 1997). The patients present with fever, diarrhoea and often enlarged liver and spleen. As the parasites are intracellular within macrophages, a large proportion of the lymphoreticular system is affected, with parasites seen in the gut lamina propria (Fig. 2.6) and lymph nodes as well as in the more familiar location of bone marrow. This disease carries a high mortality if untreated.

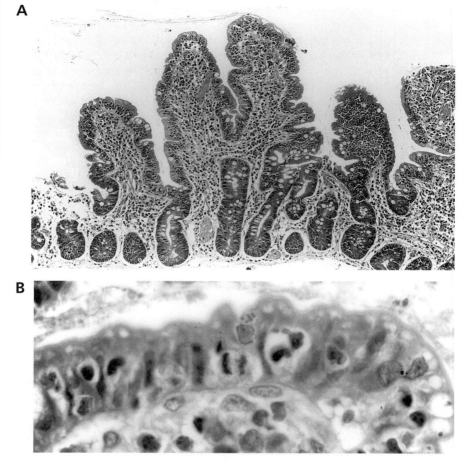

Fig. 2.5 Cyclospora infection. (**A**) Duodenal biopsy from an infected traveller with diarrhoea. There is mild villous blunting, and increased intra-epithelial lymphocytes. H&E. (**B**) Oil-immersion view showing a schizont cluster of 7 parasites in the supranuclear portion of one enterocyte. H&E.

HIV/AIDS alters the usual clinicopathological patterns of leishmaniasis and unusual skin lesions, often with very heavy parasite loads, also develop. It is, therefore, important to look for leishmanial amastigotes in all biopsies taken from HIV-infected patients.

In people who are not infected with HIV, leishmaniasis may also present with unusual and misleading manifestations. Two are notable – caseation necrosis in lymph nodes as well as caseation in the skin lesions, and post kala azar dermal leishmaniasis (PKDL). In patients with cutaneous leishmaniasis, the parasites probably go to local nodes often, but do not usually cause significant lymphadenopathy. Sometimes they can produce a granulomatous caseation in a node that is indistinguishable from that caused by tuberculosis. Leishmania amastigotes are not visible, but PCR can be conclusive diagnostically (see below).

PKDL is a recurrence of visceral leishmaniasis treated months or years previously localised to the skin and mucosae. It is particularly prevalent in north-east India, Bangladesh and Sudan (where about 50% of treated patients with visceral leishmaniasis develop PKDL; Zijlstra et al 1995, Nandy et al 1998). Clinically, there are macules or nodules, often on the upper part of the body. Skin biopsy shows a varied pattern. In the Asian pattern, there is florid lymphohistio-cytic and plasmacytic infiltration, without tuberculoid granulomas, resembling lymphoma on the low power. In Africa, granulomas without necrosis are more frequent. Parasites may be numerous or hard to find in macrophages (Majunder 1967, El Hassan et al 1992).

PCR has proved very helpful in the rapid identification and speciation of leishmania, both in fresh clinical and cultured samples, and in formalin-fixed paraffin wax-embedded tissues (de Bruijn & Barker 1992, Laskay et al 1995). In one study of cutaneous leishmaniasis, the relative sensitivities of PCR, histopathology and direct smears in the detection of amastigotes were 86%, 76% and 55%, respectively (Andresen et al 1996).

FALCIPARUM MALARIA

Malaria remains one of the major killer diseases globally, particularly among young children in Africa (Newton et al 1998). About 2,000 people are diagnosed with imported malaria each year in the UK. *Plasmodium falciparum* is the

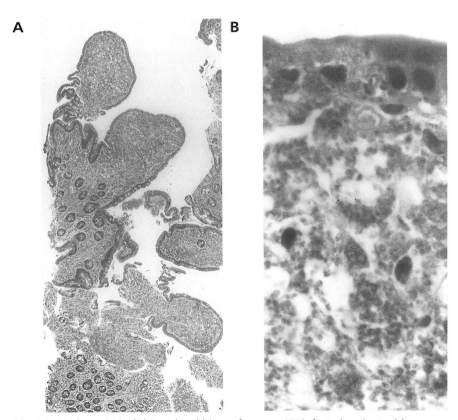

A   **B**

Fig. 2.6 Leishmaniasis. (**A**) Duodenal biopsy from an HIV-infected patient with diarrhoea. The villi are blunted and abnormally cellular. H&E. (**B**) The macrophages in the lamina propria are stuffed with Leishmania amastigotes, some of which are also seen crossing the epithelium. H&E.

commonest species (> 1000 per annum) and the most important as it has a significant case fatality rate. The other 3 species (Table 2.1) cause anaemia and fever, but not cerebral disease or significant lung disease or haemodynamic upset and so are incidental if identified histologically. Malaria causes characteristic infection of erythrocytes, with sequestration, i.e. high concentration and packing of parasitised red blood cells (PRBC), in the capillaries and venules of certain organs – brain, gut mucosa, lung. Falciparum malaria is seen in the placenta, liver, and occasional intestinal samples. In the placenta, the maternal sinuses are packed with PRBC, along with macrophages containing the haemozoin pigment (the fetal vessels do not contain parasites; Bulmer et al 1993). In liver and gut mucosa, PRBC and haemozoin-containing monocytes or macrophages are present, without associated inflammation.

The most important role for the histopathologist outside endemic areas in the evaluation of malaria is in the autopsy room; each year about 10 people die of falciparum malaria in the UK (UK malaria data from D. Bradley, Malaria Reference Centre, London School of Hygiene & Tropical Medicine, London, UK). In most cases, the infection is already known, but not always. If malaria has been treated, the morphology depends on the duration of therapy antemortem, for the parasites will be cleared from the blood vessels within a week, leaving haemozoin pigment in liver, spleen and bone marrow macrophages. The other features will be those of shock and pathological complications of terminal intensive care.

The brain in those untreated or treated for only a few days is characteristic. The meninges are congested and the brain is usually somewhat swollen though without sufficient cerebral swelling to cause herniation and cerebellar coning (Lucas et al 1996). On cutting, the grey matter is often a darker grey-brown than normal, and about half of the cases show petechial haemorrhages in the cerebral white matter and throughout the cerebellum. A rapid diagnosis can be obtained by a brain smear: take a 3–4 mm cube of cortex, squash and drag it between two glass slides, air-dry and stain with Giemsa (Fig. 2.7). In the arcades of capillaries and venules, parasitized red cells are clearly observed. Histologically, one sees dilated congested small blood vessels with sequestered PRBC, perivascular haemorrhages (composed of non-parasitized RBC), haemozoin pigment in intravascular macrophages, variable parenchymal oedema (in < 50% of cases), thrombi in small vessels (in < 30% of cases), early reactive gliosis, and a notable lack of perivascular neutrophils or lymphocytes (Marchiafava & Bignami 1894, Spitz 1946, Lucas et al 1996, Turner 1997).

The parasites are not always easy to identify in RBC as the intracellular haemozoin pigment can obscure them. They begin as small blobs of haematoxyphilic nucleus which during the 2 day malaria cycle enlarge and become ring forms – a 2 µm disc of pale cytoplasm with a peripheral curved nucleus. In a suspected case of malaria, if there is confusion between formalin pigment and haemozoin, one can remove both pigment types with picric acid, and then view the actual parasites more easily.

The morphology of fatal falciparum malaria has been known for a century. Why malaria remains pathologically fascinating is the controversy over the pathogenesis of cerebral malaria among other aspects (Newton et al 1998). There is ongoing dispute between those who assert that mechanical obstruction by sequestered PRBC is paramount, and those who assert that systemic cytokine release explains much or all of clinical malaria. Both may be correct.

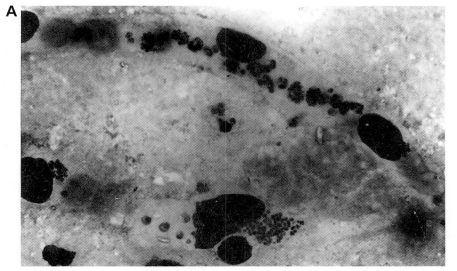

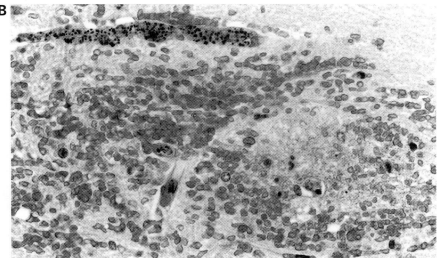

Fig. 2.7 Cerebral malaria. (**A**) Brain smear (see text). Two capillaries with red cells containing clustered parasites – schizonts prior to red cell rupture. Giemsa stain. (**B**) Histological section from the cerebellum of a child. At top is a capillary filled with small dots representing parasitised red blood cells. The centre is a petechial haemorrhage (of non-parasitised cells) caused by rupture of the vessel seen in cross-section at lower right. H&E.

Historical and recent landmarks include:

♦ the description of parasite sequestration in 1894 and the hypothesis that PRBC sludging with subsequent ischaemia causes coma (Marchiafava et al; 1894)

♦ the proposal that malaria 'toxins' lead to altered vascular permeability, cerebral oedema and coma (Maegraith 1977)

♦ the association of sequestration in cerebral malaria and the electron microscopic demonstration of knobs on sequestered PRBC (MacPherson et al 1985, Turner 1997), indicating the sites at which PRBC adhere to endothelial cells through parasite-derived ligands binding to expressed receptors on endothelial cells

- the proposal that endotoxin (tumour necrosis factor, TNF) causes much of the multi-organ clinical disease in severe falciparum malaria (Clark 1978)

- the identification of up-regulation of endothelial receptors for PRBC, particularly ICAM-1, which could be the result of TNF in the circulation (Turner et al 1994). PRBC bind to such receptors, slowing down the local circulation.

- the extension of the nitric oxide hypothesis to CM (Clark et al 1991). At its simplest, infection-stimulated macrophages secrete TNF and IL-1, which induces NO production from endothelial cells via inducible nitric oxide synthase (iNOS). NO as a vasodilator could cause systemic hypotension (seen in malaria) as well as intracerebral vasodilatation; local NO production acts as a neurotransmitter, sending 'nonsense' signals within the brain and compromising cerebral function and so coma.

There is also speculation that the haemozoin pigment itself influences release of TNF and the expression of adhesion molecules for leucocytes, and that it may directly damage endothelial cells and lead to increased permeability (Picchyangkul et al 1997). Major obstacles in our understanding the pathogenesis of cerebral malaria include: (i) the lack of a good experimental model; (ii) our inability to image the local cerebral blood flow at high resolution in malaria patients; and (iii) the fact that patients die sometime after going into coma, so the autopsy morphology is not necessarily representative of the initiating sequence of events.

HELMINTH INFECTIONS

SPARGANOSIS

Sparganosis is infection by a larval stage of a *Spirometra* spp., which wanders in the soft tissues of the body, a type of larva migrans (Carroll et al 1997). The adult worms are endemic in animals in the Far East and Africa and the life cycle involves several intermediate hosts, man being an incidental host. The worm is ribbon-like and millimetres to centimetres long. It may present as an painful migrating subcuticular or intramuscular swelling and, sometimes, may migrate to the orbit causing proptosis and even to the brain causing a focal lesion. The lag between initial infection and presentation may be years; in a recent case in the UK, the infection was acquired in China more than 20 years previously.

Skin and subcutis biopsy samples may reveal fragments of a white thin flat worm about 1 mm across, surrounded by acute and chronic inflammation and fibrosis; if the worm has migrated away, there may be an empty track with surrounding necrosis. Eosinophilia in tissues and blood is common. Histologically, the worm has a characteristic cestode tegument and calcareous bodies, and a spongy but not cystic internal structure without intestines (Fig. 2.8).

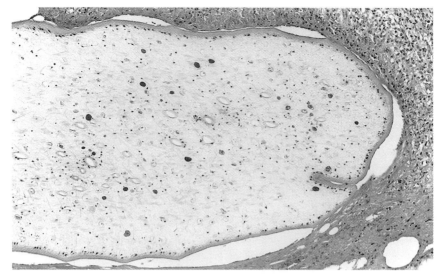

Fig. 2.8 Sparganosis – a spot-diagnosis rarity. Medium power view of the subcutis of a patient with larva migrans. There is a spongy worm seen here in cross-section, with a thin tegument. The dark dots are calcareous corpuscles; the tubule-like structures are typical of *Spirometra* larvae. There is an eosinophilic and fibrinous surrounding reaction. H&E.

CONCLUSIONS

This is a brief survey of some infections that histopathologists may encounter. Emerging infections (Schwartz et al 1995, Schwartz 1997) – newly recognised infections, re-emergence of infections that were regarded as declining to insignificance, and newly drug-resistant recognised infections – will continue to occupy an increasingly important area of pathological practice. It is only a matter of time before new diseases, such as erlichiosis and Hantavirus pulmonary syndrome, appear in the UK from endemic areas in travellers. Diagnoses such as intestinal and hepatic amoebiasis, visceral leishmaniasis, strongyloidiasis and disseminated tuberculosis are medical emergencies and urgent treatment is required. Diagnosis requires a high index of suspicion, knowledge of the histopathological features and enhanced communications with ward clinicians and microbiologists.

References

Advisory Committee on Dangerous Pathogens 1995 Categorisation of biological agents according to hazard and categories of containment. London: HSE Books

Albrecht H, Sobottka I, Emminger C et al 1997 Visceral leishmaniasis emerging as an important opportunistic infection in HIV-infected persons living in areas non-endemic for *Leishmania donovani*. Arch Pathol Lab Med 121: 189–198

Alvar J, Canavate C, Gutierrez-Solar B et al 1997 Leishmania and HIV co-infection: the first 10 years. Clin Microbiol Rev 10: 298–319

Andresen K, Gaafar A, El-Hassan A M et al 1996 Evaluation of PCR in the diagnosis of cutaneous leishmaniasis due to Leishmania major: a comparison with direct microscopy of smears and sections from lesions. Trans R Soc Trop Med Hyg 90: 133–135

Baselga E, Margall N, Barnadas M A, Coll P, de Moragas J M 1997 Detection of *Mycobacterium tuberculosis* DNA in lobular granulomatous panniculitis (erythema induratum-nodular vasculitis). Arch Dermatol 133: 457–462

Bendall R P, Lucas S B, Moody A, Tovey G, Chiodini P L 1993 Diarrhoea associated with cyanobacterium-like bodies: a new coccidian enteritis of man. Lancet 341: 590–592

BHIVA Guidelines Co-ordinating Committee 1997 British HIV Association guidelines for antiretroviral treatment of HIV seropositive individuals. Lancet 349: 1086–1092

Blenden D C, Creech W, Torres-Anjel M J 1984 Use of immunofluorescence examination to detect rabies virus antigen in the skin of humans with clinical encephalitis. J Infect Dis 154: 698–701

Bulmer J N, Rasheed F N, Francis N, Morrison L, Greenwood B M 1993 Placental malaria. 1. Pathological classification. Histopathology 22: 211–218

Burt F J, Swanepoel R, Shieh W J et al 1997 Immunohistochemical and in situ localisation of Crimean-Congo hemorrhagic fever (CCHF) virus in human tissues and implications for CCHF pathogenesis. Arch Pathol Lab Med 121: 839–846

Carr A, Marriott D, Field A, Vasak E, Cooper D A 1998 Treatment of HIV-1-associated microsporidiosis and cryptosporidiosis with combination antiretroviral therapy. Lancet 351: 256–261

Carroll C L, Connor D H. Sparganosis 1997 In: Connor D H, Chandler F W (eds) Pathology of infectious diseases. Stanford: Appleton & Lange, pp 1559–1566

Christou L G, Dalekos G N, Barbati K, Tsianos E V 1997 A 54-year old stockbreeder with ascites. Lancet 349: 994

Clark I A 1978 Does endotoxin cause both the disease and parasite death in acute malaria and babesiosis? Lancet; ii: 75–77

Clark I A, Rockett K A, Cowden W B 1991 Proposed link between cytokines, NO and human cerebral malaria. Parasitol Today 7: 205–207

Cooper C R, McGinnis M R 1997 Pathology of *Penicillium marneffei*. An emerging AIDS-related pathogen. Arch Pathol Lab Med 121: 798–804

Cowley G P, Miller R F, Papadaki L, Canning E U, Lucas S B 1997 Disseminated micro-sporidiosis (*Encephalitozoon intestinalis*) in a patient with AIDS. Histopathology 30: 386–389

Davis K J, Anderson A O, Geisbert T W et al 1997 Pathology of experimental Ebola virus infection in African green monkeys. Arch Pathol Lab Med 121: 805–819

de Bruijn M H, Barker D C 1992 Diagnosis of New World leishmaniasis: specific detection of species of the L.brasililensis comples by amplification of kinetoplast DNA. Acta Trop 52: 45–58

De Wit M Y L, Faber W R, Krieg S R et al 1991 Application of a polymerase chain reaction for the detection of *Mycobacterium leprae* in skin tissues. J Clin Microbiol 29: 906–910

Di Bisceglie A M 1998 Hepatitis C. Lancet 351: 351–355

DiSalvo A F, Fickling A M, Ajello L 1973 Infection caused by *Penicillium marneffei*: description of first natural infection in man. Am J Clin Pathol 59: 259

Duong T A 1996 Infection due to *Penicillium marneffei*, an emerging pathogen: review of 155 reported cases. Clin Infect Dis 23: 125–130

Eberhard M L, Pieniazek N J, Arrowood M J 1997 Laboratory diagnosis of *Cyclospora* infections. Arch Pathol Lab Med 121: 792–797

El Hassan A M, Ghalib H W, Zijlstra E E et al 1992 Post kala-azar dermal leishmaniasis in the Sudan: clinical features, pathology and treatment. Trans R Soc Trop Med Hyg 86: 245–248

Fine P E M, Job C K, Lucas S B, Meyers W M, Pönnighaus J M, Sterne J A C 1993 The extent, origin and implications of observer variation in the histopathological diagnosis of leprosy. Int J Lepr 61: 270–282

Hara K, Tsuzuki T, Takagi N, Shimokata K 1997 Nodular granulomatous phlebitis of the skin: a fourth type of tuberculid. Histopathology 30: 129–134

Hilmarsdottir I, Meynard J L, Rogeaux O et al 1993 Dissemianted *Penicillium marneffei* infection associated with human immunodeficiency virus: a report of two cases and a review of 35 published cases. J Acquir Immune Defic Syndr 6: 466–471

Jamil S, Keer J T, Lucas S B et al 1993 Use of the polymerase chain reaction in evaluating the efficacy of leprosy chemotherapy. Lancet 342: 264–268

Job C K, Baskaran B, Jayakumar J, Aschoff M 1997a Histopathologic evidence to show that indeterminate leprosy may be a primary lesion of the disease. Int J Lepr 65: 443–449

Job C K, Jayakumar J, Williams D L, Gillis T P 1997b Role of polymerase chain reaction in the diagnosis of early leprosy. Int J Lepr 65: 461–464

Klatser P R, van Beers S, Madjid B, Day R, De Wit M Y L 1993 Detection of *Mycobacterium leprae* nasal carriage in a leprosy endemic population. J Clin Microbiol 31: 2947–2951

Laskay T, Miko T L, Negesse Y, Solbach W, Rollinghoff M, Frommel D 1995 Detection of cutaneous Leishmania infection in paraffin-embedded skin biopsies using the polymerase chain reaction. Trans R Soc Trop Med Hyg 89: 273–275

Lucas S B 1989 Aspects of infectious disease. In: Anthony P P, MacSween R N M (eds) Recent Advances in Histopathology vol 14. Edinburgh: Churchill Livingstone, pp 281–302

Lucas S B 1990 Missing infections in AIDS. Trans R Soc Trop Med Hyg; 84 Suppl 1: 34–38

Lucas S B 1993 HIV and leprosy [editorial]. Lepr Rev 64: 97–103

Lucas S B 1994 Other viral and infectious diseases and HIV-related liver disease. In: McSween R N M, Anthony P P, Scheuer P, Burt A D (eds) Pathology of the liver. Edinburgh: Churchill Livingstone, pp 269–315

Lucas S B 1998 Histopathology. In: Davies P D O (ed) Clinical tuberculosis. London: Chapman & Hall, pp 113–127

Lucas S B, Hounnou A, Bell J E et al 1996 Severe cerebral swelling is not observed in children dying with malaria. Q J Med 89: 351–353

MacPherson G G, Warrell M J, White N J, Looareesuwan S, Warrell D A 1985 Human cerebral malaria. A quantitative ultrastructural analysis of parasitized erythrocyte sequestration. Am J Pathol 119: 385–401

Maegraith B 1977 Interdependence. Am J Trop Med Hyg 26: 344–355

Majunder T D 1967 Histopathology of Indian PKDL. Dermatol Int 6: 174–177

Marchiafava E, Bignami A 1894 On summer-autumnal malaria fevers. In: Anonymous Malaria and the parasites of malarial fevers. London: The Syndenham Society, pp 1–234

McDougall A C 1997 Recent developments in the chemotherapy of leprosy. Lepr Rev 68: 294–298

Metze K, Feiden W 1991 Rabies virus nucleoprotein in the heart. N Engl J Med 324: 1814–1815

Miller R F, Lucas S B, Pinching A J 1994 Disseminated histoplasmosis in patients with acquired immunodeficiency syndrome. Genitourin Med 70: 132–137

Mrak R E, Young L 1994 Rabies encephalitis in humans: pathology, pathogenesis and pathophysiology. J Neuropathol Exp Neurol 53: 1–10

Nambuya A, Sewankambo N K, Mugerwa J, Goodgame R W, Lucas S B 1988 Tuberculous lymphadenitis associated with human immunodeficiency virus (HIV) in Uganda. J Clin Pathol 41: 93–96

Nandy A, Addy M, Maji A K, Guha S K, Banerjee D, Chaudhuri D 1998 Recurrence of kala azar after PKDL: role of co-factors. Trop Med Int Health 3: 76–78

Newton C R J, Taylor T E, Whitten R O 1998 Pathophysiology of fatal falciparum malaria in African children. Am J Trop Med Hyg 58: 673–683

Nolte K B, Feddersen R M, Foucar K et al 1995 Hantavirus pulmonary syndrome in the USA: a pathological description of a disease caused by a new agent. Hum Pathol 26: 110–120

Noordhoek G T, van Emden J D, Kolk A H 1996 Reliability of nucleic acid amplification for detection of *Mycobacterium tuberculosis*: an international collaborative quality control study among 30 laboratories. J Clin Microbiol 34: 2522–2525

Ormerod P 1996 Tuberculosis and immigration. Br J Hosp Med 56: 209–212

PHLS CDSC 1998 AIDS and HIV-1 infection in the UK: monthly report. Commun Dis Rep CDR Wkly 8: 37–40

Pichhyangkul S, Saengkrai P, Yongvanitchit K, Heppner D G, Kyle D E, Webster H K 1997 Regulation of leukocyte adhesion molecules CD11b/CD18 and LAM-1 on phagocytic cells activated by malaria pigment. Am J Trop Med Hyg 57: 383–388

Pönnighaus J M, Fine P E M, Sterne J A C et al 1992 Efficacy of BCG vaccine against leprosy and tuberculosis in northern Malawi. Lancet 339: 636–639

Raman G V, Prosser A, Spreadbury P L, Cockcroft P M, Okubadejo O A 1988 Rabies presenting with myocarditis and encephalitis. J Infect 17: 155–158

Richter E, Greinert U, Kirsten D et al 1996 Assessment of mycobacterial DNA in cells and tissues of mycobacterial and sarcoid lesions. Am J Resp Crit Care Med 153: 375–380

Richter E, Schlütter C, Duchrow M et al 1995 An improved method for the species-specific assessment of mycobacteria in routinely formalin-fixed and paraffin-embedded tissues. J Pathol 175: 85–92

Rollin P E, Ksiazek T G 1998 Ebola haemorrhagic fever. Trans R Soc Trop Med Hyg 92: 1–2

Saboor S A, Johnson N M, McFadden J 1992 Detection of mycobacterial DNA in sarcoidosis and tuberculosis with polymerase chain reaction. Lancet 339: 1012–1015

Santa Cruz D J, Strayer D S 1982 The histopathologic spectrum of the cutaneous mycobacteriosis. Hum Pathol 13: 485–495

Schmaljohn C, Hjelle B 1997 Hantaviruses: a global disease problem. Emerg Infect Dis 3: 95–104

Schultz T F, Boshoff C H, Weiss R A 1996 HIV infection and neoplasia. Lancet 348: 587–591

Schwartz D A 1997 Emerging and re-emerging infections. Progress and challenges in the subspecialty of infectious disease pathology. Arch Pathol Lab Med 121: 776–784

Schwartz D A, Bryan R T, Hughes J M 1995 Pathology and emerging infections – quo vadimus? Am J Pathol 147: 1525–1533

Sepkowitz K A 1998 Effect of HAART on natural history of AIDS-related opportunistic infections. Lancet 351: 228–230

Spitz S 1946 The pathology of acute falciparum malaria. Milit Surg 99: 555–572

Tsui W M S, Ma K F, Tsang D N C 1992 Disseminated *Penicillium marneffei* infection in HIV-infected subject. Histopathology 20: 287–291

Turner G D H 1997 Cerebral malaria. Brain Pathol 7: 569–582

Turner G D H, Morrison H, Jones M et al 1994 An immunohistochemical study of the pathology of fatal malaria. Am J Pathol 145: 1057–1069

UNAIDS 1997 Report on the global HIV/AIDS epidemic. Geneva: UNAIDS, pp 1–13

van Nhieu J T, Nin F, Fleury-Feith J et al 1996 Identification of intracelluar stages of *Cyclospora* species by light microscopy of thick sections using H&E. Hum Pathol 27: 1107–1109

Waddell K M, Lewallen S, Lucas S B, Ateenyi-Agaba C, Herrington C S, Liomba N G 1996 Carcinoma of the conjunctiva and HIV infection in Uganda and Malawi. Br J Ophthalmol 80: 503–508

Walker D H, Dumler J S 1997 Human monocytic and granulocytic erlichiosis. Arch Pathol Lab Med 121: 785–791

Wheat L J, Slama T G, Norton J A et al 1982 Risk factors for disseminated or fatal histoplasmosis. Ann Intern Med 96: 159–163

World Health Organization 1997 Report of the third meeting of the leprosy elimination group, Geneva, 16–17th July, 1997. WHO/LEP97 6

Yachnis A T, Berg J, Martinez-Salazar A et al 1996 Disseminated microsporidiosis especially infecting the brain, heart, and kidneys. Am J Clin Pathol 106: 535–543

Zaki S R, Greer P W, Goldsmith C S et al 1996 Ebola virus hemorrhagic fever: pathologic, immunopathologic and ultrastructural studies. Lab Invest 74 133A

Zaki S R, Khan A S, Goodman R A et al 1997 Retrospective diagnosis of Hantavirus pulmonary syndrome, 1979–93. Arch Pathol Lab Med 121: 134–139

Zaki S R, Shieh W J 1996 Leptospirosis associated with an outbreak of acute febrile illness and pulmonary haemorrhage, Nicaragua 1995. Lancet 347: 535–536

Zijlstra E E, El-Hassan A M, Ismael A 1995 Endemic kala azar in eastern Sudan: post kala azar dermal leishmaniasis. Am J Trop Med Hyg 52: 299–305

J. E. Martin, V. V. Smith, P. Domizio

CHAPTER 3

Myopathies of the gastrointestinal tract

The normal motility of the gastrointestinal tract relies on proper innervation and effective contraction of smooth muscle. Loss of co-ordinated neuro-muscular function results in altered motility and abnormal bowel transit. Functional intestinal obstruction or chronic intestinal pseudo-obstruction occurs when, as a result of nerve or muscle dysfunction, intestinal peristalsis fails to overcome resistance to flow. This clinical syndrome is characterised by repeated episodes of intestinal obstruction in the absence of any mechanical blockage of the lumen.

Many nerve and muscle diseases can lead to gastrointestinal motility disorders with or without functional intestinal obstruction. The disordered physiology of these diseases has been understood for some time but only recently have advances been made in characterising the underlying structural and morphological abnormalities. Much of this information has been obtained in children from full-thickness intestinal samples taken during decompression surgery and in adults from partial or total colectomy specimens examined following surgical intervention in patients refractory to medical therapy, and from experimental models. Recent advances in laparoscopic surgery have made the deeper layers of the bowel wall more accessible to biopsy and histological examination while avoiding the morbidity associated with exploratory laparotomy. The muscularis propria and myenteric plexus can now be examined at earlier stages of the pathological process before end-stage changes develop.

In this chapter we will concentrate on newly described myopathies of the gastrointestinal tract in adults and children.

Dr P. Domizio, Department of Histopathology, St Bartholomew's Hospital, West Smithfield, London EC1A 7BE, UK
Prof. J.E. Martin, Department of Histopathology, The Royal London Hospital, London, UK
Dr V.V. Smith, Department of Histopathology, Camelia Botnar Laboratories, Great Ormond Street Hospital for Children NHS Trust, Great Ormond Street, London WC1N 3JH, UK

Table 3.1 Classification of gastro-intestinal myopathies

PRIMARY MYOPATHIES

Congenital/Early onset

Abnormal developmental (morphogenic) phenotypes
Focal absence of enteric muscle coats
Segmental fusion of enteric muscle coats
Presence of additional muscle coats

Other phenotypes
Myopathy with autophagic activity
Pink blush myopathy with nuclear crowding
Contractile protein abnormality

Myopathies with atrophy and fibrosis

Late onset

Myopathies with atrophy and fibrosis
Hollow visceral myopathies: sporadic or familial
Degenerative leiomyopathy

Autoimmune myopathy

Inclusion body myopathies
Polyglucosan body myopathy
Mitochondrial leiomyopathy

SECONDARY MYOPATHIES

Systemic disorders
Desmin myopathy
Muscular dystrophies
Mitochondrial cytopathies
Metabolic storage disorders
Amyloidosis
Progressive systemic sclerosis
Other collagen vascular disorders

Local disorders
Irradiation

CLASSIFICATION

Intestinal myopathy can be primary or secondary. Primary myopathies are due to an innate abnormality in enteric muscle and can be congenital, of early onset or of late onset. Secondary myopathies occur as part of a multisystem disease such as progressive systemic sclerosis (Schuffler & Beegle 1979, Venizelos et al 1988) and can also complicate abdominal or pelvic radiotherapy. Two main groups of congenital or early onset myopathies are recognised: those resulting from developmental (morphogenic) abnormalities in the intestinal musculature and specific phenotypes in which no developmental abnormality is apparent. A third group of fibrosing myopathies is similar to that occurring in older children and adults. A classification of enteric myopathies is given in Table 3.1.

In adults, secondary myopathies are more common than primary while in children the converse is true. Most primary myopathies in children are either congenital or of early onset; late onset forms are rare (Smith & Milla 1997).

The region of gut affected by intestinal myopathy can be segmental, multifocal or diffuse (Fitzgibbons & Chandrasoma 1987, Smith & Milla 1997, Verne & Sninsky 1995, Emanuel et al 1967, Humphry et al 1980, Yamagiwa et al 1988). In general, patients' symptoms and prognosis do not depend on the type of myopathy but on whether the disease is segmental or diffuse. Intestinal pseudo-obstruction is associated with diffuse myopathy while severe constipation is frequent in segmental disease. Symptoms of pseudo-obstruction include chronic abdominal pain, abdominal distension and bloating, early satiety, recurrent nausea and vomiting, and alternating diarrhoea and constipation. Without treatment, weight loss and malnutrition eventually ensue (Christensen et al 1990, Schuffler et al 1977, Schuffler et al 1981) It is important to clarify the extent of disease, as surgery is helpful in segmental and focal conditions but is of limited use in diffuse disorders.

Involvement of the urinary tract may accompany myopathies of the gut, usually of congenital type and less commonly of late onset type (Higman et al 1992, Schuffler et al 1988, Knafelz et al 1996). The resulting syndrome has been termed hollow visceral myopathy. Children with hollow visceral myopathy present at or before birth with hydronephrosis, megaureters and megacystis, or in the first year of life with constipation and episodes of intestinal pseudo-obstruction (Milla 1994) with or without urinary obstruction and recurrent urinary tract infections (Knafelz et al 1996). Hollow visceral myopathy in adults may present at any age. As in children, gastrointestinal symptoms such as constipation and pseudo-obstruction are associated with a varying degree of urinary symptomatology. Some patients have no urinary symptoms while others suffer urinary retention and/or recurrent urinary tract infections (Fitzgibbons & Chandrasoma 1987, Higman et al 1992, Schuffler et al 1977).

Myopathies can be sporadic or familial. Familial myopathies can show an autosomal dominant (Fitzgibbons & Chandrasoma 1987, Schuffler & Pope 1977, Rodrigues et al 1989), autosomal recessive (Smith & Milla 1997) or X-linked (Smith & Milla 1997) pattern of inheritance. In a series of 25 children with primary intestinal myopathy (Knafelz et al 1996), three were related and another four had an affected family member. There may be considerable underestimation of the number of patients who are actually related to each other, as has been found following pedigree searching of patients with neurodegenerative disorders, and a further series of founder mutations may be identified once the genetic basis of this group of disorders is clarified.

INVESTIGATIONS

Initial investigations in patients with suspected intestinal myopathy include plain abdominal X-rays, abdominal ultrasound, radio-opaque pellet radiography and contrast studies. In children with congenital disease and adults with suspected hollow visceral myopathy, micturating cystourethrography or cystometric studies can be useful. Scintigraphy may be performed for assessing colonic motility and gastric emptying. Defecography may be useful in isolated rectal evacuatory defects. Rectal suction biopsy to look for Hirschsprung's disease is important in a child or young adult with functional intestinal obstruction (Lake et al 1978).

Physiological studies such as surface electrogastrography (Devane et al 1992) and antroduodenal jejunal manometry (Fell et al 1996) are being increasingly used for gastric, colonic and anorectal motility profiling. Remote monitoring and long period ambulatory telemetry can be used to assess motility throughout the gastrointestinal tract but are still predominantly research tools.

Sensory function is frequently studied in the attempt to exclude a neuropathic element to the gastrointestinal motility disorder. Such sensory testing may include barostat visceral sensation and compliance studies which involve balloon distention of parts of the gastrointestinal tract. Recordings of cortical evoked potentials after visceral balloon distension has also been used to study central pathways of motility control. Electrophysiological studies including nerve conduction studies and evoked potentials are also used in this context.

SPECIMEN HANDLING

Pathological studies of full thickness intestinal biopsies are increasingly important in diagnosis, but few pathologists outside specialist centres have experience of these. The abnormalities in many intestinal myopathies may not be apparent on haematoxylin and eosin-stained sections; thus histochemical, immunohistochemical and ultrastructural examination may be required to establish a diagnosis. Ideally, each case should be discussed with the pathologist before a biopsy is taken so that it can be submitted in the most appropriate manner, usually as a fresh specimen. Most pathologists will have no warning, however, and will have to be content to attempt a diagnosis on formalin fixed material. Clinical information is essential in the diagnosis of this group of disorders, particularly in relation to the presence or absence of diabetes, neurological disease, sensory neuropathy and systemic sclerosis.

On receipt of the fresh specimen, it should be divided: full thickness portions should be snap-frozen for histochemistry; fixed in formal saline for routine histology; and fixed in glutaraldehyde for electron microscopy. Laparoscopic biopsies are typically 1–2 cm by 1 cm, and though categorised as full thickness, rarely include serosal fat or peritoneum. The size of non-laparoscopic specimens varies from a sleeve of full-thickness intestine about 4 cm long obtained at the time of planned decompression surgery to a total colectomy specimen.

Sampling should be thorough as myopathic changes can be patchy. In a total colectomy specimen from an adult, blocks should be taken at 5 cm intervals. In a child, the colon is relatively shorter and sequential blocks can be taken along the whole length of the colon. A laparoscopic specimen embedded in one block should be cut at several levels to look for focal changes. If there is any possibility of short segment Hirschsprung's disease a full length 'Swiss roll' strip of bowel should be taken to examine the neuronal plexuses, but this diagnosis is likely to have been excluded prior to full thickness biopsy or surgery.

The orientation of the specimen in the block is important, as the interpretation of muscle layering and thickness is dependent on good orientation of the layers of the bowel wall.

All blocks sampled should have sections stained with haematoxylin and eosin, periodic acid–Schiff and a connective tissue stain such as haematoxylin–van Gieson, trichrome or picrosirius. Additional histochemical stains useful in paediatric specimens include acid phosphatase to identify active lysosomes and acetylcholinesterase to examine intestinal innervation. Immunohistochemical stains for desmin, alpha smooth muscle actin and neurofilament proteins can give useful information, as can immunostains for other proteins involved in smooth muscle contraction, especially when changes on routine stains are not detectable or only subtle.

Electron microscopy is a key investigation in suspected gastrointestinal myopathy, giving information on myofilament structure and dense-body distribution, structural integrity and distribution of mitochondria, and the nature of inclusion bodies.

PROBLEMS IN INTERPRETATION

Artefactual vacuolation and shrinkage of muscle fibres may be produced in several ways, including heat damage during diathermy, drying of the specimen and putting the specimen into water before fixation. An artefactual feature of particular note is the mosaic pattern of fibre-staining produced by severe traction or compression during surgery. This is manifested as staining of individual myofibres in a range of pale eosinophilic shades, unlike the relatively uniform bright eosinophilia of normal fibres.

Focal fibrosis with loss of muscle may be the result of previous surgery and ischaemia but this is unlikely to cause confusion with myopathy if a good clinical history is provided. Full-thickness rectal biopsy is generally unsuitable for the diagnosis of intestinal myopathy as normal lower rectal circular muscle consists of fan-like smooth muscle bundles with prominent intramysial connective tissue separated by wide fibrous tissue septa, which therefore mimic the changes of myopathic disease.

MORPHOLOGICAL CHANGES

Morphological changes seen in intestinal myopathies include varying degrees of fibrosis, hypertrophy or atrophy of muscle fibres, vacuolation of myocytes (Schuffler et al 1977, Schuffler & Pope 1977, Faulk et al 1978, Jacobs et al 1979, Smith et al 1982, Anuras et al 1983, Milla et al 1983, Puri et al 1983, Bagwell et al 1984, Smout et al 1985, Anuras et al 1986a,b, Kaschula et al 1987, Alstead et al 1988, Schuffler et al 1988, Vargas et al 1988, Nonaka et al 1989, Rodrigues et al 1989, Martin et al 1990, Rode et al 1992), presence of intracellular inclusion bodies (Martin et al 1990, Fogel et al 1993), abnormal layering of the muscle (Emanuel et al 1967, Humphry et al 1980, Yamagiwa et al 1988, Husain et al 1992, Smith & Milla 1997) and alteration in the immunohistochemical staining pattern of myocyte contractile proteins (Smith et al 1992). Though many of these abnormalities are similar in childhood and adult myopathies, some differences have been observed. One such difference is inclusion bodies which are relatively common in adults but have not been reported in children.

Careful examination of vascular smooth muscle is important in the assessment of any enteric myopathy but is often overlooked. When changes such as inflammation, fibrosis or inclusion bodies are present in vascular smooth muscle, they are more likely to indicate a systemic disorder than a primary myopathy.

PRIMARY MYOPATHIES

CONGENITAL AND EARLY ONSET MYOPATHIES

Phenotypes with abnormal muscular development (morphogenic phenotypes)

Strictly speaking, this group of disorders falls outside the accepted classification of gastrointestinal myopathies, but it is useful to consider them since they may present as a failure of gastrointestinal motility. The number of reported patients with developmental phenotypes is so far small, but improving awareness of their existence should permit greater recognition.

Focal absence of enteric muscle coats. Focal absence of one or both layers of the muscularis propria has been reported. In the small intestine, the circular layer can be missing with a normal longitudinal layer (Humphry et al 1980), or both layers can be absent, either as single or multiple foci (Emanuel et al 1967, Husain et al 1992). Focal absence of the muscularis propria has also been reported in the colon (Gosseye et al 1985).

Segmental fusion of enteric muscle coats. Intra-uterine varicella infection at around 15 weeks' gestation can affect normal layering of intestinal muscle coats. Most commonly there is segmental fusion of the muscularis mucosae with the two layers of the muscularis propria resulting in a single muscle band (Hitchcock et al 1995, Smith & Milla 1997).

Presence of additional muscle coats. An additional oblique smooth muscle coat has been described on the outer aspect of the muscularis propria of the small bowel (Yamagiwa et al 1988) and has been seen in the adult colon (personal observation).

An additional circular muscle coat, affecting the gut either segmentally or diffusely, has also been reported (Smith & Milla 1997). The segmental form occurs in the distal small intestine where an additional circular muscle layer is present on the inner aspect of the muscularis propria. This additional layer is composed of bundles of smooth muscle cells orientated in the same plane as the normal circular muscle coat. The bundles are separated from each other and from the normal circular muscle, and a neural plexus is present between the two circular muscle layers (Fig. 3.1A). The diffuse form occurs throughout the whole gut and has an X-linked mode of inheritance. The circular muscle in these patients appears to be bisected by a misplaced neural plexus resulting in

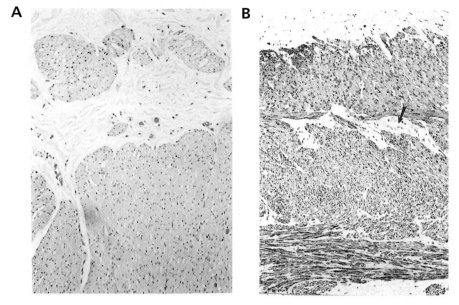

Fig. 3.1 Photomicrographs of the muscularis propria in patients with an additional circular muscle layer. **(A)** Segmental form – the additional smooth muscle bundles can be seen on the inner aspect of the muscularis propria. H & E × 100. **(B)** Diffuse form – the additional circular muscle layer is separated from the subjacent circular muscle by a misplaced neural plexus (arrow). Desmin × 100.

two distinct circular muscle layers (Fig. 3.1B). Clinically, these boys have pyloric stenosis, malrotation and a short small bowel. We have seen this phenotype in four boys, three previously described (Smith & Milla 1997) and in one other unrelated baby boy. Linkage studies in these families are currently in progress to try to establish a genetic basis for this abnormality.

Other phenotypes

Myopathy with autophagic activity. This entity, described by Smith and Milla (1997), affects the entire gut diffusely and is characterised by gross fibrous replacement and profound atrophy of smooth muscle cells in the muscularis propria. In the circular muscle there is a prominent diffuse increase in acetylcholinesterase activity and a number of myocytes show punctate acid phosphatase activity. Immunostaining for neurofilaments shows many neurofilament-positive small tangled fibres in the circular muscle coat, an abnormality associated with myopathic disease (Smith 1990). Immunostaining for contractile proteins is unremarkable even in atrophied smooth muscle cells. On ultrastructural examination, in addition to the fibrosis and myocyte atrophy, a number of smooth muscle cells show dilated active lysosomes containing electron-dense degradation products (Fig. 3.2), which correspond to the acid phosphatase activity seen on light microscopy.

Pink blush myopathy with nuclear crowding. In this phenotype (Smith & Milla 1997), there is an obvious alteration in the distribution of myocyte nuclei

Fig. 3.2 Electron micrograph of a myocyte in a patient with myopathy with autophagic activity. The myocyte shows dilated active lysosomes containing electron dense degradation products. Scale bar = 1 μm. Reproduced with permission from Wrightson Biomedical Publishing Ltd and the authors.

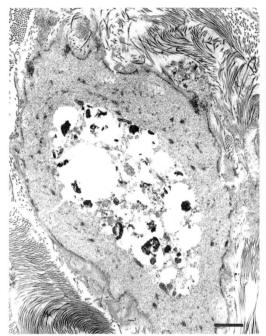

in the circular muscle, with some areas showing nuclear crowding and others showing absence of nuclei (Fig. 3.3). Connective tissue is diffusely increased in the areas where nuclei are lacking, appearing as a 'pink blush' on the picrosirius stain. Ultrastructurally, myocytes are separated from each other by accumulations of granular proteinaceous material in which there are a few collagen fibres.

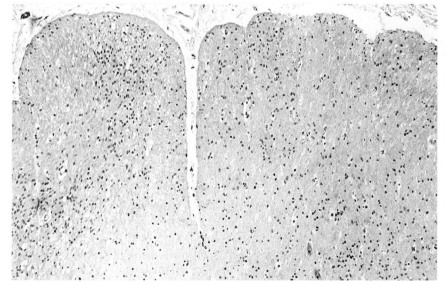

Fig. 3.3 Photomicrograph of the muscularis propria in pink blush myopathy with nuclear crowding. The circular muscle shows areas of nuclear crowding alternating with areas of reduced nuclear density. H & E × 100.

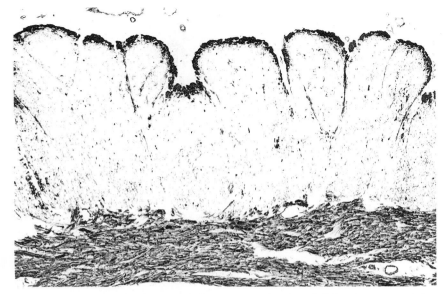

Fig. 3.4 Photomicrograph of the muscularis propria showing deficient immunostaining for alpha smooth muscle isoactin. The deficiency is present in the outer aspect of the circular muscle but not in the inner aspect of the circular muscle or the longitudinal muscle. Smooth muscle isoactin × 100.

Primary specific contractile protein abnormality in apparently normal smooth muscle. Deficient immunostaining for alpha smooth muscle isoactin in the absence of any other muscle abnormality has been reported (Smith et al 1992). The deficiency is seen only in the outer aspect of the circular muscle layer of the muscularis propria and not in the embryologically distinct inner circular muscle layer, the longitudinal muscle layer or the muscularis mucosae (Fig. 3.4). No abnormality is found on immunostaining for other contractile proteins such as beta or gamma actins, myosin, tropomyosin, caldesmon, filamin or desmin. On routine and electron microscopy there is no fibrosis, atrophy or vacuolation of myocytes and the myofilaments appear entirely normal.

Myopathies with atrophy and fibrosis

About 50% of children with congenital or early onset myopathies present with non-specific findings, such as muscular atrophy and fibrosis. These changes are identical to those described in adults with hollow visceral myopathy and are described in greater detail in the following section.

LATE ONSET GASTROINTESTINAL MYOPATHIES

Myopathies with atrophy and fibrosis

Hollow visceral myopathies The most commonly described entity in this group of disorders are the hollow visceral myopathies. Familial and sporadic forms are recognised and the pathological findings are similar in both types. By light microscopy, smooth muscle fibres in the circular and longitudinal

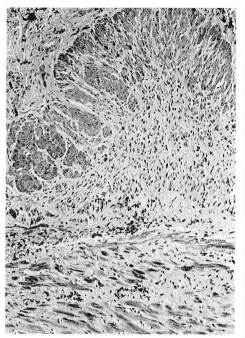

Fig. 3.5 Photomicrograph of muscularis propria in HVM showing severe fibrosis and myocyte atrophy both in the circular and longitudinal muscle layers. H&E × 100.

layers of the muscularis propria show varying degrees of atrophy, vacuolation and fibrosis (Fig. 3.5). Occasionally such changes are not obvious by light microscopy and are visible only on electron microscopy. Ultrastructural changes include myocyte damage with perinuclear vacuolation, disorientation and dissolution of myofilaments, electron lucency of myocyte cytoplasm and swelling of mitochondria (Adler et al 1989). Inclusion bodies are not a recognised finding in this disorder.

Degenerative leiomyopathy. A syndrome of degenerative leiomyopathy affecting intestinal and bladder function has been reported in young Africans from southern, central and eastern Africa (Rode et al 1992). Pathological changes such as intramuscular oedema, intracellular vacuolar change, and muscular atrophy and fibrosis have been described in this condition. It has been suggested that the underlying aetiology is a smooth muscle toxin, possibly derived from herbal medicines (Rode et al 1992), though an acquired auto-immune myopathy or myopathy with autophagic activity may be related to this condition (Smith & Milla 1997).

Auto-immune myopathy

Several authors have described inflammatory myopathies thought to have an auto-immune aetiology in which the main pathological abnormality has been dense T-cell infiltration of the muscularis propria with or without associated fibrosis (McDonald et al 1985, Davies et al 1994, Ginies et al 1996, Smith & Milla 1997). Smith and Milla (1997) described two children with T-cell myositis diffusely involving the small and large intestine associated with circulating IgG-class auto-antibodies against smooth muscle. Davies et al (1994) reported similar findings in an adult presenting with pseudo-obstruction of the small

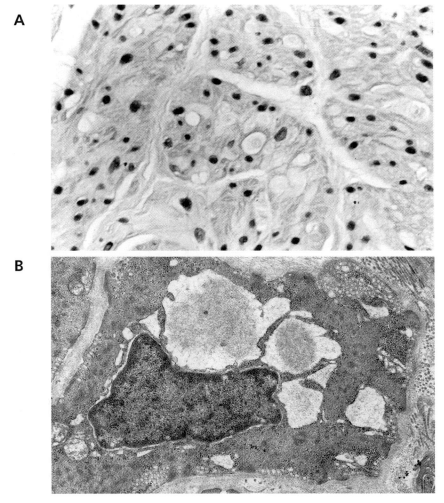

Fig. 3.6 (A) Photomicrograph and **(B)** electron micrograph of muscularis propria in polyglucosan body myopathy showing myocyte vacuolation. (A) H & E ×400, (B) ×7000.

intestine. Full thickness ileal biopsy revealed dense T-cell infiltration of the muscularis propria and subsequent autopsy examination showed diffuse involvement of the whole small and large intestine with patchy fibrosis. No circulating smooth muscle antibodies were identified, however. Immuno-suppressive treatment with prednisolone and cyclosporin has been reported to be of benefit in this condition (Ginies et al 1996, Knafelz et al 1996).

Inclusion body myopathies

Polyglucosan body myopathies. A familial myopathy affecting the smooth muscle of the internal anal sphincter has been reported in several patients (Kamm et al 1991, Martin et al 1990, Guy et al 1997) and we have seen two further cases. Patients are typically women who present with severe anal pain – proctalgia fugax – and hypertrophy of the internal anal sphincter. The

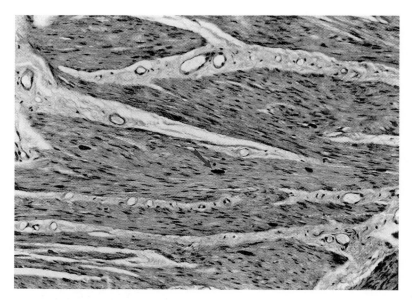

Fig. 3.7 Photomicrograph of muscularis propria in polyglucosan body myopathy showing a polyglucosan inclusion body (arrow). PAS-diastase × 250.

hypertrophic sphincter has a distinctive appearance which is evident both clinically and on imaging. Histologically, myocytes are hypertrophied and show some degree of myofilament disarray and myocyte vacuolation (Fig. 3.6), but the characteristic feature is the presence of PAS-positive, diastase-resistant ovoid inclusion bodies (Fig. 3.7). These inclusion bodies measure up to 200 µm long and have a fibrillary structure on electron microscopy (Fig. 3.8). In size, staining profile and ultrastructural appearance, they bear a striking resemblance to corpora amylacea; these polyglucosan bodies are a common feature of the ageing brain. Similar polyglucosan bodies have also been described in intestinal smooth muscle cells of elderly dogs without associated muscle dysfunction (Kamiya et al 1983). We have found similar inclusions in the muscularis propria of a man with an isolated gastric and jejunal motility disorder in the absence of other clinical or pathological findings. We have not seen them, however, in numerous small and large bowel resection specimens from elderly patients with a range of non-myopathic conditions and they are therefore unlikely to be related specifically to ageing.

Mitochondrial inclusion body myopathy. The spectrum of mitochondrial myopathy is wide and includes a number of phenotypes affecting different organs and tissues. In neurological practice, criteria for the diagnosis of mitochondrial myopathies include the presence of intracellular inclusion bodies by light microscopy, abnormal mitochondrial morphology by electron microscopy, functional disorders of mitochondrial metabolism, and abnormalities in mitochondrial proteins or genome. Similar criteria will probably apply to the diagnosis of mitochondrial myopathies in other organs, including the gastrointestinal tract, pending a comprehensive series of tests for mitochondrial genetic status and function.

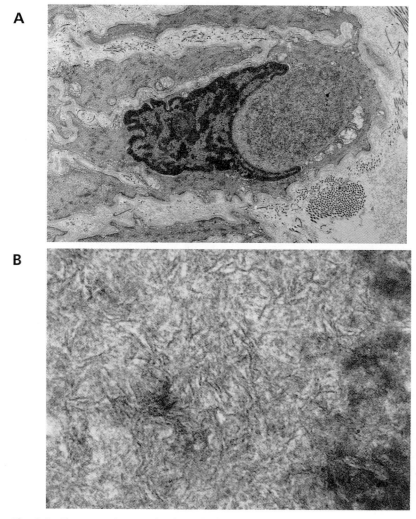

Fig. 3.8 Electron micrograph of a polyglucosan body indenting a myocyte nucleus (**A**). At greater magnification, the fibrillary structure is clearly visible (**B**). (A) ×7000, (B) ×25000.

We have recently become aware of a subgroup of gastrointestinal motility disorders that may be related to this group of diseases (Martin, unpublished data). We have found that up to 40% of adults with gastrointestinal motility disorder predominantly affecting the large bowel have intracellular inclusion bodies in myocytes of the muscularis propria (Fig. 3.9). These occur on a background of histologically normal large bowel, with no evidence of muscular hypertrophy, atrophy or fibrosis and no myocyte vacuolation or myofibrillar disarray. The inclusion bodies are seen in both layers of the muscularis propria but are particularly noticeable in longitudinally cut fibres. They are round, up to 150 μm in diameter and have amphophilic staining characteristics. They do not stain with periodic acid–Schiff, and are negative on immunostaining for structural elements such as cytoskeletal and stress proteins. We have found

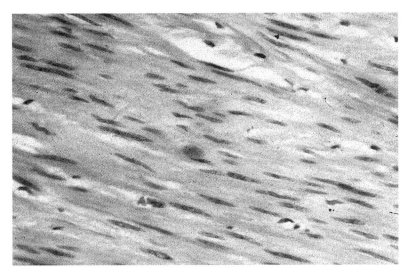

Fig. 3.9 Photomicrograph of muscularis propria in mitochondrial inclusion body myopathy showing an intracellular inclusion body. H & E × 400.

occasional single inclusions in the gut of nonagenarian patients without evidence of enteric myopathy, but have not seen them in a series of 50 small and large bowel resection specimens from younger patients with a range of non-myopathic conditions.

In some patients with these unusual inclusion bodies, ultrastructural examination has shown large aggregates of 5–10 nm fibrils within the cytoplasm. These abnormalities are different from the artefactual changes that occur in mitochondria as a result of poor fixation or peri-operative ischaemia, from which they should be distinguished. These inclusion bodies possibly represent a pathological feature secondary to the motility dysfunction or to a subclinical neuropathy rather than being a primary abnormality. As such, they might be analogous to the inclusion bodies described by Duchen et al (1980) in enteric smooth muscle of diabetic patients with autonomic neuropathy.

'SECONDARY' MYOPATHIES

Clinically apparent gastrointestinal involvement is uncommon in most of the systemic disorders listed in Table 3.1 except for oesophageal involvement in progressive systemic sclerosis. The pathological features of these disorders reflect those of the underlying disease, e.g. fibrosis, inclusion body formation or amyloid deposition.

In progressive systemic sclerosis, changes in gastrointestinal smooth muscle include atrophy and fibrosis of the inner circular muscle layer and fibrosis in the subserosa (Bevans 1945, Schuffler & Beegle 1979). Vacuolation of myocytes is not usually seen. Some authors have suggested that the histological changes can be distinguished from those of primary myopathies, especially when the clinical features are taken into account (Schuffler & Beegle 1979, Lewin et al 1989), while others have suggested that the features may overlap (Venizelos et al 1988).

Inclusion bodies in intestinal smooth muscle cells have been described in many disorders including viral infection, adult polysaccharidosis, Lafora's disease and Batten's disease. Many of these diseases are systemic and the consequences of smooth muscle dysfunction are less clinically significant than failure of other involved organs. A possible exception is desmin myopathy: in this very rare condition, cardiac and skeletal muscle cells contain cytoplasmic inclusions comprising aggregates of the intermediate filament desmin (Ariza et al 1995). Involvement of enteric smooth muscle has recently been reported in a patient with desmin myopathy in whom intestinal pseudo-obstruction was part of the clinical picture (Ariza et al 1995).

Duchen et al (1980) reported the post-mortem findings in a series of diabetic patients with autonomic neuropathy. These findings included eosinophilic inclusion bodies in the smooth muscle cells of the gastrointestinal tract. These inclusion bodies are likely to represent a secondary response to autonomic neuropathy rather than a primary disorder, but little other post-mortem data are available on smooth muscle involvement in other forms of autonomic neuropathy.

Irradiation damage causing atrophy and fibrosis can affect any part of the gastrointestinal tract, but the rectum and internal anal sphincter are particularly susceptible to damage during the course of radiotherapy for cervical and other pelvic neoplasms (Kamm 1998).

AETIOLOGY OF GASTROINTESTINAL MYOPATHIES

A better understanding of bowel wall development and of the genetic mechanisms that control normal ontogeny may help to clarify the aetiology of some of the congenital disorders of gastrointestinal motility. In the embryo, enteric muscle develops from migrating splanchnic mesoderm and the different layers form in a specific sequence (Kedinger et al 1990, Desa 1991) with a rostro-caudal gradient. Neural crest cells may also contribute to a small extent towards the enteric musculature (Peters van der Sanden 1994). In the human embryo, the circular muscle coat first appears at about the 9th week of gestation and the longitudinal muscle at about the 12th week. The muscularis mucosae does not develop until the 5th month and the innermost circular muscle, which is embryologically separate from the rest of the circular muscle, is the last muscle layer to form. Some of the developmental morphogenic abnormalities described above could result from defective genetic control of this sequential process, though other mechanisms such as congenital viral infection or intra-uterine vascular defects/accidents might also operate.

Morphogenesis of the gut is governed by a hierarchy of developmental control genes that regulate each other and their down-stream genes, as yet unidentified (Bitgood et al 1995, Roberts et al 1995, Lyons et al 1995). These genes are responsible for the correct migration of precursor cells, for the differentiation and maturation of immature cells and for the regulation of apoptosis (Glucksmann 1951, McHugh 1995). It can be postulated, for example, that genetic defects resulting in inappropriate apoptosis could lead to myopathy with autophagic activity or that genetically determined abnormalities in the extracellular matrix could be responsible for the pink blush phenotype.

Membrane proteins, intracellular proteins and extracellular matrix proteins are all important in myogenesis and the maturation of myocytes (Schofield et al 1995). An abnormality in any of the up-stream or down-stream genes could result in impairment of these functions and lead to the muscle defects seen in enteric myopathies. Skeletal muscular dystrophies are known to be associated with abnormalities in dystrophin, merosin and other sarcolemmal proteins and similar mechanisms are likely to be involved in gut leiomyodystrophies.

Many of the pathological changes described in acquired gastrointestinal myopathies can directly lead to muscular dysfunction. For example, fibrosis causes separation of myocytes and interferes with normal electrocoupling between them. It is clear that structural myocyte defects such as disorganisation of myofilaments, cytoplasmic vacuolation and alteration in the proteins involved in contraction can all affect the contractile properties of the myocyte, but functional myocyte failure may also occur in the absence of structural changes (Slater et al 1997). Even when demonstrable abnormalities are present, their aetiology is often obscure. In one group of diseases an explanation can be suggested: in the acquired auto-immune myopathies, smooth muscle dysfunction is due to auto-immune myositis causing cell damage, which may be analogous to that occurring in auto-immune enteric ganglionitis (Smith et al 1997). Some cases of myopathy with atrophy and fibrosis may represent end stages of such an auto-immune myopathic process, in which the acute phase of cellular damage and associated inflammatory response is no longer evident, similar to the autopsy findings in the case reported by Davies et al (1994).

The origin of fibrosis in enteric myopathies is not well understood but is probably not due to fibroblastic proliferation as this is almost never a feature of the fibrosing myopathies. The smooth muscle cells, however, often show ultrastructural changes consistent with myofibroblastic differentiation (Martin et al 1993). These include basement membrane around the cells, elongation, notching or convolution of the nucleus, increase in the amount of rough endoplasmic reticulum, pinocytotic vesicles near the plasma membrane, and electron-lucent cytoplasm containing prominent 6–10 nm filaments with conspicuous focal densities (Fig. 3.10). Such myofibroblast-type cells are partly surrounded by mature collagen fibres.

The concept of a mesenchymal cell with features of both fibroblasts and smooth muscle cells, the so-called myofibroblast, was introduced in 1971 (Gabbiani et al 1971, Majno et al 1971). Since then, there has been increasing awareness that myofibroblasts are a normal component of many tissues, including umbilical cord, lung and colon (Lipper et al 1980, Richman et al 1987, Adler et al 1989, Roche 1990, Schurch et al 1992). Myofibroblasts have been implicated in fibrous reactions in many pathological conditions including fibrosing conditions of the large bowel (Balazs & Kovacs 1982, Hwang et al 1986). The origin of these cells has been the subject of much debate: it has been variously suggested that they originate from fibroblasts, smooth muscle cells, pericytes and, in thrombus, from circulating blood cells (Adler et al 1989, Feigl et al 1985, Gabbiani et al 1971, Lipper et al 1980, Majno et al 1971, Hwang et al 1986, Richman et al 1987, Roche 1990, Ross & Klebanoff 1971, Schurch et al 1992). Experimental models in which oestrogen-stimulated rat myometrial cells developed ultrastructural features of fibroblasts highlight the relationship between the two cell types and suggest the presence of intermediate forms

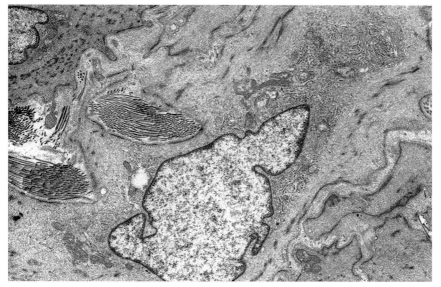

Fig. 3.10 Electron micrograph of a myofibroblast. The nucleus is notched and there is proliferation of endoplasmic reticulum in the cytoplasm, × 14000.

(Ross & Klebanoff 1971). These and other studies have also documented the production of connective tissue proteins by such transformed smooth muscle cells, observations in keeping with the concept that enteric muscle is a dynamic structure. Smooth muscle cells retain the developmental potential to modulate their phenotype to a synthetic proliferative form in response to a range of stimuli including inflammation (Martin et al 1993, McHugh 1995). The changes seen in intestinal myocytes in fibrosing enteric myopathies may, therefore, be an adaptive rather than a primary pathogenetic mechanism. The stimuli which induce such alterations, and the potential reversibility of the changes remain to be clarified.

Points of best practice

- Gut myopathies can be primary (early or late onset) or secondary.

- Myopathic features include fibrosis, hypertrophy or atrophy of muscle fibres, vacuolation of myocytes and the presence of intracellular inclusion bodies.

- Myopathic changes seen in vascular smooth muscle are more likely to indicate a systemic disorder than a primary myopathy.

- Myopathic bowel may look normal on light microscopy and only show ultrastructural changes.

- Artefactual changes may mimic myopathic features

References

Adler K B, Low R B, Leslie K O, Mitchell J, Evans J N 1989 Contractile cells in normal and fibrotic lung. Lab Invest 60: 473–485

Alstead E M, Murphy M N, Flanagan A M, Bishop A E, Hodgson H J F 1988 Familial autonomic visceral myopathy with degeneration of muscularis mucosae. J Clin Pathol 41: 424–429

Anuras S, Mitros F A, Nowak T V et al 1983 Familial visceral myopathy with external ophthalmoplegia and autosomal recessive transmission. Gastroenterology 84: 346–353

Anuras S, Mitros F A, Soper R T et al 1986a Chronic intestinal pseudo-obstruction in young children. Gastroenterology 91: 62–70

Anuras S, Mitros F A, Milano A, Kuminsky R, Decanio R, Green J B 1986b A familial visceral myopathy with dilatation of the entire gastrointestinal tract. Gastroenterology 90: 385–390

Ariza A, Coll J, Fernandes-Figueras M T et al 1995 Desmin myopathy: a multisystem disorder involving skeletal, cardiac and smooth muscle. Hum Pathol 26: 1032–1037

Bagwell C E, Filler R M, Cutz E et al 1984 Neonatal intestinal pseudo-obstruction. J Pediatr Surg 19: 732–739

Balazs M, Kovacs A 1982 The 'transitional' mucosa adjacent to large bowel carcinoma – electron microscopic features and myofibroblast reaction. Histopathology 6: 617–629

Bevans M 1945 Pathology of scleroderma with special reference to changes in the gastrointestinal tract. Am J Pathol 21: 25–51

Bitgood M J, McMahon A P 1995 Hedgehog and Bmp genes are coexpressed at many diverse sites of cell-cell interaction in the mouse embryo. Dev Biol 172: 126–138

Christensen J, Dent J, Malagelada J-R, Wingate D L 1990 Pseudo-obstruction. Gastroenterol Int 3: 107–119

Davies SE, Domizio P, Norton A J 1994 A case of the IMPPOSIBLE – inflammatory myopathy presenting as pseudo-obstruction of the small intestine with bowel loop enlargement. J Pathol 172 suppl: 110A

Desa D J 1991 Alimentary tract. In: Wigglesworth J S, Singer D B (eds) Text book of fetal and perinatal pathology, vol 2. Boston: Blackwell, pp 903–979

Devane S P, Ravelli A M, Bisset W M, Smith V V, Lake B D, Milla P J 1992 Gastric antral dys-rhythmias in children with chronic intestinal pseudo-obstruction (CIIP). Gut 33: 1477–1481

Duchen L W, Anjorin A, Watkins P J, Mackay J D 1980 Pathology of autonomic neuropathy in diabetes mellitus. Ann Intern Med 92: 301–303

Emanuel B, Gault J, Sanson J 1967 Neonatal intestinal obstruction due to absence of intestinal musculature: a new entity. J Pediatr Surg 2: 332–335

Faulk D L, Anuras S, Gardner G D, Mitros F A, Summers R W, Christensen J 1978 A familial visceral myopathy. Ann Intern Med 89: 600–606

Feigl W, Susani M, Ulrich W, Matejka M, Losert U, Sinzinger H 1985 Organisation of experimental thrombosis by blood cells. Virchows Arch 406: 133–148

Fell J E, Smith V V, Milla P J 1996 Infantile chronic idiopathic intestinal pseudo-obstruction: the role of small intestinal manometry as a diagnostic tool and prognostic indicator. Gut 39: 306–311

Fitzgibbons P L, Chandrasoma P T 1987 Familial visceral myopathy. Evidence of diffuse involvement of intestinal smooth muscle. Am J Surg Pathol 11: 846–854

Fogel S P, DeTar M W, Shimada H, Chandrasoma P T 1993 Sporadic visceral myopathy with inclusion bodies. Am J Surg Pathol 17: 473–481

Gabbiani G, Ryan G B, Majno G 1971 Presence of modified fibroblasts in granulation tissue and their possible role in wound contraction. Experientia 27: 549–550

Ginies J L, Francois H, Joseph M G, Champion G, Coupris L, Limal J M 1996 A curable cause of chronic idiopathic intestinal pseudo-obstruction in children: idiopathic myositis of the small intestine. J Pediatr Gastroenterol Nutr 23: 426–429

Glucksmann A 1951 Cell deaths in normal vertebrate autogeny. Biol Rev 26: 59–86

Gosseye S, Libotte B, Moulin D, Buts J P, Otte J B 1985 Localised absence of colonic muscul-ature: an unusual cause of perforation in a colonic esophageal transplant. Pediatr Pathol 4: 143–148

Guy R J, Kamm M A, Martin J 1997 Internal anal sphincter myopathy causing proctalgia fugax and constipation: further clinical and radiological characterisation in a patient. Eur J Hepatol 9: 221–224

Higman D, Peters P, Stewart M 1992 Familial hollow visceral myopathy with varying urological manifestations. Br J Urol 70: 435–438

Hitchcock R, Birthistle K, Carrington D, Calvert S A, Holmes K 1995 Colonic atresia and spinal cord atrophy associated with a case of fetal varicella syndrome. J Pediatr Surg 30: 1344–1347

Humphry A, Mancer K, Stephens C A 1980 Obstructive circular-muscle defect in the small bowel in a one-year-old child. J Pediatr Surg 15: 197–199

Husain A N, Hong H Y, Gooneratne S, Muraskas J, Black P R 1992 Segmental absence of small intestinal musculature. Pediatr Pathol 12: 407–415

Hwang W S, Kally J K, Shaffer E A, Hershfield N B 1986 Collagenous colitis: a disease of pericryptal fibroblast sheath? J Pathol 149: 33–40

Jacobs E, Ardichvili D, Perissino A, Gottignies P, Hanssens J-F 1979 A case of familial visceral myopathy with atrophy and fibrosis of the longitudinal muscle layer of the entire small bowel. Gastroenterology 77: 745–750

Kamiya S, Suzuki Y, Sugimura M 1983 Polyglucosan bodies in the digestive tract of the aged dog. Acta Neuropathol (Berl) 60: 297–300

Kamm M A 1998 Faecal incontinence. BMJ 316: 528–531

Kamm M A, Hoyle C H V, Burleigh D E et al 1991 Hereditary internal sphincter myopathy causing proctalgia fugax and constipation: a newly identified condition. Gastroenterology 100: 805–810

Kaschula R O C, Cywes S, Katz A, Louw J H 1987 Degenerative leiomyopathy with massive megacolon. Myopathic form of chronic idiopathic intestinal pseudo-obstruction occurring in indigenous Africans. Perspect Pediatr Pathol 11: 193–213

Kedinger M, Simon-Assmann P, Bouziges F, Arnold C, Alexandre E, Haffen K 1990 Smooth muscle actin expression during rat development and induction of fetal skin fibroblastic cells associated with intestinal embryonic epithelium. Differentiation 43: 87–97

Knafelz D, Smith V V, Milla P J 1996 The natural history and treatment of hollow visceral myopathy. J Pediatr Gastroenterol Nutr 22: 415

Lake B D, Puri P, Nixon H H, Claireaux A E 1978 Hirschsprung's disease. An appraisal of histochemically demonstrated acetylcholinesterase activity in suction rectal biopsy specimens as an aid to diagnosis. Arch Pathol Lab Med 102: 244–247

Lewin K J, Riddell R H, Weinstein W M 1983 Neuromuscular and neurologic disorders. In: Gastrointestinal pathology and its clinical implications. New York: Igaku-Shoin, pp 258–283

Lipper S, Khan L B, Reddick R L 1980 The myofibroblast. Pathol Ann 15: 409–441

Lyons K M, Hogan B L M, Robertson E J 1995 Colocalization of BMP 7 and BMP 2 RNAs suggest that these factors cooperatively mediate tissue interactions during murine development. Mech Dev 50: 71–83

Majno G, Gabbiani G, Hirschel B J, Statkov P R 1971 Contraction of granulation tissue in vitro: similarity to smooth muscle. Science 173: 548–550

Martin J E, Swash M, Kamm M A, Marher K, Cox E L, Gray A 1990 Myopathy of internal anal sphincter with polyglucosan inclusions. J Pathol 161: 221–226

Martin J E, Benson M, Swash M, Salih V, Gary A 1993 Myofibroblasts in hollow visceral myopathy: the origin of gastrointestinal fibrosis. Gut 34: 999–1001

McDonald G B, Schuffler M D, Kadin M E, Tytgat G N J 1985 Intestinal pseudo-obstruction caused by diffuse lymphoid infiltration of the small intestine. Gastroenterology 89: 882–889

McHugh K M 1995 Molecular analysis of smooth muscle development in the mouse. Dev Dyn 204: 278–290

Milla P J 1994 Clinical features of intestinal pseudo-obstruction in children. In: Kamm M A, Lennard-Jones J E (eds) Constipation. Petersfield: Wrightson, pp 251–258

Milla P J, Lake B D, Spitz L, Nixon H H, Harries J T, Fenton T R 1983 Chronic idiopathic intestinal pseudo-obstruction in infancy: a smooth muscle disease. In: Labo G, Bortolotti M (eds) Gastrointestinal motility. Verona: Cortinal International, pp 125–131

Nonaka M, Goulet O, Arahan P, Fekete C, Ricour C, Nezelof C 1989 Primary intestinal myopathy, a cause of chronic idiopathic intestinal pseudo-obstruction syndrome (CIPS): clinicopathological studies of seven cases in children. Pediatr Pathol 9: 409–424

Peters van der Sanden M J H 1994 The hind brain neural crest and the development of the enteric nervous system. PhD thesis. Rotterdam, The Netherlands: Erasmus University

Puri P, Lake B D, Gorman F, O'Donnell B, Nixon H H 1983 Megacystis-microcolon-hypoperistalsis syndrome: a visceral myopathy. J Pediatr Surg 18: 64–69

Richman P I, Tilly R, Jass J R, Bodmer W F 1987 Colonic pericrypt sheath cells: characterisation of cell type with a new monoclonal antibody. J Clin Pathol 40: 593–600

Roberts D J, Johnson R L, Burke A C, Nelson C E, Morgan B A, Tabin C 1995 Sonic hedgehog is an endodermal signal inducing Bmp-4 and Hox genes during induction and regionalization of the chick hindgut. Development 121: 3163–3174

Roche W R 1990 Myofibroblasts. J Pathol 161: 281–282

Rode H, Moore S W, Kaschula R O C, Brown R A, Cywes S 1992 Degenerative leiomyopathy in children. A clinico-pathological study. Pediatr Surg Int 7: 23–29

Rodrigues C A, Shepherd N A, Lennard-Jones J E, Hawley P R, Thompson H H 1989 Familial visceral myopathy: a family with at least 6 involved members. Gut 30: 1285–1292

Ross R, Klebanoff S J 1971 The smooth muscle cell. 1. In vivo synthesis of connective tissue proteins. J Cell Biol 50: 159–165

Schofield J N, Gorecki D C, Blake D J, Davies K, Edwards Y H 1995 Dystroglycan mRNA expression during normal and mdx mouse embryogenesis: a comparison with utrophin and the apo-dystrophins. Dev Dyn 204: 178–185

Schuffler M D, Lowe M C, Bill A H 1977 Studies of idiopathic intestinal pseudo-obstruction. 1. Hereditary hollow visceral myopathy: clinical and pathological studies. Gastroenterology 73: 327–338

Schuffler M D, Pope C E 1977 Studies of idiopathic intestinal pseudo-obstruction. 2. Hereditary hollow visceral myopathy: family studies. Gastroenterology; 73: 339–348

Schuffler M D, Beegle R G 1979 Progressive systemic sclerosis of the gastrointestinal tract and hereditary hollow visceral myopathy: two distinguishable disorders of intestinal smooth muscle. Gastroenterology 77: 664–671

Schuffler M D, Rorhman C A, Chaffee R G, Brand D L, Delaney J H, Young J H 1981 Chronic intestinal pseudo-obstruction: a report of 27 cases and review of the literature. Medicine 60: 173–196

Schuffler M D, Pagon R A, Schwartz R, Bill A H 1988 Visceral myopathy of the gastrointestinal and genitourinary tracts in infants. Gastroenterology 94: 892–898

Schurch W, Seemayer T A, Gabbiani G. Myofibroblast 1992 In: Sternberg S S (ed) Histology for pathologists. New York: Raven, pp 109–144

Slater B J, Varma J S, Gillespie J I 1997 Abnormalities in the contractile properties of colonic smooth muscle in idiopathic slow transit constipation. Br J Surg 84: 181–184

Smith J A, Hauser S C, Madara J I 1982 Hollow visceral myopathy. A light and electron microscopic study. Am J Surg Pathol 6: 269–275

Smith V V 1990 Neurofilament antibodies will differentiate muscle and nerve disorders of chronic idiopathic intestinal pseudo-obstruction. Proc R Microsc Soc 25: 52

Smith V V, Lake B D, Kamm M A, Nicholls J R 1992 Intestinal pseudo-obstruction with deficient smooth muscle alpha actin. Histopathology 21: 535–542

Smith V V, Gregson N, Foggensteiner L, Neale G, Milla P J 1997 Acquired intestinal aganglionosis and circulating autoantibodies without neoplasia or other neural involvement. Gastroenterology 112: 1366–1371

Smith V V, Milla P J 1997 Histological phenotypes of enteric smooth muscle disease causing functional intestinal obstruction in childhood. Histopathology 31: 112–122

Smout A J P M, de Wilde K, Kooyman C D, Ten Thije O J 1985 Chronic idiopathic intestinal pseudo-obstruction. Coexistence of smooth muscle and neuronal abnormalities. Dig Dis Sci 30: 282–287

Vargas J H, Sachs P, Ament M E 1988 Chronic intestinal pseudo-obstruction syndrome in pediatrics. Results of national survey by members of the North American Society of Pediatric Gastroenterology and Nutrition. J Pediatr Gastroenterol Nutr 7: 323–332

Venizelos I D, Shousha S, Bull T B, Parkins R A 1988 Chronic intestinal pseudo-obstruction in two patients. Overlap of features of systemic sclerosis and visceral myopathy. Histopathology 12: 533–540

Verne G N, Sninsky C A 1995 Chronic intestinal pseudo-obstruction. Dig Dis Sci 13: 163–181

Yamagiwa I, Ohta M, Obata K, Washio M 1988 Intestinal pseudo-obstruction in a neonate caused by idiopathic muscular hypertrophy of the entire small intestine. J Pediatr Surg 23: 866–869

Bryan F. Warren, Neil A. Shepherd

Surgical pathology of the intestines: the pelvic ileal reservoir and diversion proctocolitis

Despite its relative heterogeneity, the intestinal mucosa has only a limited repertoire of responses to changing environments and injurious agents. This is well exemplified by changes produced in the intestines as a consequence of various surgical techniques. These cause a wide range of histopathological changes that require precise clinical and endoscopic correlation if the correct diagnosis is to be made. This chapter deals with the pathology of two of the most important, contentious and potentially confusing of these iatrogenic conditions: the pelvic ileal reservoir (or ileo-anal pouch) and diversion proctocolitis. Both are associated with inflammatory changes in the mucosa of the intestine that can be misinterpreted by pathologists. There are important overlaps between the pathology of the pelvic ileal reservoir and that of diversion proctocolitis in terms of histopathological features, pathogenesis and management implications.

PATHOLOGY OF THE PELVIC ILEAL RESERVOIR

Restorative proctocolectomy with ileal reservoir, known as ileal pouch-anal anastomosis in North America, has become a leading surgical procedure for patients with ulcerative colitis and familial adenomatous polyposis (FAP) requiring total colectomy. It continues to be a popular alternative to terminal ileostomy with both surgeons and patients: it is also performed, infrequently, for other conditions such as necrotising enterocolitis in children, other polyposis syndromes (especially juvenile polyposis), intractable constipation and idiopathic megacolon. The pouch acts as a neo-rectum and hence morphological changes familiar to pathologists in the rectum also affect the

Dr Bryan F. Warren, Department of Cellular Pathology, John Radcliffe Hospital, Headington, Oxford OX3 9DU, UK
Professor Neil A. Shepherd, Department of Histopathology, Gloucestershire Royal Hospital, Great Western Road, Gloucester GL1 3NN, UK

reservoir (Warren & Shepherd 1993). Pelvic ileal reservoir construction offers new challenges for pathologists: they may be crucially involved in patient selection, intra-operative diagnosis, and diagnosis and monitoring of the mucosal changes of the reservoir (Warren & Shepherd 1992a, Mortensen 1993).

PRE-OPERATIVE ASSESSMENT AND PATIENT SELECTION

The prime indications for pelvic ileal reservoir surgery are ulcerative colitis and FAP. The pathologist's role in patient selection is relatively easy in FAP and in rarer conditions, such as juvenile polyposis (Stoltenberg et al 1997) but is less straightforward in ulcerative colitis. Correct patient selection is probably the single most important factor affecting the long-term outcome of pelvic ileal reservoir surgery (Mortensen 1993). The pathologist's role is to aid the clinicians in achieving a confident diagnosis of ulcerative colitis and to exclude a diagnosis of Crohn's disease. In most hospitals, Crohn's disease is considered a major contra-indication to reservoir surgery: it is the experience of most coloproctological surgeons that patients with ileal reservoirs constructed for Crohn's disease (often made as a retrospective diagnosis on histopathological assessment of the total colectomy specimen) do badly (Deutsch et al 1991, Mortensen 1993). Only a few coloproctologists are in favour of reservoir construction in selected patients with Crohn's disease (Grobler et al 1993, Panis et al 1996). Inadvertent pouch surgery for patients with subsequently diagnosed Crohn's disease has resulted in a 45% pouch failure rate, usually requiring reservoir excision (Sagar et al 1996). Conversely, indeterminate colitis is associated, generally, with successful reservoir function; patients have similar pouchitis rates to those with ulcerative colitis, but higher rates of pelvic sepsis (Pezim et al 1989, McIntyre et al 1995). Most surgeons would advocate pouch surgery for indeterminate colitis, though this also may be a retrospective diagnosis if reservoir surgery has been undertaken at the time of proctocolectomy (Wells et al 1991). Some patients (about 10%) with a diagnosis of indeterminate colitis at the time of proctocolectomy will subsequently be shown to have Crohn's disease and the outcome of these pouches is very variable (Wells et al 1991, Lucarotti et al 1995).

The pathologist's involvement in the management of patients having pelvic ileal reservoir surgery varies according to the operation and the number of stages of the procedure, whether chosen by the surgeon or dictated by the disease. For example, in patients with fulminant inflammatory bowel disease,

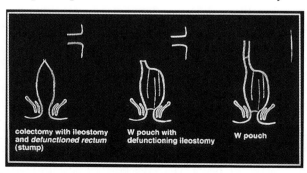

colectomy with ileostomy and *defunctioned rectum* (stump) W pouch with defunctioning ileostomy W pouch

Fig. 4.1 The three-stage pouch procedure of restorative proctocolectomy.

a colectomy with mucus fistula may be the operation of choice with a subsequent reservoir operation when the patient is in a fit state for surgery: this is the three-stage pouch procedure (Fig. 4.1; Parks & Nicholls 1978). In less urgent circumstances, a reservoir will be constructed at the time of colectomy with a temporary ileostomy and subsequent connection to the faecal stream – the two-stage pouch procedure. Some surgeons omit the temporary ileostomy – the one-stage pouch procedure (Fazio et al 1993).

In the three-stage pouch procedure, total colectomy with preservation of a rectal stump and formation of a defunctioning ileostomy are performed initially, followed by construction of a pelvic ileal reservoir anastomosed to the top of the anal canal (Fig. 4.1; Parks & Nicholls 1978). The defunctioning ileostomy is maintained for 6 weeks to allow the reservoir suture lines to heal. Subsequently, the ileostomy is closed and the faecal stream reaches the pelvic ileal reservoir.

The pathologist, with the benefit of a critical review of the clinical history, radiology and previous biopsies, will have confirmed the diagnosis of ulcerative colitis. The two-stage pouch procedure does not permit such detailed examination and here the pathologist has to make a decision pre-operatively or intra-operatively. All previous biopsies should be examined by a pathologist who is not only experienced in inflammatory bowel disease but who also understands the pelvic ileal reservoir procedure, is aware of the importance of a correct diagnosis before successful pelvic ileal reservoir surgery, and is prepared to offer an intra-operative diagnostic service.

Biopsy assessment of chronic inflammatory bowel disease

The histological features that are most reliable on multiple colonic mucosal biopsies to distinguish ulcerative colitis from Crohn's disease have been established for many years (for review *see* Jenkins et al 1997). Crypt distortion and villous surface architecture are characteristic features of ulcerative colitis and are normally present even on an initial biopsy (Talbot & Price 1987, Jenkins et al 1997), providing it has been taken more than 6 weeks after the onset of symptoms. Villous architecture is much less common and less prominent in Crohn's disease and, as with crypt architectural distortion, is absent in acute infective colitis. Mucin depletion has been claimed by some authors to be of value in distinguishing ulcerative colitis from Crohn's disease. We have not found this to be a useful criterion in fulminant ulcerative colitis in which there may be a surprising amount of mucin preservation in non-ulcerated areas. The inflammatory cell infiltrate varies in type and severity with disease activity and, thus, is not an especially useful disease discriminator. Just as the distribution of disease is a useful discriminator of disease in radiological, endoscopic and macroscopical assessment, so the distribution of inflammatory cells, in histological terms, is important in distinguishing ulcerative colitis from Crohn's disease (Jenkins et al 1997). In ulcerative colitis, the infiltrate is diffuse throughout the full thickness of the lamina propria and the full length of the biopsy, and is usually more dense in the distal large bowel.

In some cases of ulcerative colitis there may be some accentuation of the inflammatory infiltrate in the caecal mucosa. This caecal patch lesion is usually a disc-shaped area of inflammation in the caecum separated from the inflamed distal colon by normal mucosa in the ascending colon (d'Haens et al 1997). This pathology is, as yet, unexplained and may represent part of the spectrum of changes in ulcerative colitis. The changes of ulcerative colitis at this site might relate to faecal stasis, which might explain why ulcerative colitis is worse distally in most patients. Relative sparing of the rectum has been described in ulcerative colitis patients. This may be the result of enema treatment, especially steroids, but occurs occasionally in patients without a history of enema usage (Spiliadis et al 1987). Recent studies have also demonstrated that the rectal mucosa affected by unequivocal ulcerative colitis may return to normality, especially after treatment: a normal rectal biopsy can no longer be regarded as a contra-indication to the diagnosis of ulcerative colitis (Levine et al 1997).

Acute inflammation in ulcerative colitis in the form of cryptitis or crypt abscesses tends to be a diffuse process. Biopsies in ulcerative colitis may have patchy acute inflammation in two circumstances: when biopsies are taken from the interface between normal and diseased colon; and when biopsies are taken after treatment (Tanaka & Riddell 1990).

In Crohn's disease, the chronic inflammation in the lamina propria is patchy, often with a striking variability from biopsy to biopsy as well as within an individual biopsy. Acute inflammation in Crohn's disease is also very patchy with individual crypt involvement giving rise to a gland with cryptitis or a crypt abscess being flanked by normal crypts. This patchiness of inflammation, both active and chronic, at the microscopic level is very characteristic of Crohn's disease and has been proven to be the most useful diagnostic discriminator in interobserver studies (Jenkins et al 1997).

The importance of mucosal granulomas in the diagnosis of idiopathic inflammatory bowel disease is overemphasised by some pathologists. Granulomas may occur in inflammatory disease of the colonic mucosa because of mucin release from ruptured crypts, in which they take on a characteristic appearance that includes neutrophils as well as giant cells and are called cryptolytic lesions. There is some doubt about their diagnostic significance (Lee et al 1997, Warren et al 1997). We have found such lesions in several situations including ulcerative colitis, diversion colitis, pouchitis and diverticulosis-associated mucosal inflammation and think that they do not necessarily indicate a diagnosis of Crohn's disease (Warren et al 1997). Microgranulomas (defined as five or more macrophages in aggregation; Jenkins et al 1997) away from disrupted inflamed crypts may also be seen in other conditions, especially as a late result of salmonella and campylobacter enterocolitis (Day et al 1978, Price et al 1979). Tangential sectioning of a crypt base can closely resemble a microgranuloma. Mucosal microgranulomas are of most diagnostic importance when seen in the lamina propria between crypts at multiple sites, and especially when abutting the muscularis mucosae (Jenkins et al 1997). In this situation they help to substantiate the diagnosis of Crohn's disease.

INTRA-OPERATIVE ASSESSMENT

The assistance of a pathologist in assessment of disease at the time of surgery is valuable in the one-stage and two-stage pouch procedure but is rarely required in the three-stage procedure. Perhaps most useful is the intra-operative macroscopic assessment by the pathologist of the colectomy or proctocolectomy specimen before pouch construction is undertaken. Intra-operative assessment of the serosa of the small bowel by both surgeon and pathologist may substantiate a diagnosis of Crohn's disease if the characteristic changes such as serosal exudate and fat wrapping are present (Sheehan et al 1991). The colon can be opened and the mucosa assessed for evidence of diffuse disease and left-sided predominance, features of ulcerative colitis. Skip lesions, other than in the appendix or as a caecal patch lesion, fissuring, bowel wall thickening and fistulae are all changes that suggest Crohn's disease. If the macroscopic features are suggestive of Crohn's disease, a colectomy should be performed leaving a rectal stump. The pathologist can then assess the colectomy specimen microscopically before pouch surgery is undertaken.

Skip lesions have always been considered to be characteristic of Crohn's disease, but may, however, be seen in two circumstances in ulcerative colitis. The appendix in a colectomy specimen may show active chronic inflammatory bowel disease when the proximal colon is normal and there is more distal, often only left-sided active ulcerative colitis (Davison & Dixon 1990). This appendiceal skip lesion is not a contra-indication to restorative procto-colectomy, provided no clinical or microscopic features of Crohn's disease are present. Skip lesions in ulcerative colitis can also involve the caecum, the so-called caecal patch lesion of ulcerative colitis (d'Haens et al 1997). In our experience and that of others (d'Haens et al 1997), this lesion does not change the diagnosis and reservoir surgery is not contra-indicated.

In general, pathologists do not see a role for frozen section diagnosis in the assessment of inflammatory bowel disease. There is a limited role for frozen section diagnosis in the intra-operative evaluation of the large bowel during reservoir surgery.

In such limited situations we recommend frozen sections of:

1. *The largest lymph node.* The presence of well-formed sarcoid-like epithelioid cell granulomas will help to establish a diagnosis of Crohn's disease; poorly formed granulomas should be disregarded. Such changes may be mimicked by various non-specific changes in lymph nodes, especially sinus histiocytosis.

2. *A full thickness biopsy of the most severely affected area.* This will readily assess the presence and pattern of transmural inflammation. Transmural inflammation in Crohn's disease takes the form of multiple discrete lymphoid aggregates throughout the full thickness of the bowel wall, especially involving the external border of the muscularis propria. In acute severe ulcerative colitis, inflammation may be seen deep to the mucosa but the pattern is quite different: there is a diffuse infiltration of inflammatory cells throughout the wall at sites of severe ulceration and discrete lymphoid aggregates are not seen.

3. *Macroscopically normal bowel between focal lesions.* This is often the most useful sample, used to look for mucosal disease, particularly crypt architectural distortion and continuity of any excess of chronic inflammatory cells in the lamina propria. These features suggest current or previous chronic

inflammation and indicate continuous mucosal disease, making a diagnosis of ulcerative colitis more confident. When undertaking this assessment, it is crucial to be aware of the skip lesions in ulcerative colitis described previously in the appendix and in the caecum.

In the intra-operative assessment of resection specimens and frozen sections, the pathologist should be prepared to give one of three firm answers: 'definite ulcerative colitis', 'definite Crohn's disease' or 'I do not know'. The term 'indeterminate colitis' (Price 1978) should be reserved for use only after thorough microscopic examination of the resected colon with multiple paraffin wax sections: such a diagnosis is made in about 10–15% of colectomies for acute/fulminant colonic inflammatory bowel disease and does not represent incompetence on the part of the pathologist (Mortensen 1993). At this operative stage, a definite diagnosis of ulcerative colitis indicates that pouch surgery should proceed: a diagnosis of Crohn's disease will result in conservative surgery and time for definitive pathological assessment. If the pathologist is uncertain of the diagnosis at the operative stage, the surgeon should proceed to colectomy leaving the rectum in situ, ileorectal anastomosis or ileostomy, depending on the histopathological features seen in the colectomy specimen. Pouch surgery may follow if analysis of paraffin wax sections of the resected colon reveals a diagnosis of ulcerative colitis or indeterminate colitis and if other clinical features are favourable.

POSTOPERATIVE ASSESSMENT

After definitive reservoir surgery, the pathologist should assess: (i) the colect-omy or proctocolectomy specimen in a one or two stage pouch procedure; (ii) the rectal stump in a three-stage procedure; (iii) the donuts from a pouch-anal anastomosis; and (iv) the pathology and adaptation of the pelvic ileal reservoir.

The colectomy specimen

All lymph nodes should be sampled, as should the appendix and any included ileum. The last is especially important in FAP as the presence of adenomas in the terminal ileal mucosa may indicate an increased risk of neoplasia in the reservoir (Nugent et al 1993; Tytgat & Gopinath 1995). The presence of backwash ileitis in patients with ulcerative colitis does not appear to predict an increased incidence of pouchitis (Gustavsson et al 1987). At this stage, it is important to document features that may indicate a diagnosis of Crohn's disease.

The defunctioned rectum in ulcerative colitis

Defunctioning the rectum in patients with ulcerative colitis may induce florid inflammatory changes. These may be manifest clinically and endoscopically as severe active proctitis with nodularity and ulceration, often looking more severe than the original ulcerative colitis in the rectum (Fig. 4.2). Histologically, the rectal stump shows the characteristic features of ulcerative colitis together with florid lymphoid hyperplasia (the endoscopic nodularity) and, often, ulceration (frequently overlying hyperplastic lymphoid follicles; Roe et al 1993, Warren et al 1993). Fissures, mucosal granulomas and patchiness of

Fig. 4.2 The macroscopic features of the defunctioned rectum in ulcerative colitis. The luminal diameter of the rectum is reduced and there is a severe active proctitis with nodularity and ulceration.

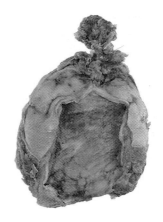

inflammation are seen in some cases: it is easy to see how these changes may be misconstrued as Crohn's disease, especially as transmural inflammation in the form of lymphoid aggregates is also a characteristic feature (Warren et al 1993). We believe that the confusing histological changes seen in rectal stumps result from a combination of diversion proctitis and pre-existing ulcerative colitis and that the pathological diagnosis of inflammatory bowel disease should be made on the macroscopic and microscopic assessment of the colectomy specimen, together with the clinical, radiological and endoscopic assessment of the whole patient (Warren et al 1993). A diagnosis of Crohn's disease should not be based solely on the histopathological appearances seen in the defunctioned rectum (Warren & Shepherd 1992a).

Donuts

Pouch-anal anastomosis may be established using a stapling gun or a handsewn anastomosis. The stapling technique produces two donuts of tissue for histopathological examination. The anorectal donut, if sectioned properly, will provide information on the exact histological level of the pouch-anal anastomosis. This normally includes columnar cuff mucosa from the top of the anal canal but, in some patients' anastomoses, may include anal transitional zone mucosa, and the pathologist should make some comment on its presence or absence. Donut assessment may require some modification of laboratory handling technique: maximal information about epithelial types present is obtained by cutting the donut radially and submitting all pieces for histological examination. There is no place for processing a donut whole, as serial sectioning to produce a 'full face' slice of the tissue block will usually cut through any columnar cuff or transitional mucosa which may be present. If dysplasia or malignancy is present in the colectomy specimen, it is particularly important to examine cuff mucosa in the donut for dysplasia. A considerable number of patients with dysplasia or malignancy in the colectomy specimen will develop dysplasia or malignancy in their retained columnar cuff (Ziv et al 1994). The ileal donut should be examined for any features that might suggest Crohn's disease.

THE PELVIC ILEAL RESERVOIR BEFORE ILEOSTOMY REVERSAL

In the few months that elapse between reservoir construction and closure of the defunctioning ileostomy, there is rarely any endoscopic or histological assessment of the reservoir. Many surgeons prefer not to biopsy a newly formed reservoir. However, occasional patients develop a discharge per anum from the pouch with endoscopic evidence of inflammation. Histologically, the pouch shows changes similar to those seen in late onset pouchitis and this has been called 'preclosure pouchitis' (Warren & Shepherd 1993). Its relationship to late onset pouchitis is, as yet, unclear, as follow-up is relatively short and cases are rare. Ischaemia has been proposed as a possible mechanism but this is unlikely as neither preclosure pouchitis nor pouchitis are recognised in familial adenomatous polyposis and yet mucosal ischaemia would be expected as frequently in pouch construction for familial adenomatous polyposis as for ulcerative colitis (Warren & Shepherd 1993). A type of diversion ileitis has also been proposed as an aetiology for preclosure pouchitis in a similar manner to diversion colitis. Nevertheless, preclosure pouchitis seems to be rare though most pouches do not transmit a faecal stream when a covering ileostomy is used. Furthermore, diversion pouchitis has different histological features, akin to those of diversion proctitis (Fig. 4.3; Warren & Shepherd 1992b). The cause of preclosure pouchitis remains obscure, but it certainly does not appear to represent Crohn's disease (Warren & Shepherd 1993).

ADAPTIVE CHANGES IN THE FUNCTIONING RESERVOIR MUCOSA

Once the reservoir is established, it shows a form of mucosal adaptation (Shepherd et al 1987, de Silva et al 1991a, Setti Carraro et al 1994, Veress et al 1996). Varying degrees of chronic inflammation and architectural abnormality (villous flattening or partial villous atrophy) are found in over 90% of established pelvic ileal reservoirs (Fig. 4.4; Shepherd et al 1987). When villous atrophy is severe there is crypt hyperplasia though there is no intra-epithelial lymphocytic infiltrate that characterises coeliac disease (Shepherd et al 1987, de Silva et al 1991a). These adaptive changes are almost universal: they have

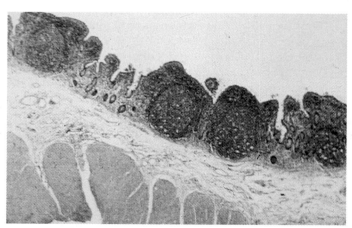

Fig. 4.3 The histology of diversion pouchitis. The most notable change at this power is florid lymphoid follicular hyperplasia. H & E × 15.

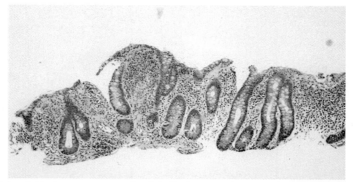

Fig. 4.4 A relatively severe case of pelvic ileal reservoir mucosal adaptation. There is subtotal villous atrophy with diffuse chronic inflammation. Crypt hyperplasia is prominent but there is no increase in intra-epithelial lymphocytes. H & E × 40.

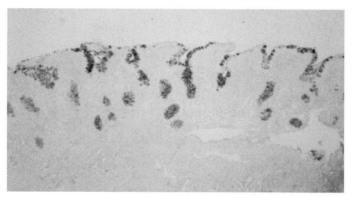

Fig. 4.5 High iron diamine (HIDAB) mucin histochemistry in ileal reservoir mucosa. Instead of the blue (light grey) staining sialomucin of the small intestine, there is predominance of brown/black (black) staining sulphomucin, typical of the left colon and rectum. H & E × 40.

been shown to be more pronounced in patients with ulcerative colitis than those with familial adenomatous polyposis but are seen in most patients with both diagnoses (Shepherd et al 1987). It is important not to equate such common inflammatory changes with a diagnosis of pouchitis.

The adaptive changes have been called colonic phenotypic change (Shepherd et al 1993) or colonisation (O'Connell et al 1986) since the villous atrophy and crypt hyperplasia produces an appearance resembling normal colon (Shepherd et al 1987, de Silva et al 1991a). These alterations may be due to changed faecal flora. The close similarity to colonic mucosa is supported by mucin histochemistry (Fig. 4.5; Shepherd et al 1987, Campbell et al 1994), immunohistochemistry (de Silva et al 1991a, Shepherd et al 1993), lectin histochemistry (Bahia et al 1993), mucin biochemistry (Corfield et al 1992) and electron microscopy (Warren & Shepherd 1993). Pouches retain some properties of small bowel mucosa, evidenced by retention of disaccharidase activity (de Silva et al 1991a). Because of this, the term 'colonic phenotypic change' is preferred to 'colonic metaplasia'.

Two recent studies have classified the adaptive changes in patients with ulcerative colitis into three groups: it appears that the amount of inflammatory/adaptive change is remarkably consistent within individuals and with time

Fig. 4.6
A biopsy from a patient with pouchitis. Villous atrophy is marked with diffuse chronic inflammation and crypt hyperplastic change prominent. The surface epithelium is attenuated and infiltrated by polymorphs. Crypt abscesses were present elsewhere. The changes seen here are characteristic of the severe mucosal adaptation that occurs in the group of patients who suffer from recurrent pouchitis. H & E × 100.

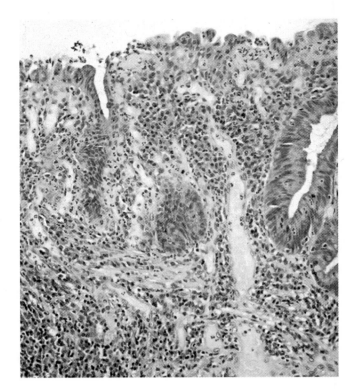

(Setti-Carraro et al 1994, Veress et al 1995). Firstly about half of patients with ulcerative colitis maintain a relatively healthy reservoir mucosa throughout the life of the pouch with minor villous changes, moderate chronic inflammation and minimal active inflammation. A second group of about 40% of patients shows intermittent inflammatory changes with reasonable architectural recovery. The third group of between 10–20% of patients have a flat and chronically inflamed mucosa with exacerbations of active inflammation. It is these patients who suffer from long-term recurrent pouchitis (Setti-Carraro et al 1994, Veress et al 1995). Biopsies taken within the first 6 months of reservoir construction will determine which of the three groups an individual patient falls into and this should therefore give a useful guide to those patients who demand the most rigorous surveillance (Setti-Carraro et al 1994). However, the exact implication for these three groups in terms of selection of reservoir patients for endoscopic and biopsy surveillance remains uncertain at present.

POUCHITIS

Pouchitis is the commonest and most important complication of restorative proctocolectomy (Mortensen & Madden 1993). It remains the most enigmatic condition in terms of pathogenesis, management and prognosis. Many of the uncertainties about this disease arise from poor understanding of normality and a lack of agreed criteria for the diagnosis of pouchitis (Warren & Shepherd 1993; Sandborn 1994). The term itself, despite its widespread usage, is a poor one that is open to misinterpretation. In the past, the term pouchitis has been

Fig. 4.7
Ulcer-associated cell lineage/ pseudopyloric metaplasia in the reservoir mucosa of a patient with pouchitis. The pale glands of the lineage contrast with the ileal epithelium above. H&E ×40.

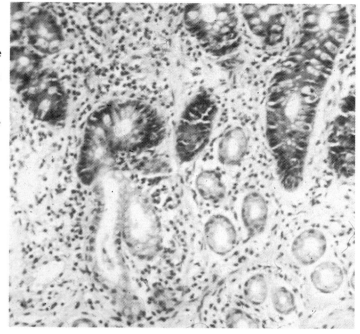

too loosely applied: many different inflammatory diseases causing active inflammation in the reservoir have been called pouchitis. The term should be reserved for those patients with an acute-on-chronic, relapsing inflammatory and ulcerating condition of the functioning reservoir with characteristic clinical, endoscopic and pathological features (Nicholls 1989, Mortensen & Madden 1993). Problems with definition account for the wide range of prevalence rates of pouchitis from different centres and differing response rates to treatment (Shepherd 1995). Because of the confusion over terminology, 'chronic relapsing pouchitis' may be a more appropriate term for this condition. Symptomatology includes diarrhoea, often bloody, abdominal pain, urgency, discharge, bloating and systemic symptoms: the clinical features are not dissimilar to those of the disease for which pouch surgery was performed, ulcerative colitis. Endoscopic examination in patients with pouchitis reveals increased vascularity, contact bleeding and ulceration, typical features of active idiopathic chronic inflammatory bowel disease (Tytgat 1989).

Several conditions cause active inflammation in the reservoir, but the pathological hallmarks of pouchitis are acute inflammation and focal ulceration, occurring on a background of marked chronic inflammation and villous atrophy (Fig. 4.6; Shepherd et al 1987). As one would expect from a chronic ulcerating condition of the small bowel, ulcer-associated cell lineage/pseudopyloric metaplasia (Fig. 4.7) is a characteristic marker of the disease (Warren & Shepherd 1993). The overall histological appearances of pouchitis bear a close likeness to those of ulcerative colitis and are unlike those of Crohn's disease. The ulceration in pouchitis is usually superficial: deep ulceration with mucosal erosion is unusual and should raise suspicions of a more specific pathology such as Crohn's disease or ischaemic enteritis. Pathological scoring systems (Table 4.1) have been used to define pouchitis by

Table 4.1 Scoring system for pathological changes in the pelvic ileal reservoir mucosa (from Shepherd et al 1987)

	Score
ACUTE CHANGES	
Acute inflammatory cell infiltrate	
None	0
Mild and patchy infiltrate in the surface epithelium	1
Moderate with crypt abscesses	2
Severe with crypt abscesses	3
Ulceration	
None	0
Mild superficial	1
Moderate	2
Extensive	3
Maximum total	6
CHRONIC CHANGES	
Chronic inflammatory cell infiltrate	
None	0
Mild and patchy	1
Moderate	2
Severe	3
Villous atrophy	
None	0
Minor abnormality of villous architecture	1
Partial villous atrophy	2
Major villous atrophy	3
Maximum total	6

the acute inflammatory score incorporating marked active inflammation with ulceration, the latter usually being a *sine qua non* for the pathological diagnosis (Moskowitz et al 1986, Shepherd et al 1987, Setti-Carraro et al 1994). Once these clinical, endoscopic and histopathological characteristics are present, the diagnosis is effectively established. When so defined, the prevalence of pouchitis varies between 10–20% of patients, though there are great variations in prevalence rates reported. Like ulcerative colitis in the colorectum, in which the majority of patients have disease limited to the distal colon and rectum and in whom the disease may be time-limited, similar cases also occur in pouchitis and so the diagnosis may still be valid even though the presentation is finite.

What is the cause of pouchitis?

There are several different theories about the cause of pouchitis (Warren & Shepherd 1993, Sandborn 1994). Suggested mechanisms have included stasis, bacterial changes with or without mucolysis, mucosal ischaemia, mucosal prolapse, Crohn's disease, mucosal disease as a result of a lack of small intestinal nutrients, and recurrent ulcerative colitis in a reservoir with colonic phenotypic change. The hypothesis that stasis and bacterial changes cause pouchitis is supported by the relative success of metronidazole and some other antibiotics in the treatment of pouchitis (Moskowitz et al 1986, Madden et al

1994). The mucosal changes that most pouches show represent a response of the ileal mucosa to the altered environment and are probably due to stasis and changes in the bacterial flora of the ileum. Studies of serial mucosal biopsies indicate that these changes occur soon after exposure to the faecal stream and, once present, the mucosa appears to reach a steady state in terms of inflammation, architectural abnormality, histochemistry and proliferation (de Silva et al 1991a, Warren & Shepherd 1993, Setti-Carraro et al 1994). Such changes are probably the precursors for subsequent acute inflammatory changes that occur in pouchitis. The pathological changes (and endoscopic abnormalities) are particularly severe in the posterior and inferior parts of the pouch suggesting that contact with static faecal residue is a major determinant of these changes (Shepherd et al 1993). Despite this, no consistent changes in bacterial flora have been demonstrated in patients with pouchitis. The inverse relation between villous atrophy and volatile fatty acids suggests that anaerobic bacteria may have a protective role and intramural counts of aerobic facultative bacteria have been found to be raised in patients with pouchitis (Nasmyth et al 1989, McLeod et al 1994, Ruseler-van Embden et al 1994, Sandborn et al 1995). Current evidence indicates that stasis and bacteriological changes are important in the production of chronic mucosal changes and adaptation, but that additional factors are required to produce pouchitis (Warren & Shepherd 1993).

It is clearly possible for Crohn's disease to affect a reservoir, particularly if it was constructed on the basis of a wrong initial diagnosis, but there is no evidence that Crohn's disease is the cause of chronic relapsing pouchitis (Subramani et al 1993). A focal area of active inflammation may occur in reservoir mucosa as a result of a mass, especially an inflammatory mass in association with pelvic sepsis, in the wall or outside the reservoir. This is secondary pouchitis and does not predicate a diagnosis of Crohn's disease or chronic relapsing pouchitis. Mucosal ischaemia has been demonstrated in reservoir mucosa but it seems most unlikely that this could account for pouchitis (Sandborn 1994). The remarkable variation in the prevalence of pouchitis among different surgeons and centres suggests the possibility of environmental factors (e.g. bacterial factors) or surgical factors (such as over-long efferent limbs causing faecal pooling), but the most likely explanation is the use of different definitions. It has been suggested that pouchitis can develop because of a deficiency of epithelial nutrients in the reservoir. Diversion colitis is thought to be due to a deficiency of short chain fatty acids, particularly butyrates (an important colonic epithelial cell nutrient), because of a lack of faecal flora in the diverted colon (Harig et al 1991). A proposed corollary for pouchitis is that glutamine, an important small intestinal epithelial cell nutrient, is deficient. The glutamine deficiency would explain the occurrence of pouchitis-like syndromes in reservoirs not exposed to the faecal stream such as before ileostomy reversal (preclosure pouchitis) and in the diverted reservoir (diversion pouchitis). One trial has shown benefit with glutamine enemas in pouchitis (Wischmeyer et al 1993), but others have not reported success.

The most favoured hypothesis for the cause of pouchitis is that it represents a re-emergence of ulcerative colitis in reservoirs with colonic metaplasia/colonic phenotypic change (Warren & Shepherd 1993, Luukonnen et al 1994). Most

Surgical pathology of the intestines: the pelvic ileal reservoir and diversion proctocolitis

accept that pouchitis is essentially a disease of patients with ulcerative colitis, though one report describes pouchitis occurring in a patient with FAP (Kmiot et al 1990). Patients with ulcerative colitis show more inflammatory change in their reservoirs than patients with FAP (Shepherd et al 1987) and there are intriguing associations between ulcerative colitis, extra-intestinal manifestations and pouchitis – especially primary sclerosing cholangitis and arthritis (Lohmuller et al 1990, Penna et al 1996). Similarities in the immunopathology of pouchitis and ulcerative colitis have also been reported (de Silva et al 1991b, Shepherd & Warren 1993). Like ulcerative colitis, pouchitis shows a strong negative association with smoking (Merrett et al 1996). Although there is no evidence of a link between the prevalence of pouchitis and pre-existing backwash ileitis (Gustavsson et al 1989) or the extent of colitis in the proctocolectomy specimen (Samarasekara et al 1996), re-emergence of ulcerative colitis in ileal mucosa which has undergone phenotypic change remains the most favoured hypothesis for the pathogenesis of pouchitis (Warren & Shepherd 1993, Sandborn 1994). The most contentious aspect is the significance of colonic phenotypic change in the mucosa. As already indicated, current evidence suggests that colonic metaplasia is not complete in the reservoir: it is this area of reservoir mucosal pathophysiology that needs further research.

OTHER DISEASE IN THE PELVIC ILEAL RESERVOIR

Crohn's disease and mimicry of Crohn's disease in the pouch

Patients who have pouch surgery for Crohn's disease are at risk of developing the changes of Crohn's disease in their reservoir (Lucarotti et al 1995). Histologically these changes resemble Crohn's disease elsewhere in the gut. Diagnostic care is required because any of the histological features of Crohn's disease may be seen in the reservoir in patients who do not have Crohn's disease. For instance, granulomas are a characteristic feature of reservoir mucosa, usually seen in the centre of lymphoid follicles, both associated with and without pouchitis (Fig. 4.8; Shepherd 1990a). Granulomas may also be seen in the mucosa as a result of ruptured crypts and deep within the wall in relation to suture material (Warren & Shepherd 1992a). Vertical fissures resembling those of Crohn's disease may be seen in pouch mucosa in relation to ruptured deep crypt abscesses and at anastomosis lines (Tytgat 1989), a feature also seen in the defunctioned rectum in ulcerative colitis (Warren et al 1993). Fistulae may occur soon after reservoir construction, particularly at suture lines (Tytgat 1989). Crohn's-like complications of the pelvic ileal reservoir may also include anal strictures, peri-anal abscesses and colovaginal fistulae: all of these may occur in patients with an unequivocal pre-operative diagnosis of ulcerative colitis (Goldstein et al 1997). We strongly believe that, as in the case of the diverted rectum in idiopathic inflammatory bowel disease (Warren et al 1993), the diagnosis of Crohn's disease should never be made on the histological appearances of the reservoir alone. A change in diagnosis at this stage has grave consequences for the patient and should always be substantiated by examination of the original proctocolectomy specimen or by further examination and investigation of the remaining alimentary tract (Warren & Shepherd 1993, Goldstein et al 1997).

Fig. 4.8
Small granulomas, such as this one, are a relatively common feature of the ileal reservoir mucosa, especially within lymphoid follicles. Alone, they certainly do not imply a diagnosis of Crohn's disease. H&E ×100.

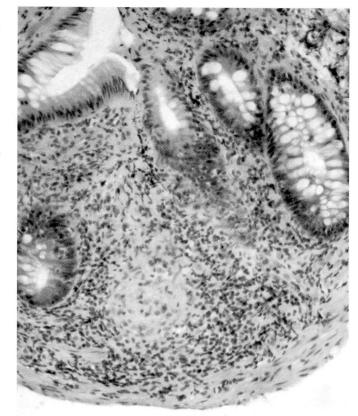

Mucosal ischaemia

Mucosal ischaemia occurs in a small number of patients soon after reservoir construction (Hosie et al 1989). This could be responsible for high fluid output that develops in a small group of patients soon after construction and before ileostomy reversal (Warren & Shepherd 1993). Mild ischaemic changes are seen endoscopically (Tytgat 1989) and histologically (Shepherd 1990a) in patients with pouches. This may be due to traction on the mesenteric vasculature or local impairment of the mucosal microcirculation as a consequence of surgery. Ischaemia, however, is a most unlikely cause of pouchitis. Pouchitis primarily affects those patients with preceding ulcerative colitis and not those with FAP or other colonic disease, yet the surgical techniques are identical for the different conditions. The histological features of chronic relapsing pouchitis bear little resemblance to those of mucosal ischaemia (Shepherd 1990a).

Mucosal prolapse

The pelvic ileal reservoir is a neorectum which may develop many of the disorders of a normal rectum. The clinical, endoscopic and histological features of mucosal prolapse are occasionally observed in the reservoir mucosa, usually on the anterior wall. The endoscopic appearance is of an anterior strip or patch of inflammation or ulceration, whilst the rest of the pouch is normal.

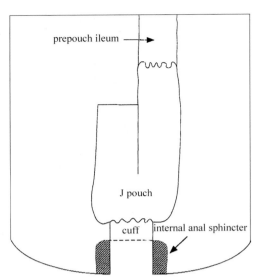

Fig. 4.9 The relationship of the reservoir to the prepouch ileum and the columnar cuff.

Histopathological examination is important to distinguish this condition from pouchitis. The histological features are those of mucosal prolapse as seen elsewhere and include fibromuscular obliteration of the lamina propria, with smooth muscle fibres in the lamina propria and disrupted muscularis mucosae (Warren & Shepherd 1993). The condition has been referred to anterior strip pouchitis. Some American authors have used the term strip pouchitis to refer to inflammation in the residual columnar cuff in the anal canal. To avoid confusion we believe that the latter condition should be referred to as cuffitis (Thompson-Fawcett, Warren & Mortensen 1999).

Polyps in the pelvic ileal reservoir

Inflammatory polyps, especially at anastomosis lines, are the commonest polypoid lesion in the reservoir: these are usually of little consequence apart from endoscopically mimicking more significant polyps. Patients with FAP may develop adenomatous polyps in the pouch mucosa with consequent malignant potential (Nugent et al 1993, Tytgat & Gopinath 1995). These patients should be screened, endoscopically on a regular basis. Rarely, patients with juvenile polyposis may also develop recurrent ileal polyposis within the reservoir (Stoltenberg et al 1997). Polypoid mucosal prolapse has been described in the reservoir (Blazeby et al 1994), as have inflammatory fibroid polyps (Tysk et al 1994): both are probably a direct consequence of the surgery and may be associated with significant symptomatology. Polyps may cause alarm because of the belief that they may represent premalignant dysplasia, as in the DALM (dysplasia-associated lesion or mass) lesions of ulcerativè colitis. All polyps should be examined histologically.

Prepouch ileitis and cuffitis

Some patients with symptoms suggestive of pouchitis will have no endoscopic or histological evidence of pouchitis. A small number of these patients will

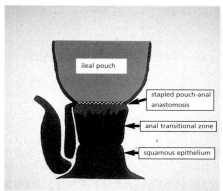

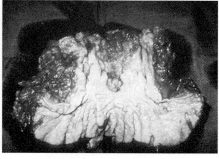

Fig. 4.10 The columnar cuff and its relationship to the reservoir and the anal canal. The cuff is that irregular mucosal area immediately below the pouch-anal anastomosis.

Fig. 4.11 A resected anal canal and columnar cuff from a patient with ulcerative colitis who had previously had a pelvic ileal reservoir constructed. Centrally at the upper border of the specimen, in the cuff, is an ulcerating adenocarcinoma, a poignant reminder of the neoplastic potential of the remaining rectal-type mucosa in patients with both ulcerative colitis and FA.

have active inflammation in the ileal mucosa proximal to the pouch, prepouch ileitis, or in the columnar cuff mucosa distal to the pouch, cuffitis (Fig. 4.9). These conditions may go unnoticed endoscopically unless the endoscopist makes a special effort to examine these areas. Prepouch ileitis is a diffuse mucosal acute and chronic inflammation with ulceration and crypt distortion of the ileum proximal to the reservoir. It has been most commonly seen in patients who also have pouchitis, but may be seen in isolation. There are histological similarities to prestomal ileitis. In some patients it may be related to reservoir outlet obstruction and in others to obstruction at the ileal-pouch anastomosis, but the condition is not always obviously related to obstruction. Prepouch ileitis is rare and most pouch patients have an entirely normal ileal mucosa proximal to the reservoir (Shepherd et al 1993).

The amount of columnar cuff, that part of the upper anal canal/lower rectum remaining adjacent to the ileal-anal anastomosis, varies primarily according to the surgical technique (Fig. 4.10). In a hand sewn pouch-anal anastomosis this mucosa is stripped, usually incompletely as the junctions between columnar, transitional and squamous epithelia are indistinct (Thompson-Fawcett & Mortensen 1996). In the double stapled pouch-anal anastomosis, columnar cuff mucosa is always retained, but varies considerably in amount as not all anastomoses are at the intended level of the upper border of the internal anal sphincter (Thompson-Fawcett et al 1998). This columnar cuff mucosa is likely to develop persistent or recurrent active inflammation in patients with ulcerative colitis. If the active inflammation is severe enough, this may give rise to the clinical syndrome of cuffitis. This diagnosis implies a clinical presentation of urgency with intra-anal burning in association with endoscopic and pathological evidence of active inflammation in the cuff mucosa. Scoring systems similar to those of pouchitis have been used to define the condition (Thompson-Fawcett et al 1999).

The remaining columnar cuff has important neoplastic potential, especially when there is cuffitis (Fig. 4.11). Patients with FAP and patients with ulcerative colitis who had dysplasia and carcinoma in their proctocolectomy specimens are most at risk: neoplasia has been shown to develop relatively quickly in the cuff mucosa (King et al 1989, Stern et al 1990, Ziv et al 1994, von Herbay et al 1996, Sequens 1997). Retained columnar cuff is unlikely to have any influence on the occurrence of pouchitis but is a significant cause of long-term morbidity in the pelvic reservoir.

LONG-TERM SURVEILLANCE

The concept of proctocolectomy is to remove all potentially neoplastic tissue in ulcerative colitis and FAP. In fact, the surgery neither removes all colorectal mucosa (see columnar cuff, above) nor eradicates the neoplastic potential, particularly in FAP, in which adenomas may form in the ileal mucosa of the reservoir (Nugent et al 1993, Tytgat & Gopinath 1995). Neoplastic change in the reservoir arises principally in remaining rectal mucosa (the cuff) at the lower aspect of the reservoir. Colonic phenotypic change in ileal mucosa, in combination with inflammatory change and associated epithelial hyper-proliferation, suggests that there is potential for increased neoplastic risk of the ileal mucosa in the reservoir (Shepherd 1990b). In the experience of most groups, dysplasia and carcinoma in the ileal reservoir mucosa of ulcerative colitis patients are extremely rare. However, workers in Sweden have intensively studied patients over many years with multiple endoscopies and biopsies and demonstrated relatively high rates of dysplasia in patients with ulcerative colitis: in their studies about 10% of patients with reservoir developed the most florid inflammatory changes with severe villous atrophy. It is this group that is subject to pouchitis and 71% of patients in this group had dysplasia including one with high grade dysplasia (Veress et al 1996, Gullberg et al 1997).

These studies would suggest that there is potential for neoplastic change in the ileal mucosa of the pelvic ileal reservoir in patients with ulcerative colitis. For management purposes, it seems that the highest risk is with those patients with the most severe pathological changes, those most likely to develop pouchitis. As these patients can be identified within 6 months of ileostomy reversal (Setti-Carraro et al 1994), they should be selected for the most comprehensive surveillance. Management for reservoir mucosal dysplasia should be similar to that for ulcerative colitis. Low grade dysplasia and changes indefinite for dysplasia should be managed by close surveillance with mucosal biopsies taken from multiple sites in the reservoir. High grade dysplasia with a lesion or mass (DALM) may be an indication for pouchectomy though accurate imaging may allow ablative therapy such as laser or photodynamic therapy to eradicate the neoplastic epithelium (Shepherd 1995).

Currently we should maintain a balanced attitude toward neoplastic risk in the pouch. Dysplasia, in native ileal mucosa, has only been described from one centre (Veress et al 1995) and no one else has yet reported such dysplastic changes. One conundrum of the pelvic ileal reservoir is its dissimilarity, in terms of the prevalence and severity of pouchitis, and, ostensibly, neoplastic risk, with Kock's continent abdominal reservoir. In the latter it has been shown that in the majority of patients, the ileal mucosa returns almost to normal when the reservoir has been established for 20 years (Helander et al 1990), although there is one recent report of carcinoma arising in the ileal mucosa of a Kock pouch (Cox et al 1997). Why the presence of the anal mechanism should have, apparently, such a great influence on long term inflammatory, metaplastic and neoplastic potential of the pelvic reservoir, compared to that of the continent abdominal reservoir, is perplexing. Remaining columnar cuff and differing alterations in the micro-environment would seem possible explanations but investigations are certainly not conclusive. For now all patients with a pelvic ileal reservoir require comprehensive clinical and endoscopic follow-up, with extensive biopsy sampling, until we know more of the risks of neoplastic change in the reservoir (Shepherd 1995).

CONCLUSION

The evolution and success of the pelvic ileal reservoir have created a unique in vivo model for ulcerative colitis, in pouchitis, and an uncertain neoplastic potential. We believe patients and doctors should remain optimistic about the future of pelvic ileal reservoirs, but should also be aware of the potential risks of the pathological mucosal changes. For this reason, we believe all patients with reservoir should undergo regular surveillance (Warren & Shepherd 1992).

DIVERSION PROCTOCOLITIS

Morson and Dawson (1972) first described inflammation in the diverted colon and Glotzer and his colleagues (1981) coined the term diversion colitis and provided the first detailed account of the disease. Diversion colitis is an iatrogenic inflammation of the large bowel, induced by diversion of the faecal stream. Colon is most often excluded from the faecal stream during Hartmann's operation for obstruction of the sigmoid colon and/or rectum, usually for carcinoma or complicated diverticular disease. Diversion is also performed for paediatric conditions like Hirschsprung's disease. Inflammatory bowel disease may also be an indication for diversion: in Crohn's disease it can ameliorate the disease and in ulcerative colitis, the rectum is defunctioned during the three-stage ileal pouch procedure (*see above*; Fig. 4.2). Diversion proctocolitis is associated with characteristic macroscopic and histological features, but symptomatology is very variable. Pathological changes occur in most diverted large intestines, but not all patients suffer symptoms. Rectal bleeding, mucous diarrhoea and abdominal pain are all described but are not consistent features of the disease.

AETIOLOGY OF DIVERSION PROCTOCOLITIS

Despite much literature suggesting the opposite, the cause of diversion colitis remains uncertain. Harig and colleagues (1989) first suggested that butyrate, the preferred metabolic substrate for colonic epithelial cell growth and differentiation and produced by bacteria within the faecal stream, was deficient in the diverted colon and rectum and that this deficiency was the cause of diversion pathology. In support of this theorem, they induced clinical

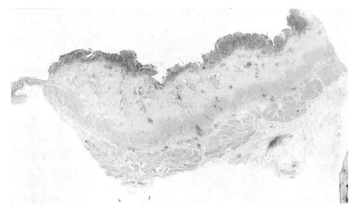

Fig. 4.12 A wholemount of the wall of a defunctioned rectum in ulcerative colitis. There is notable lymphoid follicular hyperplasia of the mucosa and, even at this power, transmural inflammation in the form of lymphoid aggregates is apparent. The submucosa and muscularis propria appear thickened.

remission of the disease by the instillation of butyrate enemas (Harig et al 1989). Against this evidence is the result of the only controlled trial of butyrate, which showed no significant improvement compared to controls (Guillemot et al 1991). The same group observed reduction of strict anaerobes in the defunctioned intestine and have suggested that this altered microflora might directly induce inflammation (Neut et al 1989). More recently, they have suggested that increased nitrate-reducing bacteria may be a factor in the induction of inflammation (Neut et al 1997). The exact aetiopathogenesis of inflammation in diversion proctocolitis remains uncertain and further research is needed.

MACROSCOPIC AND MICROSCOPIC PATHOLOGY OF DIVERSION PROCTOCOLITIS

The histological features of the disease vary according to the nature of the disease for which the bowel was diverted (Yeong et al 1991, Warren & Shepherd 1992b). For instance, the appearances of the rectum, defunctioned after total colectomy in chronic ulcerative colitis, are very different from those of the diverted colon in Crohn's disease (Warren & Shepherd 1992b). The most characteristic histological feature of diversion is lymphoid follicular hyperplasia (Yeong et al 1991; Fig. 4.12). This is apparent endoscopically as the nodularity that is so characteristic of the disease, especially in children (Drut & Drut 1992). The nodules may show overlying aphthoid ulceration and this should not be taken to represent Crohn's disease (Lusk et al 1984). Most diverted intestines show mucosal abnormality, but the severity and pattern of the disease are very variable and not predictable from the length of time the bowel has been diverted (Komorowski 1990, Geraghty & Talbot 1991). There is a histological spectrum from mild chronic inflammation and crypt architectural distortion to florid active inflammation mimicking active chronic idiopathic inflammatory bowel disease, especially ulcerative colitis (Komorowski 1990, Ma et al 1990, Geraghty & Talbot 1991). Occasionally well-defined epithelioid cell granulomas can be observed in the mucosa of diversion colitis (Ma et al 1990, Warren & Shepherd 1992b) and, alone, should not be taken as evidence of Crohn's disease.

The histological changes of diversion are apparent within 3 months of defunctioning (Roe et al 1993) and are rapidly restored to normal by re-anastomosis (Geraghty & Talbot 1991). Nevertheless diversion proctocolitis is accompanied by involution which may be dramatic and may preclude re-anastomosis (Roe et al 1993). It is not usually possible to predict those cases likely to undergo involution. Involution is accompanied by an excess of adipose tissue in the submucosa and subserosa with thickening of the muscularis propria. Often the mucosa shows gross atrophy in addition to the more standard inflammatory changes. Florid neuronal hyperplasia may be a feature of diversion and multiple microcarcinoids have been described in the diverted colon (Griffiths & Dixon 1992). However, there appears to be little evidence of any increased malignant potential.

DIVERSION IN CHRONIC INFLAMMATORY BOWEL DISEASE

One curiosity of diversion disease, and indeed of chronic idiopathic inflammatory bowel disease, is the fact that the pathological features (and, usually, the clinical features) of ulcerative colitis frequently worsen after the faecal stream is diverted, while the pathological changes in Crohn's disease improve when the colon is defunctioned. In addition to the changes that mimic Crohn's disease, namely transmural inflammation, granulomas and fissures (Warren et al 1993), the defunctioned rectum in ulcerative colitis shows florid lymphoid follicular hyperplasia, disruptive crypt abscesses and surface ulceration (Fig. 4.12). A characteristic additional feature is the presence of summit-type lesions with pseudomembrane formation that closely mimic pseudomembranous colitis (Warren et al 1993). It may be that these features represent a combination of the original inflammatory bowel disease, often altered by diversion-type pathological features, with mucosal ischaemia to account for the mimicry of pseudomembranous colitis.

The rectum is diverted in ulcerative colitis to facilitate subsequent pouch surgery, not necessarily with the hope of improving the disease. In Crohn's disease, the colon is diverted with disease amelioration very much in mind. About two-thirds of patients with Crohn's colitis will achieve sustained clinical remission subsequent to diversion (Harper et al 1985, Winslet et al 1993). It may also be effective for peri-anal Crohn's disease that fails to respond to other measures (Harper et al 1982), though occasionally peri-anal disease may rapidly worsen (Williamson & Hughes 1994). Reconnection of the faecal stream induces recurrent disease in about 40% of those diverted for Crohn's colitis. Systematic pathological review of the diverted colon in Crohn's disease has not been undertaken but some notable observations have been made. The colon shows considerable reduction in luminal diameter, a feature that may also be seen in diversion of the colon and rectum, performed upon normal bowel or that affected by ulcerative colitis. This involution may provide difficulties for the surgeon attempting re-anastomosis. Histologically, there is reduction in ulceration and both acute and chronic inflammation. Granulomas are usually regarded as transient features in Crohn's disease and this has been used to explain why Crohn's granulomas do not often contain calcified bodies unlike those in sarcoidosis, in which the granulomas are thought to be a long-standing characteristic. A distinctive feature of diverted Crohn's colitis is the presence of granulomas containing calcified Schaumann bodies (Warren & Shepherd 1992a).

When Crohn's colitis relapses after re-anastomosis subsequent to a period of diversion, often the only course of action is total proctocolectomy. The interpretation of the histopathology of such a resected specimen requires caution. Partial resolution of the Crohn's colitis with the superimposed histological changes of diversion colitis may produce changes indistin-guishable from ulcerative colitis. The danger here is that the preceding clinico-pathological and radiological evidence for Crohn's colitis may be overlooked. Fortunately most cases will have transmural inflammation in the form of lymphoid aggregates or granulomas, particularly deep within the wall. We strongly recommend that all resection specimens and biopsies are reviewed before a change of diagnosis is made in patients with idiopathic inflammatory bowel disease who have undergone these forms of surgery.

CONCLUSIONS

None of the pathological features that many would consider pathognomonic for the different types of idiopathic inflammatory bowel disease are entirely specific. For instance the diffuse chronic inflammation, crypt architectural distortion and crypt abscesses of ulcerative colitis can be just as readily seen in diversion colitis. Similarly all the pathological changes of Crohn's disease can be mimicked in the diverted rectum affected by ulcerative colitis. The pelvic ileal reservoir may also demonstrate apparent endoscopic and histopatho-logical changes of Crohn's disease in a patient with no evidence, whatever, of Crohn's disease. Previous surgery induces pathological changes that confuse and complicate the pathological picture. We believe that only by paying close attention to the clinical, endoscopic and pathological features, in what are often complex clinico-pathological circumstances, can the pathologist accurately interpret the information available to him and reach the appropriate pathological diagnosis.

ACKNOWLEDGEMENT

We are grateful to Professor Richard Sequens for Figure 4.11.

References

Bahia S S, McMahon R F, Hobbiss J, Taylor T V, Stoddart R W 1993 Pelvic ileo-anal reservoirs: a lectin histochemical study. Histochem J 25: 392–400

Blazeby J M, Durdey P, Warren B F 1994 Polypoid mucosal prolapse in a pelvic ileal reservoir. Gut 35: 1668–1669

Campbell A P, Merrett M N, Kettlewell M, Mortensen N J, Jewell D P 1994 Expression of colonic antigens by goblet and columnar epithelial cells in ileal pouch mucosa: their association with inflammatory changes and faecal stasis. J Clin Pathol 47: 834–838

Corfield A P, Warren B F, Bartolo D C, Wagner S A, Clamp J R 1992 Mucin changes in ileoanal pouches monitored by metabolic labelling and histochemistry. Br J Surg 79: 1209–1212

Cox C L, Butts D R, Roberts M P, Wessels R A, Bailey H R 1997 Development of invasive adenocarcinoma in a long-standing Kock continent ileostomy: report of a case. Dis Colon Rectum 40: 500–503

Davison A M, Dixon M F 1990 The appendix as a skip lesion in ulcerative colitis. Histopathology 16: 93–95

Day D W, Mandall B K, Morson B C 1978 The rectal biopsy appearances of *Salmonella* colitis. Histopathology 2: 117–131

de Silva H J, Millard P R, Kettlewell M, Mortensen N, Prince C, Jewell D P 1991a Mucosal characteristics of pelvic ileal pouches. Gut 32: 61–65

de Silva H J, Jones M, Prince C, Kettlewell M, Mortensen N J, Jewell D P 1991b Lymphocyte and macrophage subpopulations in pelvic ileal pouches. Gut 32: 1160–1165

Deutsch A A, McLeod R S, Cullen J, Cohen Z 1991 Results of the pelvic pouch procedure in patients with Crohn's disease. Dis Colon Rectum 23: 475–477

D'Haens G, Geboes K, Peeters M, Baert F, Ectors N, Rutgeerts P 1997 Patchy cecal inflammation associated with distal ulcerative colitis: a prospective endoscopic study. Am J Gastroenterol 92: 1275–1279

Drut R, Drut R M 1992 Hyperplasia of lymphoglandular complexes in colon segments in Hirschsprung's disease: a form of diversion colitis. Pediatr Pathol 12: 575–581

Fazio V W, Tjandra J J, Lavery I C 1993 Techniques of pouch construction. In: Nicholls R J, Bartolo D C C, Mortensen N J Mc C (eds) Restorative proctocolectomy. Oxford: Blackwell, pp 18–33

Geraghty J M, Talbot I C. 1991 Diversion colitis: histological features in the colon and rectum after defunctioning colostomy. Gut 32: 1020–1023

Glotzer D J, Glick M E, Goldman H 1981 Proctitis and colitis following diversion of the fecal stream. Gastroenterology 80: 438–441

Goldstein N S, Sanford W W, Bodzin J H 1997 Crohn's-like complications in patients with ulcerative colitis after total proctocolectomy and ileal pouch-anal anastomosis. Am J Surg Pathol 21: 1343–1353

Griffiths A P, Dixon M F 1992 Microcarcinoids and diversion colitis in a colon defunctioned for 18 years. Report of a case. Dis Colon Rectum 35: 685–688

Grobler S P, Hosie K B, Affie E, Thompson H, Keighley M R 1993 Outcome of restorative proctocolectomy when the diagnosis is suggestive of Crohn's disease. Gut 34: 1384–1388

Guillemot F, Colombel J F, Neut C et al 1991 Treatment of diversion colitis by short-chain fatty acids. Prospective and double-blind study. Dis Colon Rectum 34: 861–864

Gullberg K, Stahlberg D, Liljeqvist L et al 1997 Neoplastic transformation of the pelvic pouch mucosa in patients with ulcerative colitis. Gastroenterology 112: 1487–1492

Gustavsson S, Weiland L H, Kelly K A 1987 Relationship of backwash ileitis to ileal pouchitis after ileoanal anastomosis. Dis Colon Rectum 30: 25–28

Harig J M, Soergel K H, Komorowski R A, Wood C M 1989 Treatment of diversion colitis with short-chain-fatty acid irrigation. N Engl J Med 320: 23–28

Harper P H, Kettlewell M G, Lee E C 1982 The effect of split ileostomy on perianal Crohn's disease. Br J Surg 69: 608–610

Harper P H, Lee E C, Kettlewell M G, Bennett M K, Jewell D P 1985 Role of the faecal stream in the maintenance of Crohn's colitis. Gut 26: 279–284

Helander K G, Ahren C, Philipson B M, Samuelsson B M, Ojerskog B O 1990 Structure of mucosa in continent ileal reservoirs 15 to 19 years after construction. Hum Pathol 21: 1235–1238

Hosie K, Sagamuchi M, Tudor R, Gourevitch D, Kmiot W, Keighley M R B 1989 Pouchitis after restorative proctocolectomy is associated with mucosal ischaemia. Gut 30: A1471–A1472

Jenkins D, Balsitis M, Gallivan S et al 1997 Guidelines for the initial biopsy diagnosis of suspected chronic idiopathic inflammatory bowel disease. The British Society of Gastroenterology Initiative. J Clin Pathol 50: 93–105

King D W, Lubowski D Z, Cook T A 1989 Anal canal mucosa in restorative proctocolectomy for ulcerative colitis. Br J Surg 76: 970–972

Kmiot W A, Williams M R, Keighley M R B 1990 Pouchitis following colectomy and ileal reservoir construction for familial adenomatous polyposis. Br J Surg 77: 1283

Komorowski R A 1990 Histologic spectrum of diversion colitis. Am J Surg Pathol 14: 548–554

Lee F D, Maguire C, Obeidat W, Russell R I 1997 Importance of cryptolytic lesions and pericryptal granulomas in inflammatory bowel disease. J Clin Pathol 50: 148–152

Levine T S, Tzardi M, Mitchell S, Sowter C, Price A B 1996 Diagnostic difficulty arising from rectal recovery in ulcerative colitis. J Clin Pathol 49: 319–323

Lohmuller J L, Pemberton J H, Dozois R R, Ilstrup D 1990 The relationship between pouchitis after pouch-anal anastomosis and extra-intestinal manifestations of chronic ulcerative colitis. Ann Surg 211: 622–629

Lucarotti M E, Freeman B J, Warren B F, Durdey P 1995 Synchronous proctocolectomy and ileoanal pouch formation and the risk of Crohn's disease. Br J Surg 82: 755–756

Lusk L B, Reichen J, Levine J S 1984 Aphthous ulceration in diversion colitis. Clinical implications. Gastroenterology 87: 1171–1173

Luukkonen P, Jarvinen H, Tanskanen M, Kahri A 1994 Pouchitis – recurrence of the inflammatory bowel disease? Gut 35: 243–246

Ma C K, Gottlieb C, Haas P A 1990 Diversion colitis: a clinico-pathological study of 21 cases. Hum Pathol 21: 29–36

Madden M V, McIntyre A S, Nicholls R J 1994 Double-blind crossover trial of metronidazole versus placebo in chronic unremitting pouchitis. Dig Dis Sci 39: 1193–1196

McIntyre P B, Pemberton J H, Wolff B G, Dozois R R, Beart Jr R W 1995 Indeterminate colitis. Long-term outcome in patients after ileal pouch-anal anastomosis. Dis Colon Rectum 38: 51–54

McLeod R S, Antonioli D, Cullen J et al 1994 Histologic and microbiologic features of biopsy samples from patients with normal and inflamed pouches. Dis Colon Rectum 37: 26–31

Merrett M N, Mortensen N, Kettlewell M, Jewell D P 1996 Smoking may prevent pouchitis in patients with restorative proctocolectomy for ulcerative colitis. Gut 38: 362–364

Morson B C, Dawson I M P 1972 Inflammatory disorders. In: Gastrointestinal pathology. Oxford: Blackwell, p 485

Mortensen N J Mc C 1993 Patient selection for restorative proctocolectomy. In: Nicholls R J, Bartolo D C C, Mortensen N J Mc C. Restorative proctocolectomy. Oxford: Blackwell, pp 7–17

Mortensen N J Mc C, Madden M V 1993 Pouchitis – acute inflammation in ileal pouches. In: Nicholls R J, Bartolo D C C, Mortensen N J Mc C (eds) Restorative proctocolectomy. Oxford: Blackwell, pp 119–131

Moskowitz R L, Shepherd N A, Nicholls R J 1986 An assessment of inflammation in the reservoir after restorative proctocolectomy with ileoanal ileal reservoir. Int J Colorect Dis 1: 167–174

Nasmyth D G, Godwin P G R, Dixon M F, Williams N S, Johnston D 1989 Ileal ecology after pouch-anal anastomosis or ileostomy. A study of mucosal morphology, fecal bacteriology, fecal volatile fatty acids and their interrelationship. Gastroenterology 96: 817–824

Neut C, Colombel J F, Guillemot F et al 1989 Impaired bacterial flora in human excluded colon. Gut 30: 1094–1098

Neut C, Guillemot F, Colombel J F 1997 Nitrate-reducing bacteria in diversion colitis: a clue to inflammation?. Dig Dis Sci 42: 2577–2580

Nicholls R J 1989 Clinical diagnosis. In: Pouchitis Workshop. Int J Colorect Dis 5: 213–216

Nugent K P, Spigelman A D, Nicholls R J, Talbot I C, Neale K, Phillips R K S 1993 Pouch adenomas in patients with familial adenomatous polyposis. Br J Surg 80: 1620

O'Connell P R, Rankin D R, Weiland L H, Kelly K A 1986 Enteric bacteriology, absorption, morphology and emptying after ileal pouch anal anastomosis. Br J Surg 73: 909–914

Panis Y, Poupard B, Nemeth J, Lavergne A, Hautefeuille P, Valleur P 1996 Ileal pouch/anal anastomosis for Crohn's disease. Lancet 347: 854–857

Parks A G, Nicholls R J 1978 Proctocolectomy without ileostomy for ulcerative colitis. BMJ ii: 85–88

Penna C, Dozois R R, Tremaine W, Sandborn W, LaRusso N, Schleck C, Ilstrup D 1996 Pouchitis after ileal pouch-anal anastomosis for ulcerative colitis occurs with increased frequency in patients with associated primary sclerosing cholangitis. Gut 38: 234–239

Pezim M E, Pemberton J H, Beart R W et al 1989 Outcome of indeterminate colitis following ileal pouch-anal anastomosis. Dis Colon Rectum 32: 653–658

Price A B 1978 Overlaps in the spectrum of non specific inflammatory bowel disease – 'colitis indeterminate'. J Clin Pathol 31: 567–577

Price A B, Jewkes J, Sanderson P J 1979 Acute diarrhoea: campylobacter colitis and the role of the rectal biopsy. J Clin Pathol 32: 990–997

Roe A M, Warren B F, Brodribb A J, Brown C 1993 Diversion colitis and involution of the defunctioned anorectum. Gut 34: 382–385

Ruseler-van Embden J G H, Schouten W R, van Lieshout L M C 1994 Pouchitis: result of microbial imbalance? Gut 35: 658–664

Sagar P M, Dozois R R, Wolff B G 1996 Long term results of ileal pouch-anal anastomosis in patients with Crohn's disease. Dis Colon Rectum 39: 893–898

Samarasekera D N, Stebbing J F, Kettlewell M G, Jewell D P, Mortensen N J 1996 Outcome of restorative proctocolectomy with ileal reservoir for ulcerative colitis: comparison of distal colitis with more proximal disease. Gut 38: 574–577

Sandborn W 1994 Pouchitis following ileal pouch-anal anastomosis: definition, pathogenesis, and treatment. Gastroenterology 107: 1856–1860

Sandborn W, Tremaine W, Batts K P et al 1995 Fecal bile acids, short-chain fatty acids, and bacteria after ileal pouch-anal anastomosis do not differ in patients with pouchitis. Dig Dis Sci 40: 1474–1483

Sequens R 1997 Cancer in the anal canal (transitional zone) after restorative proctocolectomy with stapled ileal pouch-anal anastomosis. Int J Colorectal Dis 12: 254–255

Setti Carraro P, Talbot I C, Nicholls R J 1994 Longterm appraisal of the histological appearances of the ileal reservoir after restorative proctocolectomy for ulcerative colitis. Gut 35: 1721–1727

Sheehan A L, Warren B F, Gear M W L, Shepherd N A 1992 Fat-wrapping in Crohn's disease: pathological basis and relevance to surgical practice. Br J Surg 79: 955–958

Shepherd N A 1990a The pelvic ileal reservoir: pathology and pouchitis. Neth J Med 37: S57–S64

Shepherd N A 1990b The pelvic ileal reservoir: apocalypse later? BMJ 301: 886–887

Shepherd N A 1991 Pathological mimics of chronic inflammatory bowel disease. J Clin Pathol 44: 726–733

Shepherd N A 1995 Pouchitis and neoplasia in the pelvic ileal reservoir. Gastroenterology 109: 1381–1383

Shepherd N A, Healey C J, Warren B F, Richman P I, Thomson W H F, Wilkinson S P 1993 Distribution of mucosal pathology and an assessment of colonic phenotypic change in the pelvic ileal reservoir. Gut 34: 101–105

Shepherd N A, Jass J R, Duval I, Moskowitz R L, Nicholls R J, Morson B C 1987 Restorative proctocolectomy with ileal reservoir: pathological and histochemical study of mucosal biopsy specimens. J Clin Pathol 40: 601–607

Spiliadis C A, Spiliadis C A, Lennard-Jones J E 1987 Ulcerative colitis with relative sparing of the rectum. Clinical features, histology and prognosis. Dis Colon Rectum 30: 334–336

Stern H, Walfisch S, Mullen B, McLeod R, Cohen Z 1990 Cancer in an ileoanal reservoir: a new late complication? Gut 31: 473–475

Stoltenberg R L, Madsen J A, Schlack S C, Harms B A, Jacoby R F 1997 Neoplasia in ileal pouch mucosa after total proctocolectomy for juvenile polyposis: report of a case. Dis Colon Rectum 40: 726–730

Subramani K, Harpaz N, Bilotta J et al 1993 Refractory pouchitis: does it reflect underlying Crohn's disease? Gut 34: 1539–1542

Talbot I C, Price A B 1987 Biopsy pathology in colorectal disease. London: Chapman and Hall, p 127

Tanaka M, Riddell R H 1990 The pathological diagnosis and differential diagnosis of Crohn's disease. Hepatogastroenterology 37: 18–31

Thompson H 1990 Histopathology of Crohn's disease. In: Allan R N, Keighley M R B, Alexander-Williams J, Hawkins C (eds) Inflammatory bowel diseases. Edinburgh: Churchill Livingstone, pp 263–285

Thompson-Fawcett M W, Mortensen N J 1996 Anal transitional zone and columnar cuff in restorative proctocolectomy. Br J Surg 83: 1047–1055

Thompson-Fawcett M W, Warren B F, Mortensen N J Mc C 1998 A new look at the anal transitional zone; with reference to the columnar cuff and restorative proctocolectomy. Br J Surg 85: 1517–1521

Thompson-Fawcett M W, Warren B F, Mortensen N J Mc C 1999 Cuffitis and inflammatory changes in the columnar cuff, anal transitional zone and ileal reservoir after a stapled pouch anastomosis. Dis Colon Rectum In press

Surgical pathology of the intestines: the pelvic ileal reservoir and diversion proctocolitis

Tysk C, Schnurer L B, Wickbom G 1994 Obstructing inflammatory fibroid polyp in pelvic ileal reservoir after restorative proctocolectomy in ulcerative colitis. Dis Colon Rectum 37: 1034–1037

Tytgat G N J 1989 The role of endoscopy in pouch monitoring and pouchitis. In: Pouchitis Workshop. Int J Colorectal Dis 5: 210–213

Tytgat G N, Gopinath N 1995 Recurrent polyps in the ileo-anal pouch or rectum in familial adenomatous polyposis. Eur J Cancer 31: 1154–1158

Veress B, Reinholt F P, Lindquist K, Lofberg R, Liljeqvist L 1995 Long-term histomorphological surveillance of the pelvic ileal pouch: dysplasia develops in a subgroup of patients. Gastroenterology 109: 1090–1097

von Herbay A, Stern J, Herfarth C 1996 Pouch-anal cancer after restorative proctocolectomy for familial adenomatous polyposis. Am J Surg Pathol 20: 995–999

Warren B F, Shepherd N A 1992a The role of pathology in pouch surgery. Int J Colorectal Dis 7: 68–75

Warren B F, Shepherd N A 1992b Diversion proctocolitis. Histopathology 21: 91–94

Warren B F, Shepherd N A 1993 Pouch pathology. In: Nicholls R J, Bartolo D C C, Mortensen N J Mc C (eds) Restorative proctocolectomy. Oxford: Blackwell, pp 147–162

Warren B F, Shepherd N A, Bartolo D C, Bradfield J W 1993 Pathology of the defunctioned rectum in ulcerative colitis. Gut 34: 514–516

Warren B F, Shepherd N A, Price A B, Williams G T 1997 Importance of cryptolytic lesions and pericryptal granulomas in inflammatory bowel disease. J Clin Pathol 50: 880–881

Wells A D, McMillan I, Price A B, Ritchie J K, Nicholls R J 1991 Natural history of indeterminate colitis. Br J Surg 78: 178–181

Williamson M E. Hughes L E 1994 Bowel diversion should be used with caution in stenosing anal Crohn's disease. Gut 35: 1139–1140

Winslet M C, Andrews H, Allan R N, Keighley M R 1993 Fecal diversion in the management of Crohn's disease of the colon. Dis Colon Rectum 36: 757–762

Wischmeyer P, Pemberton J H, Phillips S F 1993 Chronic pouchitis after ileal pouch-anal anastomosis: responses to butyrate and glutamine suppositories in a pilot study. Mayo Clin Proc 68: 978–981

Yeong M L, Bethwaite P B, Prasad J, Isbister W H 1991 Lymphoid follicular hyperplasia – a distinctive feature of diversion colitis. Histopathology 19: 55–61

Ziv Y, Fazio V W, Sirimarco M T, Lavery I C, Goldblum J R, Petras R E 1994 Incidence, risk factors and treatment of dysplasia in the anal transitional zone after ileal pouch-anal anastomosis. Dis Colon Rectum 37: 1281–1285

Sezgin M. Ismail

CHAPTER

5

Drug-induced changes in the female genital tract

Over the past decade, it has become clear that prolonged treatment of breast cancer with tamoxifen has complex and unexpected effects on the female genital tract. The same period has seen the introduction of gonadotrophin releasing hormone (GnRH) agonists and increasing interest in long-term hormone replacement therapy for prevention of menopausal symptoms and postmenopausal osteoporosis.

TAMOXIFEN

For over 20 years, tamoxifen has been extensively used as an adjuvant treatment for breast cancer. Its use is associated with reduced mortality from breast cancer and increased tumour-free survival (Early Breast Cancer Trialists' Collaborative Group 1992, 1988). It has been observed that tamoxifen-treated women have a reduced risk of cancer in the contralateral breast (Early Breast Cancer Trialists' Collaborative Group 1992, 1998, Fisher et al 1989, Fornander et al 1989). This observation led to several large scale, randomized placebo-controlled trials in Europe and the USA in order to evaluate the role of tamoxifen in breast cancer prevention among asymptomatic women deemed at risk of breast cancer. The American study found a 49% reduction in invasive breast cancer among tamoxifen treated women when compared to the placebo group (Fisher et al 1998), but the rate of endometrial cancer was increased in the tamoxifen group. Prelonged tamoxifen therapy has other significant side effects on the female genital tract.

PHARMACOLOGY OF TAMOXIFEN

Tamoxifen is a non-steroidal triphenylethylene derivative with a chemical structure very similar to that of the synthetic oestrogen diethylstilboestrol (Furr

Dr S. M. Ismail, Department of Pathology, University of Wales College of Medicine, Heath Park, Cardiff CF4 4XN, UK

& Jordan 1984). Its effects on breast cancer were originally thought to be due purely to competitive inhibition and downregulation of oestrogen receptors and the drug was, therefore, categorised as an anti-oestrogen. It has recently become clear that tamoxifen also has effects independent of oestrogen receptor on breast cancer including effects on local growth control mechanisms (Butta et al 1992, Huynh et al 1993, Noguchi et al 1993) and apoptosis (Perry et al 1995, Kang et al 1996).

Tamoxifen has partial oestrogen agonist activity in the human female genital tract and, like oestrogens, induces maturation of postmenopausal cervicovaginal squamous epithelial cells and proliferation of endometrial epithelial and stromal cells. Its other effects, such as the unusual morphology of tamoxifen-stimulated endometrium, cannot be explained purely on the basis of oestrogen-like activity. These phenomena could be mediated by tamoxifen-induced changes in local growth control mechanisms (Huynh & Pollak 1993, Huynh & Pollak 1994, Laatikainen et al 1995, Boettgertong & Makela 1996). In addition, the drug may affect the function of the hypothalamic-pituitary-ovarian axis particularly in premenopausal women (Groom & Griffiths 1976, Sherman et al 1979, Patterson 1981, Jordan et al 1987, Jordan et al 1991) and may have direct effects on cell membranes (Cabot et al 1995, Charlier et al 1996, Gundimeda et al 1996, Song et al 1996, Cabot et al 1997, Duh et al 1997).

In view of the uterine effects of tamoxifen, the experimental evidence showing that this drug is a carcinogen in laboratory rodents is interesting. Tamoxifen administration to female rats causes liver cell adenomas and carcinomas in a high proportion of treated animals (Williams et al 1993). The incidence, severity and multiplicity of the hepatic lesions are related to dose and duration of tamoxifen treatment. In the context of hepatic carcinogenesis, tamoxifen has initiating (Ghia & Mereto 1989) and promoting (Tager et al 1986, Dragan et al 1991) effects. The genotoxic potential of tamoxifen has been confirmed by studies which found that tamoxifen administration produces DNA adducts in the liver of treated rats (Han & Liehr 1992, White et al 1992, Li 1997), hamsters (Han & Liehr 1992) and mice (White et al 1992). The concentration of adducts was related to dose and duration of tamoxifen treatment (Han & Liehr 1992, White et al 1992, Li 1997). To date no tamoxifen-induced DNA adducts have been detected in the uterus of experimental animals. It is not clear whether tamoxifen has genotoxic effects on human endometrium: evidence to date is contradictory (Carmichael et al 1996, Hemminki et al 1996) but its potential tumour promoting effect is well established.

EFFECTS ON THE UTERINE CERVIX AND VAGINA

In 1977, Ferrazzi et al (1977) noted unexpected oestrogenic changes in squamous epithelial cells from cervical smears of postmenopausal patients with breast cancer treated with tamoxifen. These changes regressed on cessation of tamoxifen therapy and were, therefore, attributed to the drug. These findings have been repeatedly confirmed (Boccardo et al 1981, Eells et al 1990, Lahti et al 1994). Most recently, Lahti et al (1994) found that 89% of tamoxifen-treated postmenopausal women had oestrogenic changes in their cervical smears which were not associated with increased concentrations of serum oestradiol.

In postmenopausal women, prolonged tamoxifen therapy is associated with an increased incidence of proliferative endometrial abnormalities including endometrial hyperplasia (Neven et al 1989, Neven et al 1990, De Muylder et al 1991, Lahti et al 1993, Ismail 1994), unusual endometrial polyps (Nuovo et al 1989, Corley et al 1992, Lahti et al 1993, Ismail 1994, Silva et al 1994, Hann et al 1997) and malignant endometrial neoplasms (Fornander et al 1989, Fisher et al 1994,1998, Van Leeuwen et al 1994, Fornander & Wilking 1995). The effects of tamoxifen on the premenopausal female genital tract are less certain. One study compared 73 tamoxifen-treated breast cancer patients with 122 breast cancer patients not treated with this drug and found a statistically significant increase in endometrial polyps in postmenopausal women; no such increase was demonstrated in premenopausal women (McGonigle et al 1996).

The incidence of tamoxifen-associated endometrial pathology is difficult to estimate because of a lack of uniformity in pathological interpretation and confusion in the use of pathological terminology. Nevertheless, hysteroscopic follow-up studies suggest that some 50% of tamoxifen-treated women develop endometrial lesions (Neven et al 1990, DeMuylder et al 1991) over a period ranging from 6–36 months of tamoxifen exposure. Endometrial polyps are variously reported as 3× (Lahti et al 1993), 8× (Neven et al 1989) and 11× (Ismail 1994) more frequently in tamoxifen-treated women than in untreated controls.

Fornander et al (1989) were the first to show a statistically significant increase in endometrial cancer in postmenopausal patients with breast cancer treated with tamoxifen. This classic study included 1846 postmenopausal women with early breast cancer, of whom 931 were randomised to receive 40 mg/day of tamoxifen. There were 13 invasive endometrial carcinomas in the tamoxifen-treated group over a median follow-up of 4.5 years. Two cases of corpus cancer were reported in the placebo group, one a uterine leiomyosarcoma and the other a malignant mixed Müllerian tumour. The risk ratio for corpus cancer was 6.4 (95% confidence interval 1.4–28).

Other large studies have confirmed that women with breast cancer who are treated with tamoxifen are at increased risk of endometrial carcinoma when compared with breast cancer patients who are not treated with this drug (Fisher et al 1994, 1998, Van Leeuwen et al 1994, Rutqvist et al 1995, Early Breast Cancer Trialists' Collaborative Group 1998, Fischer et al 1998). Reported risk ratios have ranged from 1.3 (95% CI 0.7–2.4; Van Leeuwen et al 1994) to 7.5 (95% CI 1.7–32.7; Fisher et al 1994). Most recently, the NSABP P-1 study reported findings in a group of 13,388 women considered at increased risk of breast cancer which were randomizedto receive either placebo (n=6707) or 20 mg/day tamoxifen(n=6681) for 5 years (Fisher et al 1998). The risk of endometrial cancer was increased in the tamoxifen group (risk ratio = 2.5; 95% CI 1.35–4.97).

Pathological features of tamoxifen-treated endometrium

On pathological examination, tamoxifen-treated endometrium shows an overlapping spectrum of morphological abnormalities including endometrial hyperplasia, polyps arising on a background of endometrial hyperplasia, cancers arising in polyps and invasive endometrial neoplasms (Ismail 1994).

In endometrial hyperplasia associated with tamoxifen (Ismail 1994) there is grossly visible thickening of the endometrium, cystic dilatation of the endometrial glands and variable proliferative activity in epithelial cells. The endometrial glands show focal architectural abnormalities with irregular branching and crowding. There may be epithelial metaplasias similar to those seen in tamoxifen-associated polyps, but cytological atypia is unusual. The endometrial stroma in tamoxifen-associated endometrial hyperplasia is characterised by collagen bundles between stromal cells. This low grade cystic hyperplasia with stromal collagenization and epithelial metaplasia appears to be characteristic of tamoxifen.

Endometrial polyps that occur in tamoxifen-treated women are unusually large and often multiple, either synchronously or metachronously (Nuovo et al 1989, Corley et al 1992, Ismail 1994). Most arise on a background of hyperplasia (Ismail 1994). On microscopic examination, the polyps are composed of architecturally complex endometrial glands surrounded by abundant fibrotic or myxoid stroma. Many polyps show some degree of ulceration and some undergo extensive ischaemic necrosis. In well-preserved polyps there is proliferative activity in epithelial and stromal cells, patchy stromal condensation around glands and an admixture of epithelial metaplasias including mucinous, clear cell, papillary oxyphil cell, squamoid and apocrine metaplasias. Tamoxifen-associated endometrial polyps are distinguished from Müllerian adenosarcoma by the patchy rather than generalised periglandular condensation, relative scarcity of stromal mitoses and absence of cytological atypia and atypical mitoses in stromal cells.

Endometrial polyp-cancers, defined as endometrial carcinoma arising in a polyp, are rare in the general population: a study of 1100 endometrial polyps that predated the availability of tamoxifen included only 4 cases (Peterson & Novak 1956). Two endometrial polyp-cancers were observed by Nuovo et al (1989) among 7 women with tamoxifen associated endometrial polyps. Another study found three endometrial polyp-cancers in a group of 19 tamoxifen-treated women with breast cancer (Ismail 1994). This high prevalence of endometrial polyp-cancer among tamoxifen-treated women suggests that endometrial polyps are an important intermediate stage in the development of endometrial carcinoma in tamoxifen-treated women.

The risk of endometrial carcinoma is probably related to the cumulative dose of tamoxifen. Fornander et al (1989) found that women who received tamoxifen for 5 years had a significantly greater cumulative frequency of uterine cancer than those who discontinued tamoxifen after 2 years of treatment. Van Leeuwen et al (1994) similarly found a significant trend of increasing risk of endometrial cancer with increasing duration and cumulative dose of tamoxifen. All the endometrial cancers in another study occurred in women who had received a cumulative tamoxifen dose of more than 35 g (Ismail 1994).

The link between endometrial cancer and prolonged tamoxifen treatment is no longer seriously disputed, but there is considerable controversy about the pathological features of tamoxifen-associated endometrial cancer (Fornander et al 1993, Magriples et al 1993, Barakat et al 1994, Van Leeuwen et al 1994, Evans et al 1995). Some authors have suggested that tamoxifen-treated women are at increased risk of developing uterine cancers with a poor prognosis (Magriples et al 1993, Evans et al 1995) because of high tumour grade or unfavourable histological subtype.

A retrospective study compared the histological features of uterine cancers which developed in 15 patients who had received 40 mg/day of tamoxifen (mean duration of treatment 4.2 years, range 3 months to 10 years) with those in 38 patients with breast cancer not treated with tamoxifen (Magriples et al 1993). In this study, low grade tumours were defined as grade I and II endometrioid carcinoma; high grade tumours included grade III endometrioid carcinoma, papillary serous, clear cell and malignant mixed Müllerian tumours. Of tamoxifen-treated women, 67% had high grade endometrial cancer compared with 24% in the untreated group. Five of the tamoxifen-treated women died of endometrial cancer and only one in the untreated group. The authors concluded that women receiving tamoxifen were more likely to develop endometrial cancer with a poor prognosis than would be expected by chance.

Evans et al (1995) reported 6 cases of endometrial carcinosarcoma that occurred in tamoxifen-treated women of whom 5 had been maintained on tamoxifen for at least 6 years. They suggested a causal link between prolonged tamoxifen treatment and this subtype of endometrial carcinoma which is associated with a poor prognosis. Silva et al (1994) reviewed the clinical and pathological features of uterine corpus cancers that developed in 72 women following treatment for breast cancer. Of these patients, 57 had received no tamoxifen and 15 had been treated with tamoxifen (20 mg/day, mean duration of treatment 2–66 months). Both groups had an unexpectedly high incidence of clear cell carcinoma of the endometrium and uterine leiomyosarcoma and this was statistically significant. There was also a relatively high incidence of endometrial carcinoma of serous type in both groups. Serous endometrial carcinoma, which is associated with a particularly poor prognosis, was the commonest subtype of endometrial carcinoma among the 15 tamoxifen-treated women. The difference between the tamoxifen and non-tamoxifen recipients was statistically significant but, despite the poor prognosis expected of serous endometrial carcinoma, there was no significant difference in tumour stage or clinical outcome between the two groups. This may reflect the small size of the study or a tendency among this group of pathologists to overdiagnose serous endometrial carcinoma or both.

Other studies have not supported the suggestion that tamoxifen is associated with endometrial cancers that have a poor prognosis (Fornander et al 1993, Barakat et al 1994, Fisher et al 1994,1998, Van Leeuwen et al 1994). Van Leeuwen et al (1994) found no significant difference in stage, morphology and prevalence of death from endometrial cancer in 98 women with tamoxifen-associated endometrial cancer and 285 breast cancer patients not treated with tamoxifen who subsequently developed endometrial cancer. Interestingly, they found an excess of well-differentiated tumours in tamoxifen-users (52%) compared with non-users (32%).In the NSABP P-1 study, all 36 endometrial cancers which occurred in the tamoxifen group were FIGO Stage 1 (Fisher et al 1998). In conclusion, to date there is no clear link between tamoxifen therapy and poor prognosis endometrial cancer.

TAMOXIFEN AND ENDOMETRIAL CARCINOGENESIS

The spectrum of pathological findings seen in tamoxifen treated endometria suggests that endometrial polyps represent an intermediate step in the development of endometrial carcinomas in tamoxifen-treated women. There have been several studies demonstrating an association between endometrial polyps and endometrial carcinoma (Hertig & Sommers 1949, Peterson & Novak 1956, Armenia 1967). 55% of sporadic endometrial polyps show cytogenetic abnormalities (Dal Cin et al 1995) and similar cytogenetic abnormalities have been recently reported in tamoxifen-associated endometrial polyps (Dal Cin et al 1998).

The significance of the stromal and epithelial alterations found in tamoxifen-associated endometrial hyperplasia and polyps is uncertain. Experimental evidence suggests that endometrial epithelial proliferation is mediated by the endometrial stroma (Cooke et al 1997) and that stromal fibroblasts induce epithelial metaplasia (Obinata et al 1994). Stromal alterations in tamoxifen-treated endometria may, therefore, reflect functional alterations, related to promotion of epithelial growth, polypogenesis and epithelial metaplasia in tamoxifen-associated endometrial polyps.

The different epithelial metaplasias that occur in tamoxifen-associated endometrial polyps and hyperplasia are of particular interest in the context of carcinogenesis. Metaplasia is generally regarded as a non-neoplastic process that is usually secondary to injury. However, there is an important link between metaplasia and neoplasia in many organs, e.g. the stomach (Stemmermann 1994) and the oesophagus (Speechler & Goyal 1986). Genomic alterations have been reported in metaplasias (Tahara et al 1994, Michael et al 1997). It is, therefore, not surprising that tamoxifen-associated endometrial polyps characterised by unusual stromal changes and epithelial metaplasias also have a high prevalence of focal endometrial carcinoma arising within them.

OTHER GYNAECOLOGICAL EFFECTS OF TAMOXIFEN

Other uterine abnormalities that have been reported in association with tamoxifen include postmenopausal adenomyosis (Cohen et al 1995) and small numbers of stromal neoplasms including three cases of endometrial stromal sarcoma (Fisher et al 1989, Beer et al 1995, Eddy & Mazur 1997) and six cases of Müllerian adenosarcoma (Clement et al 1996). Patients with breast cancer, whether treated with tamoxifen or not, have an increased risk of uterine sarcoma (Silva et al 1994), and so the link between tamoxifen and uterine sarcoma remains not proven.

Prolonged tamoxifen use is also associated with ovarian cysts (Cohen et al 1994, Kedar et al 1994, Hochner-Celnikier et al 1995, Shushan et al 1996). These have been reported as occurring in both premenopausal (Cohen et al 1994, Hochner-Celnikier et al 1995) and postmenopausal (Kedar et al 1994, Shushan et al 1996) women receiving tamoxifen. In premenopausal women, these ovarian cysts may be associated with hyperoestrogenism (Cohen et al 1994, Hochner-Celnikier et al 1995). The pathology of these ovarian cysts is poorly documented, but those occurring in premenopausal women have been variously reported as luteinized or follicular cysts (Shushan et al 1996), benign unilateral corpus luteum cysts (Hochner-Celnikier et al 1995) or bilateral 'simple' functional cysts (Cohen et al 1994) which were presumably luteinised follicle cysts. The ovarian cysts in tamoxifen-treated postmenopausal women may represent cystic ovarian tumours (Cohen et al 1996) or endometriotic cysts (Hajjar et al 1993, Cohen et al 1994, Ismail & Maulik G 1997).

To date eight cases of tamoxifen-associated endometriosis have been reported in English language journals of which five were in premenopausal (Ford et al 1988, Cano et al 1989, Buckley 1990, Morgan et al 1994)l and three in postmenopausal women (Hajjar et al 1993, Cohen et al 1994, Ismail & Maulik G 1997). The oestrogen-dependent disease endometriosis is common among premenopausal women and very rare in postmenopausal women. Its association with tamoxifen therapy in the premenopausal age group may be coincidental. However, its occurrence in postmenopausal women treated with tamoxifen, a partial oestrogen agonist, suggests a causative link between the drug and the disease. It is not clear whether the drug induces endometriosis de novo or permits re-activation of pre-existing endometriosis.

The three tamoxifen-treated postmenopausal women with endometriosis had unusual pathological features. One developed intestinal and pelvic endo- metriosis that infiltrated the cervix, vagina, rectum and sigmoid colon (Hajjar et al 1993). Another patient had a cystic ovarian mass with mucinous contents, friable masses on its serosal surface and apparent infiltration of adjacent structures (Ismail & Maulik 1997). On microscopic examination, this was shown to be an endometriotic cyst which showed features identical to those described in tamoxifen-treated endometrium including epithelial metaplasias and polyp formation. Most ominously, Cohen et al (1994) reported a case of ovarian endometrioid carcinoma which occurred in a tamoxifen-related endometriotic cyst, raising the possibility that prolonged tamoxifen therapy may be associated with an increased risk of carcinoma arising in endometriotic foci.

HORMONE REPLACEMENT THERAPY

Hormone replacement therapy (HRT) has long been used in perimenopausal and postmenopausal women to alleviate vasomotor symptoms and to treat problems such as atrophic vaginitis. More recently, its long term use has been advocated to reduce the likelihood of osteoporosis and coronary artery disease in postmenopausal women.

Early HRT regimens consisted of oestrogens alone, but the majority of treated women now receive an oestrogen combined with a progestogen. There is considerable variation in prescribing schedules for combined HRT, but there are two commonly used regimens: sequential (cyclic) and continuous. In Europe, sequential HRT regimens usually comprise continuous oestrogen (usually 1–2 mg/day of oestradiol) with a progestogen added for 10–12 days per cycle or calendar month (Whitehead et al 1990). In continuous combined HRT regimens, a progestogen is administered with oestrogen throughout the cycle. In the US, sequential HRT would comprise 0.625 mg/day of conjugated equine oestrogens and a progestogen (usually 5–10 mg/day of medroxypro- gesterone acetate) for 10–14 days a month; continuous HRT would comprise 0.625 mg/day of conjugated equine oestrogens administered with continuous medroxyprogesterone acetate at a dose of 2.5–5 mg/day (Grady & Ernster 1997).

Reports on the gynaecological effects of hormone replacement therapy have almost exclusively been written by epidemiologists who have established the causal link between prolonged use of unopposed oestrogens and endometrial cancer. By contrast, the lack of pathological interest in HRT has led to a lack of understanding of the mechanisms of oestrogen-induced endometrial carcinogenesis.

UNOPPOSED OESTROGEN THERAPY

The association between endogenous hyperoestrogenism and endometrial hyperplasia was well documented during the 1940s and 1950s prior to the widespread availability of unopposed oestrogen therapy (Gusberg 1947, Mansell & Hertig 1955, Jackson & Dockerty 1957). Since the 1970s, epidemiological studies have established an undoubted link between exogenous oestrogen use and endometrial carcinoma (Smith et al 1975, Ziel & Finkle 1975, Mack et al 1976, Weiss et al 1976, Antunes et al 1979, Shapiro et al 1980, Spengler et al 1981, Shapiro et al 1985, Paganini-Hill et al 1989, Rubin et al 1990, Brinton et al 1993). The reported risk ratios for endometrial carcinoma among oestrogen treated women have ranged from 3.5 (Shapiro et al 1985) to 10 (Paganini-Hill et al 1989). The risk ratios for developing endometrial carcinoma increase with increasing daily dose and duration of therapy (Smith et al 1975, Shapiro et al 1980, Spengler et al 1981, Shapiro et al 1985, Paganini-Hill et al 1989). The large cohort study of Paganini-Hill et al (1989) found that women who had used oestrogen replacement therapy had a relative risk of endometrial cancer of 10 compared to non-users, and that women who had used oestrogens for 15 or more years had a relative risk of 20. Women who received oestrogen replacement therapy for one or more years remain at increased risk of endometrial carcinoma for many years after cessation of oestrogen therapy (Mack et al 1976, Shapiro et al 1985, Paganini-Hill et al 1989, Rubin et al 1990, Brinton et al 1993). In Paganini-Hill's series, women who had last used oestrogens 15 or more years previously still had an increased risk of developing endometrial carcinoma (relative risk = 5.8, 95% CI = 2.0–17) (Paganini-Hill et al 1989).

Endometrial carcinoma associated with exogenous oestrogen therapy tends to occur in younger women who present at an earlier tumour stage, with a lower grade tumour and less myometrial invasion than endometrial carcinoma not associated with oestrogen use (Collins et al 1980, Hulka et al 1980, Chu et al 1982). Survival rates from endometrial carcinoma are higher in women with a history of prior oestrogen use than among non-users (Collins et al 1980, Chu et al 1982, Schwartzbaum et al 1987). The possibility has been raised that these findings may be caused by overdiagnosis of endometrial carcinoma among oestrogen-treated women, but an independent review by three expert pathologists of the pathological material from the Ziehl and Finkle (1975) study confirmed the diagnosis of endometrial carcinoma in 99% of cases (Gordon et al 1977). Furthermore, endometrial carcinoma which develops on a background of ovarian disease causing endogenous oestrogenic stimulation is also more frequently early stage, low grade and superficially invasive than those which occur in women without ovarian disease (McDonald et al 1977). Pathological studies, though based on relatively few cases, also support an association between oestrogen use and endometrial carcinoma with a good prognosis (Robboy & Bradley 1979, Silverberg et al 1980). However, no pathological features were noted which were specifically associated with oestrogen use (Robboy & Bradley 1979, Silverberg et al 1980).

Unopposed oestrogen therapy is also associated with endometrial hyperplasia (Whitehead et al 1979, Paterson et al 1980, Gelfand & Ferenczy 1989, Woodruff et al 1994, The Writing Group for the PEPI Trial 1996). There is considerable variation in the reported incidence of oestrogen-associated endometrial hyperplasia, but this appears closely related to the dose of oestrogen (Whitehead et al 1979, Paterson et al 1980, Gelfand & Ferenczy 1989, Woodruff et al 1994, The Writing Group for the PEPI Trial 1996). Whitehead et al (1979) found that simple endometrial hyperplasia occurred in 12% and atypical hyperplasia in 6% of women receiving low dose oestrogens. Patients in the high dose group received twice the daily dose ingested by those in the low dose group. The incidence of simple hyperplasia in the high dose group was 23% and atypical hyperplasia occurred in 9% of women in this group. Paterson et al (1980) reported that endometrial hyperplasia occurred in 14.8% of women receiving high dose oestrogens and 7% of those receiving low dose oestrogens. In another study (Gelfand & Ferenczy 1989), 42% of all patients who received oestrogens had developed endometrial hyperplasia after 12 months of treatment but the incidence of hyperplasia was lower in the low dose (30%) than in the high dose group (57%).

The findings of two large, prospective, randomized, double-blind studies have recently been documented (Woodruff et al 1994, The Writing Group for the PEPI Trial 1996). The Menopause Study Group found that 20% women receiving unopposed oestrogen therapy developed endometrial hyperplasia (not otherwise specified) after twelve months of treatment (Woodruff et al 1994). The three-year PEPI Study reported simple endometrial hyperplasia in 27.7%, complex hyperplasia in 22.7% and atypical hyperplasia in 11.8% of women who were treated with oestrogens alone (The Writing Group for the PEPI Trial 1996). In contrast, women randomised to the placebo group in this study showed an incidence of simple endometrial hyperplasia of 0.8%, complex hyperplasia of 0.8% and atypical hyperplasia of zero.

COMBINED OESTROGEN/PROGESTOGEN THERAPY

Modern HRT regimens combine oestrogens with progestogens to minimise the undesirable endometrial side effects of long term oestrogen therapy. Progestogen used for 10 or more days per month reduces the excess risk of endometrial carcinoma (Hammond et al 1979, Persson et al 1989, Voigt et al 1991, Beresford et al 1997, Pike et al 1997) and hyperplasia (Whitehead et al 1979, Paterson et al 1980, Gelfand & Ferenczy 1989, Woodruff et al 1994) associated with long term oestrogen use.

Two recent blinded studies (Woodruff et al 1994, The Writing Group for the PEPI Trial 1996) in which a large number of subjects were randomised to oestrogen only or oestrogen with progestogen treatment, confirmed reports from previous studies (Whitehead et al 1979, Paterson et al 1980, Gelfand & Ferenczy 1989) that the addition of progestogen significantly reduced the incidence of endometrial hyperplasia. The Menopause Study Group reported endometrial hyperplasia in ≤ 1% women who received medroxyprogesterone acetate in addition to conjugated oestrogens compared with 20% of women treated with oestrogens alone (Woodruff et al 1994). Women who were randomised to receive progestogens in addition to conjugated oestrogens in the PEPI Trial had rates of endometrial hyperplasia which were similar to those of the placebo group (The Writing Group for the PEPI Trial 1996). Furthermore, the biopsy results of 34 of 36 women who developed oestrogen-induced endometrial hyperplasia during the trial reverted to normal when oestrogens were discontinued and progestogen therapy administered (The Writing Group for the PEPI Trial 1996). It appears, therefore, that the addition of progestogens eliminates, at least for 3 years, the increased risk of endometrial hyperplasia associated with long-term oestrogen treatment. It is not at present clear whether this protective effect of progestogens continues unabated for longer periods of treatment.

The addition of progestogen to oestrogens has been repeatedly shown to reduce the risk of endometrial carcinoma associated with long term oestrogen therapy (Hammond et al 1979, Persson et al 1989, Voigt et al 1991, Brinton et al 1993, Beresford et al 1997, Pike et al 1997). Some authors (Hammond et al 1979, Persson et al 1989) have reported a lower risk of endometrial carcinoma in women receiving combined oestrogen/progestogen HRT than in non-users of HRT while others (Brinton et al 1993, Voigt et al 1991) found a non-significant small increase in endometrial cancer risk associated with the use of combined oestrogen/progestogen therapy. The two most recent reports on this subject are broadly in agreement about the protective effect of added progestogen but differ in some details. In a population-based case-control study, Beresford et al (1997) investigated the risk of endometrial cancer in relation to sequential combined HRT. When compared with non-users, the relative risk of endometrial cancer was 4.0 (95% CI 3.1–5.1) among women who used unopposed oestrogen and 1.4 (1.0–1.9) among those who used a sequential oestrogen/progestogen regime. The relative risk of endometrial cancer was 3.1 (1.7–5.7) in women who used progestogen for fewer than 10 days a cycle and 1.3 (0.8–2.2) in women who used progestogen for 10 days or more. Interestingly, women who received combined sequential HRT for 5 or more years were at increased risk of endometrial cancer compared to non-users (relative risk 2.5, 95% CI 1.1–5.5) even if they used 10 or more days of progestogen per cycle.

The population based case-control study of Pike et al (1997) investigated the risk of endometrial cancer in relation to sequential and continuous combined HRT. These authors found no significant increase in endometrial cancer risk among women receiving continuous combined HRT and sequential HRT with 10 or more days of progestogen per month. In contrast, women who used sequential HRT with less than 10 days progestogen per month had an increased risk of endometrial cancer which was similar in magnitude to that of unopposed oestrogen users.

There are few systematic studies of endometrial findings in women receiving HRT (Whitehead et al 1982, Whitehead & Fraser 1987, Moyer et al 1993, Piegsa et al 1997). Whitehead and colleagues studied endometrial histology in women receiving a variety of sequential combined HRT regimens (Whitehead et al 1982, Whitehead & Fraser 1987). All endometrial biopsies taken during the oestrogen only phase of treatment showed proliferative activity (Whitehead et al 1982). On the sixth day of combined oestrogen-progestogen treatment, 3–30% had an insufficient endometrial sample, 20–30% had inactive endometrium, 40–80% had weak secretory changes and 10% or less had proliferative endometrium (Whitehead et al 1982, Whitehead & Fraser 1987).

Moyer et al (1993) studied the endometrium of 157 women who received combined sequential HRT for at least 5 years. Four of these women developed irregular bleeding; on further investigation three were found to have endometrial polyps and one had a submucosal leiomyoma. An endometrial biopsy was attempted in the remaining 153 women but no tissue was obtained in 87 cases and the material was inadequate in 13 cases. Hysteroscopic examination of these women showed endometrial atrophy. Adequate endometrial tissue was obtained from the remaining 53 women. These biopsies showed normal endometrial glands and stroma with weak secretory changes and scanty proliferative activity. Interestingly, proliferative activity was significantly lower in women receiving progestogen for 9 days or more per cycle than in those receiving a shorter duration of progestogen. Prolonged combined sequential HRT was associated with benign endometrial or uterine pathology in 3%, endometrial atrophy in 65% and endometrium showing weak secretory and proliferative changes in 32% of subjects.

Similar findings were reported in a recent small study of the endometrial effects of continuous combined HRT (Piegsa et al 1997). The 40 women in this study were followed up for a mean duration of 2.9 years. Four women developed benign endometrial pathology: one had pseudodecidual change, two developed benign endometrial polyps and one had a submucosal leiomyoma. In the remaining cases, the endometrial biopsy was inadequate in 15 cases, inactive or atrophic in 18 cases secretory in 2 cases and proliferative in 1 case.

Very little information is available about the pathological features of endometrial carcinoma associated with combined hormone replacement therapy. McGonigle et al (1994) studied 25 women who developed endometrial cancer while receiving HRT. In 14 women, the endometrial cancer developed on a background of endometrial hyperplasia. Twenty-three patients had stage I disease and two had stage IIIA disease. None had lymph node metastases. In 23 cases, the tumour was low grade and showed less than 50% myometrial invasion. Two patients had a grade 3 papillary serous carcinoma of the endometrium. Twenty-five tumours showed mucinous changes, which were extensive in 18 and focal in 7 cases. All the patients remained alive and disease-free after a mean follow-up of 26 months.

GONADOTROPHIN RELEASING HORMONE AGONISTS

Normal functions of the female genital tract are controlled by the hypothalamic-pituitary-ovarian axis. Gonadotrophin releasing hormone (GnRH) is secreted at intervals by the hypothalamus and binds to specific receptors on the surface of anterior pituitary gonadotrophs. The internalisation of the GnRH-receptor complex triggers intracellular signalling mechanisms culminating in the release of the gonadotrophins luteinising hormone and follicle stimulating hormone. These control the secretion of oestrogen and progesterone by ovarian follicles (Schally 1978, Schriock 1989).

GnRH is a 10 amino acid peptide. Replacement of the amino acid in position 6, position 10 or both results in GnRH analogues with longer half life and greater receptor affinity than GnRH. This group of drugs includes buserelin, goserelin, leuproreline and nafarelin. Treatment with GnRH agonists results in a transient elevation in gonadotrophin levels followed, in 10–14 days, by a fall in gonadotrophin levels. This results in suppression of ovulation and ovarian hormone secretion. This inhibitory effect persists for the duration of treatment but normal ovarian function returns after cessation of treatment (West & Baird 1987).

In gynaecological practice, GnRH analogues are used for the treatment of endometriosis (Henzl et al 1988, Dlugi et al 1990, Kennedy et al 1990, Venturini et al 1990), uterine leiomyomas (Filicori et al 1983, West et al 1987, Matta et al 1989, Stjernquist 1997) and in assisted reproduction. Treatment with GnRH analogues for up to 6 months has been shown to reduce the size of endometriotic foci and to improve the symptoms associated with endometriosis. However, recurrence of endometriotic symptoms is common after cessation of treatment (Shriock 1989).

Pre-operative treatment of uterine leiomyomas with GnRH analogues reduces uterine size by approximately 50%. This may be related at least in part to the GnRH induced reduction in uterine blood flow (Matta et al 1988). Regrowth of leiomyomas with recurrence of symptoms is commonly seen after cessation of treatment (Matta et al 1989). For this reason, GnRH analogues do not constitute a definitive treatment for uterine leiomyomas. They are, however, used to shrink large leiomyomas prior to surgery in order to minimize intraoperative technical problems. They are also useful in women with leiomyomas and significant pre-operative anaemia.

GnRH analogues suppress serum concentrations of oestradiol to postmenopausal levels within 2 weeks (West & Baird 1987) and induce amenorrhoea within 8 weeks. There are associated menopausal changes in the lower female genital tract with atrophy of the endometrium, cervix and vagina and patients commonly complain of vaginal dryness.

Williamson et al (1988) investigated the effects of goserelin on the ovaries. The ovaries of 23 women treated with goserelin for advanced breast cancer were compared with ovaries from 34 untreated patients with breast cancer. There were two statistically significant differences between treated and untreated ovaries: fewer goserelin-treated ovaries contained corpora lutea (13% versus 58%), and more goserelin-treated ovaries contained follicle cysts (78% versus 50%) than did untreated ovaries.

Several groups have investigated the morphological changes induced by GnRH agonists in uterine leiomyomas (Upadhyaya et al 1990, Gutmann et al 1994, Crow et al 1995). A small study comparing 9 goserelin-treated cases with 7 untreated cases found that treated leiomyomas were undistinguishable from untreated ones in 6 cases, while two treated leiomyomas were densely cellular and one showed a dense lymphocytic infiltrate (Crow et al 1995). Gutmann et al (1994) reported that there were no morphological differences between leiomyomas treated with leuprolide acetate and untreated leiomyomas while Upadhyaya et al (1990) found a significant reduction in cellularity of leuprolide treated leiomyomas. Thus, there is, at present, no consensus on the morphological basis of the shrinkage seen in leiomyomas treated with GnRH analogues.

Points of best practice

- *Tamoxifen* Prolonged use of tamoxifen in postmenopausal women is associated with an increase in incidence of endometrial carcinoma, hyperplasia and polyps. These show unusual morphological features. Other abnormalities reported in association with tamoxifen include ovarian follicle cysts in premenopausal and perimenopausal women, and adenomyosis and endometriosis in postmenopausal women.

- *Unopposed oestrogen therapy* Prolonged use of unopposed oestrogen therapy is associated with an increased incidence of simple, complex and atypical hyperplasia and endometrial carcinoma. No specific morphological features have been attributed to oestrogen-induced endometrial lesions.

- *Combined oestrogen/progestogen therapy* The addition of progestogen eliminates the risk of endometrial hyperplasia and significantly reduces the risk of endometrial carcinoma associated with unopposed oestrogens. Endometrial biopsies from treated women show atrophy in many cases but may also show weak secretory or proliferative activity.

- *GnRH analogues* These produce endometrial, cervical and vaginal atrophy. Ovaries of treated women contain follicle cysts and tend to lack stigmata of ovulation.

References

Antunes C M F, Stolley P D, Rosenshein N B et al 1979 Endometrial cancer and estrogen use. Report of a large case-control study. N Engl J Med 300: 9–13

Armenia C S 1967 Sequential relationship between endometrial polyps and carcinoma of the endometrium. Obstet Gynecol 30: 524–529

Barakat R R, Wong G, Curtin J P, Vlamis V, Hoskins W J 1994 Tamoxifen use in breast cancer patients who subsequently develop corpus cancer is not associated with a higher incidence of adverse histologic features. Gynecol Oncol 55: 164–168

Beer T W, Buchanan R, Buckley C H 1995 Uterine stromal sarcoma following tamoxifen treatment. J Clin Pathol 48: 596

Beresford S A A, Weiss N S, Voigt L F, McKnight B 1997 Risk of endometrial cancer in relation to oestrogen combined with cyclic progestagen therapy in postmenopausal women. Lancet 349: 458–461

Boccardo F, Bruzzi P, Rubagotti A, Nicolò G, Rosso R 1981 Estrogen-like action of tamoxifen on vaginal epithelium of breast cancer patients. Oncology 30: 281–285

Brinton L A, Hoover R N and the Endometrial Cancer Collaborative Group 1993 Estrogen replacement therapy and endometrial cancer risk: unresolved issues. Obstet Gynecol 81: 265–271

Buckley C H 1990 Tamoxifen and endometriosis. Case report. Br J Obstet Gynaecol 97: 645–646

Butta A, MacLennan K, Flanders K C et al 1992 Induction of transforming growth factor β1 in human breast cancer in vivo following tamoxifen treatment. Cancer Res 52: 4261–4264

Cabot M C, Zhang Z C, Giuliano A E 1995 Tamoxifen elicits rapid transmembrane lipid signal responses in human breast cancer cells. Breast Cancer Res Treat 36: 299–306

Cabot M C, Zhang Z C, Cao H T et al 1997 Tamoxifen activates cellular phospholipase C and D and elicits protein kinase C translocation. Int J Cancer 70: 567–574

Cano A, Matallin P, Legua V, Tortajada M, Bonilla-Musoles F 1989 Tamoxifen and the uterus and endometrium. Lancet i: 376

Carmichael P L, Ugwumadu A H N, Neven P, Hewer A J, Poon G K, Phillips D H 1996 Lack of genotoxicity of tamoxifen in human endometrium. Cancer Res 56: 1475–1479

Charlier C, Bruyneel E, Lechanteur C, Bracke M, Mareel M, Castronovo V 1996 Enhancement of tamoxifen-induced E-cadherin function by Ca^{2+} channel antagonists in human breast cancer MCF7/6 cells. Eur J Pharmacol 317: 413–416

Chu J C, Schweid A I, Weiss N S 1982 Survival among women with endometrial cancer; a comparison of estrogen users and nonusers. Am J Obstet Gynecol 143: 569–573

Clement P B, Oliva E, Young R H 1996 Müllerian adenocarcinoma of the uterine corpus associated with tamoxifen therapy: A report of six cases and a review of tamoxifen associated endometrial lesion. Int J Gynecol Pathol 15: 222–229

Cohen I, Altaras M M, Lew S, Tepper R, Beyth Y, Ben-Baruch G 1994 Ovarian endometrioid carcinoma and endometriosis developing in a postmenopausal breast cancer patient during tamoxifen therapy: a case report and review of the literature. Gynecol Oncol 55: 443–447

Cohen I, Beyth Y, Tepper R et al 1995 Adenomyosis in postmenopausal breast-cancer patients treated with tamoxifen – a new entity. Gynecol Oncol 58: 86–91

Cohen I, Beyth Y, Tepper R et al 1996 Ovarian tumors in postmenopausal breast cancer patients treated with tamoxifen. Gynecol Oncol 60: 54–58

Cohen I, Rosen D J D, Altaras M, Beyth Y, Shapira J, Yigael D 1994 Tamoxifen treatment in premenopausal breast cancer patients may be associated with ovarian overstimulation, cystic formations and fibroid overgrowth. Br J Cancer 69: 620–621

Collins J, Donner A, Allen L H, Adams O 1980 Oestrogen use and survival in endometrial cancer. Lancet ii: 961–964

Cooke P S, Buchanan D L, Young P et al 1997 Stromal estrogen receptors mediate mitogenic effects of estradiol on uterine epithelium. Proc Natl Acad Sci USA 94: 6535–6540

Corley D, Rowe J, Curtis M T, Hogan W M, Noumoff J S, LiVolsi V A 1992 Postmenopausal bleeding from unusual endometrial polyps in women on chronic tamoxifen therapy. Obstet Gynecol 79: 111–116

Crow J, Gardner R L, McSweeney G, Shaw R W 1995 Morphological changes in uterine leiomyomas treated by GnRH agonist goserelin. Int J Gynecol Pathol 14: 235–242

Dal Cin P, Vanni R, Marras S et al 1995 Four cytogenetic subgroups can be identified in endometrial polyps. Cancer Res 55: 1565–1568

Dal Cin P, Timmerman D, Van Den Burghe I et al 1998 Genomic changes in endometrial polyps associated with tamoxifen show no evidence for its action as an external carcinogen. Cancer Res 58: 2278–2281

De Muylder X, Neven P, De Somer M, Van Belle Y, Vanderick G, De Muylder E 1991 Endo-metrial lesions in patients undergoing tamoxifen therapy. Int J Gynaecol Obstet 36: 127–130

Dlugi A M, Miller J D, Knittle J, Lupron Study Group 1990 Lupron depot (leuprolide acetate for depot suspension) in the treatment of endometriosis: a randomized, placebo-controlled, double-blind study. Fertil Steril 54: 419–427

Dragan Y P, Xu Y D, Pitot H C 1991 Tumor promotion as a target for estrogen/antiestrogen effects in rat hepatic carcinogenesis. Prev Med 20: 15–26

Duh J L, Yu R, Jiao J J et al 1997 Activation of signal transduction kinases by tamoxifen. Pharmaceut Res 14: 186–189

Early Breast Cancer Trialists' Collaborative Group 1992 Systemic treatment of early breast cancer by hormonal, cytotoxic or immune therapy. 133 randomized trials involving 31,000 recurrences and 24,000 deaths among 75,000 women. Lancet 339: 1–15

Early Breast Cancer Trialists' Collaborative Group 1988 Effects of adjuvant tamoxifen and of cytotoxic therapy on mortality in early breast cancer: an overview of 61 randomized trials among 28,896 women. N Engl J Med 319: 1681–1692

Early Breast Cancer Trialists' Collaborative Group 1998 Tamoxifen for early breast cancer: an overview of the randomized trials. Lancet 351: 1451–1467

Eddy G L, Mazur M T 1997 Endolymphatic stromal myosis associated with tamoxifen use. Gynecol Oncol 64: 262–264

Eells T P, Alpern H D, Grzywacz C, MacMillan R W, Olson J E 1990 The effect of tamoxifen on cervical squamous maturation in Papanicolaou stained cervical smears of postmenopausal women. Cytopathology 1: 263–268

Evans M J, Langlois N E I, Kitchener H C, Miller I D 1995 Is there an association between long-term tamoxifen treatment and the development of carcinosarcoma (malignant mixed Müllerian tumor) of the uterus? Int J Gynecol Cancer 5: 310–313

Ferrazzi E, Cartei G, Mattarazzo R, Fiorentino M. Oestrogen-like effect of tamoxifen on vaginal epithelium. BMJ 1: 1351–1352

Filicori M, Hall D A, Loughlin J S, Rivier J, Vale W, Crowley W F 1983 A conservative approach to the management of uterine leiomyomata: pituitary desensitization by luteinizing hormone-releasing hormone analog. Am J Obstet Gynecol 147: 726–727

Fisher B, Costantino J P, Redmond C K et al 1994 Endometrial cancer in tamoxifen-treated breast cancer patients: findings from the National Surgical Adjuvant Breast and Bowel Project (NSABP) B-14. J Natl Cancer Inst 86: 527–537

Fisher B, Costantino J P, Redmond C et al 1989 A randomized clinical trial evaluating tamoxifen in the treatment of patients with node negative breast cancer who have estrogen-receptor-positive tumors. N Engl J Med 320: 479–484

Fisher B, Costantino J P, Wickerham D L, et al 1998 Tamoxifen for prevention of breast cancer: Report of the National Surgical Adjuvant Breast and Bowel Project (NSABP) P-1 Study. J Natl Cancer Inst 90: 1371–1388

Ford M R W, Turner M J, Wood C, Soutter W P 1988 Endometriosis developing during tamoxifen therapy. Am J Obstet Gynecol 158: 1119

Fornander T, Hellström A C, Moberger B 1993 Descriptive clinicopathologic study of 17 patients with endometrial cancer during or after adjuvant tamoxifen in early breast cancer. J Natl Cancer Inst 85: 1850–1855

Fornander T, Rutqvist L E, Cedermark B et al 1989 Adjuvant tamoxifen in early breast cancer: occurrence of new primary cancers. Lancet i: 117–120

Furr B J A, Jordan V C 1984 The pharmacology and clinical uses of tamoxifen. Pharmacol Ther 25: 127–205

Gelfand M M, Ferenczy A 1989 A prospective 1-year study of estrogen and progestin in postmenopausal women: effects on the endometrium. Obstet Gynecol 74: 398–402

Ghia M, Mereto E 1989 Induction and promotion of γ-glutamyltranspeptidase-positive foci in the liver of female rats treated with ethinyl estradiol, clomiphene, tamoxifen and their associations. Cancer Lett 46: 195–202

Gordon J, Reagan J W, Finkle W D, Ziel H K 1977 Estrogen and endometrial carcinoma. An independent pathology review supporting original risk estimate. N Engl J Med 297: 570–571

Grady D, Ernster V L 1997 Hormone replacement therapy and endometrial cancer: are current regimens safe? J Natl Cancer Inst 89: 1088–1089

Groom G V, Griffiths K 1976 Effect of the anti-oestrogen tamoxifen on plasma levels of luteinizing hormone, follicle-stimulating hormone, prolactin, oestradiol and progesterone in normal pre-menopausal women. J Endocrinol 70: 421–428

Gundimeda U, Chen Z H, Gopalakrishna R 1996 Tamoxifen modulates protein-kinase-C via oxidative stress in estrogen receptor-negative breast cancer cells. J Biol Chem 271: 13504–13514

Gusberg S B 1947 Precursors of corpus carcinoma. Estrogens and adenomatous hyperplasia. Am J Obstet Gynecol 54: 905–927

Gutmann J N, Thornton K L, Diamond M P, Carcangiu M L 1994 Evaluation of leuprolide acetate treatment on histopathology of uterine myomata. Fertil Steril 61: 622–626

Hajjar L R, Kim W S, Nolan G H, Turner S, Raju U R 1993 Intestinal and pelvic endometriosis presenting as a tumor and associated with tamoxifen therapy: report of a case. Obstet Gynecol 82: 642–644

Hammond C B, Jelovsek F R, Lee K L, Creasman W T, Parker R T 1979 Effects of long-term estrogen replacement therapy. II. Neoplasia. Am J Obstet Gynecol 133: 537–547

Han X, Liehr J G 1992 Induction of covalent DNA adducts in rodents by tamoxifen. Cancer Res 52: 1360–1363

Hann L E, Giess C S, Bach A M, Tao Y, Baum H J, Barakat R R 1997 Endometrial thickness in tamoxifen-treated patients:correlation with clinical and pathologic findings. Am J R0entgenol 168: 657–661

Hemminki K, Rajaniemi H, Lindahl B, Moberger B 1996 Tamoxifen induced DNA adducts in endometrial samples from breast cancer patients. Cancer Res 56: 4374–4377

Henzl M R, Corson S L, Moghissi K, Buttram V C, Berqvist C, Jacobson J 1988 Administration of nasal nafarelin as compared with oral danazol for endometriosis: a multicenter double-blind comparative clinical trial. N Engl J Med 318: 485–489

Hertig A T, Sommers S C 1949 Genesis of endometrial carcinoma I. Cancer 8: 946–956

Hochner-Celnikier D, Anteby E, Yagel S 1995 Ovarian cysts in tamoxifen-treated premenopausal women with breast cancer – a management dilemma. Am J Obstet Gynecol 172: 1323–1324

Hulka B S, Kaufman D G, Fowler W C, Grimson R C, Greenberg B G 1980 Predominance of early endometrial cancers after long-term estrogen use. JAMA 244: 2419–2422

Huynh H T, Pollak M 1993 Insulin-like growth factor-1 gene expression in the uterus is stimulated by tamoxifen and inhibited by the pure antiestrogen ICI-182780. Cancer Res 23: 5585–5588

Huynh H T, Tetenes E, Wallace L, Pollak M 1993 In vivo inhibition of insulin-like growth factor-1 gene-expression by tamoxifen. Cancer Res 53: 1727–1730

Huynh H T, Pollak M 1994 Uterotrophic actions of estradiol and tamoxifen are associated with inhibition of uterine insulin-like growth-factor binding protein-3 gene expression. Cancer Res 54: 3115–3119

Hyder S M, Stancel G M, Chiapetta C, Murthy L, Boettgerirtong H L, Makela S 1996 Uterine expression of vascular endothelial growth factor is increased by estradiol and tamoxifen. Cancer Res 56: 3954–3960

Ismail S M 1994 Pathology of endometrium treated with tamoxifen. J Clin Pathol 47: 827–833

Ismail S M, Maulik T G 1997 Tamoxifen-associated postmenopausal endometriosis. Histopathology 30: 187–191

Jackson R L, Dockerty M B 1957 The Stein Leventhal syndrome: analysis of 43 cases with special reference to association with endometrial carcinoma. Am J Obstet Gynecol 73: 161–173

Jordan V C, Fritz N F, Langan-Fahey S, Thompson M, Tormey D C 1991 Alteration of endocrine parameters in premenopausal women with breast cancer during long-term adjuvant therapy with tamoxifen as the single agent. J Natl Cancer Inst 83: 1488–1491

Jordan V C, Fritz N F, Tormey D C 1987 Endocrine effects of adjuvant chemotherapy and long-term tamoxifen administration on node-positive patients with breast cancer. Cancer Res 47: 624–630

Kang Y, Cortina R, Perry R R 1996 Role of c-myc in tamoxifen-induced apoptosis in estrogen-independent breast cancer cells. J Natl Cancer Inst 88: 279–284

Kedar R P, Bourne T H, Powles T J et al 1994 Effects of tamoxifen on uterus and ovaries of postmenopausal women in a randomised breast cancer prevention trial. Lancet 343: 1318–1321

Kennedy S H, Williams I A, Brodribb J, Barlow D H, Shaw R W 1990 A comparison of nafarelin acetate and danazol in the treatment of endometriosis. Fertil Steril 53: 998-1003

Laatikainen T J, Tomas E I, Voutilainen R J 1995 The expression of insulin-like growth factor and its binding-protein messenger-RNA in the endometrium of postmenopausal patients with breast cancer receiving tamoxifen. Cancer 76: 1406–1410

Lahti E, Guillermo B, Kauppila A, Apaja-Sarkkinen M, Taskinen P J, Laatikainen T 1993 Endometrial changes in postmenopausal breast cancer patients receiving tamoxifen. Obstet Gynecol 81: 660–664

Lahti E, Vuopala S, Kauppila A, Blanco G, Ruokonen A, Laatikainen T 1994 Maturation of vaginal and endometrial epithelium in postmenopausal breast cancer patients receiving long-term tamoxifen. Gynecol Oncol 55: 410–414

Li D, Dragan Y, Jordan V C, Wang M, Pitot H C 1997 Effects of chronic administration of tamoxifen and toremifene on DNA adducts in rat liver, kidney and uterus. Cancer Res 57: 1438–1441

Mack T M, Pike M C, Henderson B E et al 1976 Estrogens and endometrial cancer in a retirement community. N Engl J Med 294: 1262–1267

Magriples U, Naftolin F, Schwartz P E, Carcangiu M L 1993 High-grade endometrial carcinoma in tamoxifen-treated breast cancer patients. J Clin Oncol 11: 485–490

Mansell H, Hertig A T 1955 Granulosa-theca cell tumors and endometrial carcinoma: a study of their relationship and a survey of 80 cases. Obstet Gynecol 6: 385–394

Matta W H M, Shaw R W, Nye M 1989 Long-term follow up of patients with uterine fibroids after treatment with the LHRH agonist buserelin. Br J Obstet Gynaecol 96: 200–206

Matta W H M, Stabile I, Shaw R W, Campbell S 1988 Doppler assessment of uterine blood flow changes in patients with fibroids receiving the gonadotropin-releasing hormone agonist buserelin. Fertil Steril 49: 1083–1085

McDonald T W, Malkasian G D, Gaffey T A 1977 Endometrial cancer associated with feminizing ovarian tumor and polycystic ovarian disease. Obstet Gynecol 49: 654–658

McGonigle K F, Karlan B Y, Barbuto D A, Leuchter R S, Lagasse L D, Judd H L 1994 Development of endometrial cancer in women on estrogen and progestin hormone replacement therapy. Gynecol Oncol 55: 126–132

McGonigle K F, Lantry S A, Odommaryon T L, Chai A, Vasilev S A, Simpson J F 1996 Histopathologic effects of tamoxifen on the uterine epithelium of breast cancer patients – analysis by menopausal status. Cancer Lett 101: 59–66

Michael D, Beer D G, Wilke C W, Miller D E, Glover T W 1997 Frequent deletions of FHIT and FRA3B in Barrett's metaplasia and esophageal adenocarcinomas. Oncogene 15: 1653–1659

Morgan M A, Gincherman Y, Mikuta J J 1994 Endometriosis and tamoxifen therapy. Int J Gynecol Obstet 45: 55–57

Moyer D L, de Lignieres B, Driguez P, Pez J P 1993 Prevention of endometrial hyperplasia by progesterone during long-term estradiol replacement: influence of bleeding pattern and secretory changes. Fertil Steril 59: 992–997

Neven P, De Muylder X, Van Belle Y, Vanderick G, De Muylder E 1989 Tamoxifen and the uterus and endometrium. Lancet i: 375.

Neven P, De Muylder X, Van Belle Y, Vanderick G, De Muylder E 1990 Hysteroscopic follow-up during tamoxifen treatment. Eur J Obstet Gynecol Reprod Biol 35: 235–238

Noguchi S, Motomura K, Inaji H, Imaoka S, Koyama H 1993 Downregulation of trans-forming growth-factor-alpha by tamoxifen in human breast cancer. Cancer 72: 131–136

Nuovo M A, Nuovo G J, McCaffrey R M, Levine R U, Barron B, Winkler B 1989 Endometrial polyps in postmenopausal patients receiving tamoxifen. Int J Gynecol Pathol 8: 125–131

Obinata A, Akimoto Y, Kawamata T, Hirano H 1994, Induction of mucous metaplasia in chick embryonic skin by retinol-pretreated embryonic chick or quail dermal fibroblasts through cell-cell interaction – correlation of a transient increase in retinoic acid receptor-beta messenger-RNA in retinol-treated dermal fibroblasts with their competence to induce dermal mucous metaplasia. Dev Growth Different 36: 579–587

Paganini-Hill A, Ross R K, Henderson B E 1989 Endometrial cancer and patterns of oestrogen replacement therapy: Br J Cancer 59: 445–447

Paterson M E L, Wade-Evans T, Sturdee D W. Thom M H, Studd J W W 1980 Endometrial disease after treatment with oestrogens and progestogens in the climacteric. BMJ 280: 822–824

Patterson J S 1981 Clinical aspects and development of antioestrogen therapy: a review of the endocrine effects of tamoxifen in animals and man. J Endocrinol 89: 67P–75P

Perry R R, Kang Y, Greaves B 1995 Effects of tamoxifen on growth and apoptosis of estrogen-dependent and independent human breast cancer cells. Ann Surg Oncol 2: 238–245

Persson I, Adami H O, Bergkvist L et al 1989 Risk of endometrial cancer after treatment with oestrogens alone or in conjunction with progestogens: results of a prospective study. BMJ 298: 147–151

Peterson W F, Novak E R 1956 Endometrial polyps. Obstet Gynecol 8: 40–49

Piegsa K, Calder A, Davis J A, McKay-Hart D, Wells M, Bryden C 1997 Endometrial status in post-menopausal women on long-term continuous hormone replacement therapy (Kliofem). A comparative study of endometrial biopsy, outpatient hysteroscopy and transvaginal ultrasound. Eur J Obstet Gynecol Reprod Biol 72: 175–180

Pike M C, Peters R K, Cozen W et al 1997 Estrogen-progestin replacement therapy and endometrial cancer. J Natl Cancer Inst 89: 1110–1116

Robboy S J, Bradley R 1979 Changing trends and prognostic features in endometrial cancer associated with exogenous estrogen therapy. Obstet Gynecol 54: 269–277

Rubin G L, Peterson H B, Lee N C, Maes E F, Wingo P A, Becker S 1990 Estrogen replacement therapy and the risk of endometrial cancer: remaining controversies. Am J Obstet Gynecol 162: 148–154

Rutqvist L E, Johansson H, Signomklao T, Johansson U, Fornander T, Wilking N 1995 Adjuvant tamoxifen therapy for early stage breast cancer and second primary malignancies. J Natl Cancer Inst 87: 645–651

Schally A V 1978 Aspects of hypothalamic regulation of the pituitary gland: its implications for the control of reproductive processes. Science 202: 18–28

Schriock E D 1989 GnRH agonists. Clin Obstet Gynecol 32: 550–563

Schwartzbaum J A, Hulka B S, Fowler W C, Kaufman D G Hoberman D 1987 The influence of exogenous estrogen use on survival after diagnosis of endometrial cancer. Am J Epidemiol 126: 851–860

Shapiro S, Kaufman D W, Sloane D et al 1980; Recent and past use of conjugated estrogens in relation to adenocarcinoma of the endometrium. N Engl J Med 303: 485–489

Shapiro S, Kelly J P, Rosenberg L et al 1985 Risk of localized and widespread endometrial cancer in relation to recent and discontinued use of conjugated estrogens. New Engl J Med 313: 969–972

Sherman B M, Chapler F K, Crickard K, Wycoff D 1979 Endocrine consequences of continuous antiestrogen therapy with tamoxifen in premenopausal women. J Clin Invest 64: 398–404

Shushan A, Peretz T, Uziely B, Lewin A, Moryosef S 1996 Ovarian cysts in premenopausal and postmenopausal tamoxifen-treated women with breast cancer. Am J Obstet Gynecol 174: 141–144

Silva E G, Tornos C S, Follen-Mitchell M 1994 Malignant neoplasms of the uterine corpus in patients treated for breast carcinoma: the effects of tamoxifen. Int J Gynecol Pathol 13: 248–258

Silverberg S G, Mullen D, Faraci J A et al 1980 Endometrial carcinoma: clinico-pathologic comparison of cases in postmenopausal women receiving and not receiving exogenous estrogens. Cancer 45: 3018–3026

Smith D C, Prentice R, Thompson D J et al 1975 Association of exogenous estrogen and endometrial carcinoma. N Engl J Med 293: 1164–1167

Song J B, Standley P R, Zhang F et al 1996 Tamoxifen (estrogen antagonist) inhibits voltage-gated calcium current and contractility in vascular smooth muscle from rats. J Pharmacol Exp Ther 277:1444-53

Spechler S J, Goyal R K 1986 Barrett's oesophagus. N Engl J Med 315: 362–371

Spengler R F, Clarke R A, Woolever C A, Newman A M, Osborn R W 1981 Exogenous estrogens and endometrial cancer; a case control study and assessment of potential biases. Am J Epidemiol 114: 497–506

Stemmermann G N 1994 Intestinal metaplasia of stomach – a status report. Cancer 74: 556–564

Stjernquist M 1997 Treatment of uterine fibroids with GnRH-analogues prior to hysterectomy. Acta Obstet Gynecol Scand 76 (Suppl 164): 94–97

Tahara E, Kuniyasu H, Yasui W, Yokozaki H 1994 Gene alterations in intestinal metaplasia and gastric cancer. Eur J Gastroenterol Hepatol 6: S97–S102

The Writing Group for the PEPI Trial 1996 Effects of hormone replacement therapy on endometrial histology in postmenopausal women. The Postmenopausal Estrogen/Progestin Interventions (PEPI) Trial. JAMA 275: 370–375

Upadhyaya N B, Doody M C, Googe P B 1990 Histopathological changes in leiomyomata treated with leuprolide acetate. Fertil Steril 54: 811–814

Van Leeuwen F E, Benraadt J, Coebergh J W W et al 1994 Risk of endometrial cancer after tamoxifen treatment of breast cancer. Lancet 343: 448–452

Venturini P L, Fasce V, Anserini P, Costantini S, Cucuccio S, de Cecco L 1990 Treatment of endometriosis with goserelin depot, a long-acting gonadotropin-releasing hormone agonist analogue: endocrine and clinical results. Fertil Steril 54: 1021–1027

Voigt L F, Weiss N S, Chu J, Daling J R, McKnight B, Van Belle G 1991 Progestagen supplementation of exogenous oestrogens and risk of endometrial cancer. Lancet 338: 274–277

Weiss N S, Szekely D R, Austin D F 1976 Increasing incidence of endometrial cancer in the United States. N Engl J Med 294: 1259–1262

West C P, Baird D T 1987 Suppression of ovarian activity by Zoladex depot (ICI 118630), a long acting LHRH analogue. Clin Endocrinol 26: 213–220

West C P, Lumsden M A, Lawson S, Williamson J, Baird D T 1987 Shrinkage of uterine fibroids during therapy with Zoladex (ICI 118630): a luteinizing hormone releasing hormone agonist administered as a monthly subcutaneous depot. Fertil Steril 48: 45–51

White I N H, de Matteis F, Davies A et al 1992 Genotoxic potential of tamoxifen and analogues in female Fischer F344/n rats and C57BL/6 mice and in human MCL-5 cells. Carcinogenesis 13: 2197–2203

Whitehead M I, Fraser D 1987 The effects of estrogens and progestogens on the endometrium. Modern approach to treatment. Obstet Gynecol Clin North Am 14: 299–320

Whitehead M I, Hillard T C, Crook D 1990 The role and use of progestogens. Obstet Gynecol 75: 59S–76S

Whitehead M I, King R J B, McQueen J, Campbell S 1979 Endometrial histology and biochemistry in climacteric women during oestrogen and progestogen therapy. J R Soc Med 72: 322–327

Whitehead M I, Townsend P T, Pryse-Davies J et al 1982 Actions of progestins on the morphology and biochemistry of the endometrium of postmenopausal women receiving low-dose estrogen therapy. Am J Obstet Gynecol 142: 791–795

Williams G M, Iatropoulos M J, Djordjevic M V, Kaltenberg O P 1993 The triphenylethylene drug tamoxifen is a strong liver carcinogen in the rat. Carcinogenesis 14: 315–317

Williamson K, Robertson J F R, Ellis I O, Elston C W, Nicholson R I, Blamey R W 1988 Effect of LHRH agonist Zoladex on ovarian histology. Br J Surg 75: 595–596

Woodruff J D, Pickar J H, for The Menopause Study Group 1994 Incidence of endometrial hyperplasia in postmenopausal women taking conjugated estrogens (Premarin) with medroxyprogesterone acetate or conjugated estrogens alone. Am J Obstet Gynecol 170: 1213–1223

Yager J D, Roebuck B D, Paluscyk T L, Memoli V A 1986 Effects of ethinyl estradiol and tamoxifen on liver DNA turnover and new synthesis and appearance of gamma glutamyl transpeptidase positive foci in female rats. Carcinogenesis 7: 2007–2014

Ziel H K, Finkle W D 1975 Increased use of endometrial carcinoma among users of conjugated estrogens. N Engl J Med 293: 1167–1170

Drug-induced changes in the female genital tract

Amanda Herbert   Ian D. Buley   Robert P. Hasserjian &
Thomas Krausz   David MacVicar   Stephen R.D. Johnston

Cytopathology of metastatic neoplasia

Some organs, such as the lungs and the lymph nodes, are more commonly affected by metastases than by primary neoplasia and so knowledge of the advances made in the diagnostic cytopathology of metastatic neoplasia is important. Advances have come from a better characterisation of the cytological features of metastases, improved imaging techniques which permit specimens to be taken with greater precision and ease, and recognition of the molecular changes in metastatic cells that have a bearing on better patient management.

SECTION i

Amanda Herbert

Cytology of metastatic neoplasia in the lung

The lung is a common site for metastasis in disseminated malignancy to the extent that it is more often involved by metastasis than by primary cancer (Johnson & Elson 1991). Cytological diagnosis of metastatic cancer is less commonly used, but may be important to exclude a second primary, decide the origin of metastasis in patients with multiple primaries,or exclude benign pulmonary lesions mimicking metastasis (Sterrett et al 1995). Metastases are more likely to be seen in brushings or sputum if the bronchial epithelium is infiltrated but a wider range of metastases is accessible with fine needle aspiration cytology (FNAC). Breast and colorectal carcinomas are probably the most frequent lung metastases seen in practice but many other tumours have a predeliction to metastasise to lung. These include prostatic, renal, bladder and head and neck carcinomas as well as melanoma, lymphoma, testicular

Dr A. Herbert, Histopathology Department, North Wing, St Thomas' Hospital, London SE1 7EH, UK

Table 6i.1 Patterns of metastasis in lung

Multiple lesions	
Cannon-ball	Colorectal and renal carcinoma, melanoma, and sarcoma
Miliary	Renal and ovarian carcinoma, melanoma, and medullary carcinoma of thyroid
Diffuse parenchymal infiltration	
Lymphangitic	Lung and breast carcinoma, lymphoma
Intravascular	GI tract and liver carcinoma, choriocarcinoma
Lepidic	Well differentiated adenocarcinoma of prostate and pancreas
Lesions mimicking lung cancer (excluding BACC)	
Solitary	Renal and colorectal carcinoma, melanoma, and sarcoma
Endobronchial	Renal and colorectal carcinoma, and sarcoma

tumours and sarcomas. It is equally important to recognize that unusual tumours occasionally arise as primaries in the lung, such as lymphoma, melanoma, sarcoma and germ cell tumours. The diagnosis of metastasis can usually be established by a combination of the cytological appearance, clinical history and pattern of metastasis. Immunocytochemistry may be helpful, but requires cell blocks or spare slides to be prepared at the time the aspirate is taken. A small panel of antibodies may be needed because of the lack of specificity of many individual antibodies (Colby et al 1995).

As with any cytological diagnosis, essential information about the gross appearances of the tumour may be discovered from the radiology. Different types of primary extrapulmonary tumours have different patterns of spread in the lung (Table 6i.1).

PATTERNS OF SPREAD OF DISSEMINATED MALIGNANCY IN THE LUNG

MULTIPLE LESIONS

Metastatic colorectal and renal cell carcinoma, melanoma and sarcoma typically present with multiple round 'cannon ball' lesions. A miliary pattern of spread may be seen in melanoma and renal cell carcinoma and occasionally in ovarian carcinoma and medullary carcinoma of thyroid (Colby et al 1995). In a patient with a known primary, these radiological appearances may be diagnostic and usually will not require histological or cytological confirmation. However, it may be necessary to identify the site of origin in a patient with multiple primary tumours, and FNAC has made a wider spectrum of metastases available for cytological confirmation.

DIFFUSE PARENCHYMAL INFILTRATION

Diffuse infiltration may be seen in disseminated tumours with a 'lymphangitis carcinomatosa' intravascular or lepidic pattern of growth. Lymphangitic spread is most common with breast, lung and gastro-intestinal carcinomas but may also be seen in disseminated lymphoma. Metastatic tumour embolisation is most often seen with adenocarcinoma, particularly from breast, stomach and pancreas, but is also typical of choriocarcinoma (Colby et al 1995). Lymph-angitic and intravascular metastases are unlikely to be seen in cytological specimens though the airways may be involved eventually, when malignant cells may be seen in sputum cytology.

In diffuse parenchymal metastasis, cytological diagnosis is most likely be helpful in tumours with a lepidic pattern of spread. With this pattern of spread (which describes the 'butterfly-wing' pattern of shadowing seen on chest X-rays), well differentiated adenocarcinoma lines the alveolar walls and is readily exfoliated in sputum or bronchiolar-alveolar lavage (BAL) specimens. This is the pattern of spread of bronchio-alveolar cell carcinoma (BACC), from which metastases may be difficult if not impossible to distinguish cytologically. A lepidic pattern of growth may be seen with any well differentiated adeno-carcinoma, particularly pancreatic and prostatic carcinoma (Sterrett et al 1995), and is also described in colorectal carcinoma (Colby et al 1995). Although three-dimensional papillary clusters of cells are typical of well differentiated adenocarcinoma in sputum and BAL specimens, these tumours presents a surprisingly different appearance in FNAC: the uniform population of cells tends to consist of flat monolayered sheets of cells with inconspicuous papillary clusters (Sterrett et al 1995). With either cell pattern, it may be difficult to be certain that the cell population is malignant. Diagnosis depends on cellularity, a monotonous cell pattern and absence of cilia rather than nuclear atypia. Immunocytochemistry is potentially helpful in distinguishing BACC from metastasis, though antibodies against surfactant apoprotein and Clara cell protein are not yet widely available. They are expressed in about 40% of BACC and other pulmonary adenocarcinomas and are rarely expressed in other forms of malignancy (Linnoila et al 1992).

METASTASES MIMICKING LUNG CANCER

Solitary pulmonary metastases, which are less common than multiple metastases, are most likely to mimic primary lung cancer and are sometimes investigated in the absence of information about a previous tumour. Cytological diagnostic procedures will be the same as for primary lung cancer: bronchoscopic specimens for central lesions and FNAC for peripheral ones. Solitary metastases may be seen in any of the carcinomas which spread to the lung as well as in melanoma, testicular tumours, sarcoma and lymphoma. Some of these metastases may be recognised cytologically, as described below, but the clinical history and previous histology and cytology will be needed to establish a diagnosis. It is important to exclude a second primary, particularly in patients with previously resected primary tumours of head and neck or bladder, which are related to cigarette smoking. A second primary in the lung is likely, especially when the original tumour was well differentiated and there was no evidence of local recurrence after treatment. Histologically, these tumours may be similar to lung cancer but head and neck squamous cell carcinomas tend to be better differentiated and a stratified papillary pattern occasionally may be recognised cytologically in metastatic bladder cancer. Metastasis from carcinoma of the uterine cervix is unusual now that there is a comprehensive screening programme. Cervical cancer typically occurs in a younger age group than lung cancer and there is likely to be clinical evidence

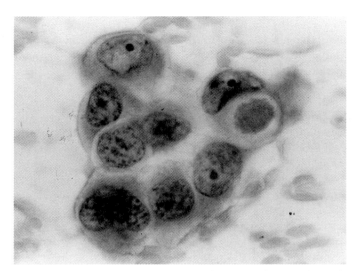

Fig. 6i.1 Cohesive adenocarcinoma cells with uniform nuclei and an intracytoplasmic mucin vacuole. Bronchial brushing from a woman aged 65 years with a history of breast carcinoma. Papanicolaou stain.

of local spread. It is equally important to exclude a benign pulmonary lesion, since it is easy to assume that a metastasis is present in a patient with previous malignancy (Cahan et al 1978, Askin 1993). As with almost all cytological diagnoses, the first objective is to establish whether or not there is evidence of malignancy.

Particularly with solitary lesions, endobronchial metastasis most closely mimics lung cancer and may produce similar symptoms, radiological findings and bronchoscopic appearances (Colby et al 1995). Endobronchial metastasis is well recognized in renal cell and colorectal carcinoma and also occurs in other forms of carcinoma and sarcoma. This pattern of spread is the most likely to produce malignant cells in sputum or bronchial brushings. Any solitary, multiple or diffuse metastatic process may eventually infiltrate bronchial mucosa and up to half of all metastases are found to have done so at autopsy (Colby et al 1995).

CYTOLOGICAL PATTERNS SUGGESTING METASTASIS

Unless there is a known clinical history, the cytological diagnosis of metastatic malignancy depends on a high index of suspicion when malignant cells do not conform to the usual spectrum of appearances in lung cancer. Final diagnosis always requires clinicopathological correlation and sometimes requires ancillary tests such as immunocytochemistry. Common types of metastatic malignancy sometimes may be recognizable by their cytological appearances, but this is less likely with poorly differentiated tumours.

BREAST CARCINOMA

Breast cancer is one of the commonest metastases to mimic lung cancer. It is seen in cytological specimens when diffuse infiltration involves airways, usually as a

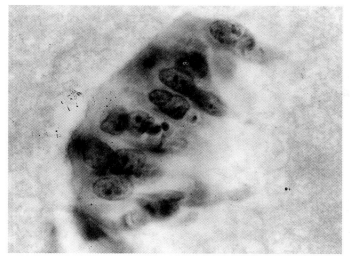

Fig. 6i.2 Cohesive group of malignant columnar cells with palisaded oval nuclei and a flat apical cytoplasmic border. Bronchial brushing from man aged 80 years with a history of colorectal carcinoma resected 12 years before. Papanicolaou stain.

terminal event. In the better differentiated tumours breast carcinoma may be recognized by its cohesive clusters of small glandular cells, usually with relatively uniform nuclei and a smooth border to the cell group (Johnson & Elson 1991). The cell groups in sputum and BAL may be similar to those seen in pleural fluids. Nuclei may be moulded but have a more regular chromatin pattern and better defined nuclear membranes than oat cell carcinoma cells. The cells may be difficult to distinguish from exfoliated bronchiolar cells as well as from well differentiated pulmonary adenocarcinoma; the presence of intracytoplasmic mucin vacuoles favours a breast origin (Fig. 6i.1).

Poorly differentiated tumours may be difficult to distinguish from lung cancer and immunocytochemistry using a panel of antibodies may be helpful. Oestrogen receptor protein, S100 and gross cystic disease fluid protein are more likely to be expressed by breast carcinoma and carcino-embryonic antigen (CEA) is more likely to be expressed by lung cancer (Raab et al 1993).

COLORECTAL CARCINOMA

Colorectal carcinoma may produce multiple lesions and mimic primary lung cancer. The diagnosis may be suggested by palisaded columnar cells with oval nuclei and apical mucin secretion (Sterrett et al 1995). The cytoplasmic border of the cell group tends to be linear (Fig. 6i.2). Typically these well differentiated cell groups are associated with necrosis as these lesions may cavitate, which is unusual in primary lung adenocarcinoma.

RENAL CELL CARCINOMA

Renal cell carcinoma has a predeliction for infiltrating mucosal surfaces and may produce solitary or multiple metastases. The diagnosis is suggested by pleomorphic malignant cells with round eccentric nuclei, prominent nucleoli

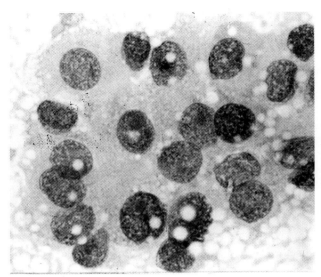

Fig. 6i.3 Malignant cells with large pleomorphic nuclei and copious vacuolated cytoplasm. FNAC from man aged 71 years with a history of renal cell carcinoma resected 10 years before. May-Grünwald-Giemsa stain.

and abundant finely vacuolated cytoplasm (Fig. 6i.3). Eosinophilic basement membrane material and fibrovascular papillary cores may also suggest this diagnosis (Trott 1995).

MELANOMA

Melanoma is usually recognizable, even without a clinical history, and is most often seen as multiple metastases. It may present a variety of cytological patterns, occasionally closely mimicking carcinoma (Sterrett et al 1995). It is usually characterized by a free cell pattern, pleomorphic nuclei with prominent nucleoli, the presence of double nuclei, and spindle cell forms. Melanin may or not be seen as irregular blue/green granules on Romanowsky stains or brown with Papanicolaou stain. Melanoma may very rarely present as a primary lung tumour but may be diagnosed only after an extensive search for a primary tumour in a more usual site (Colby et al 1995).

LYMPHOMA

Non-Hodgkin's lymphoma (NHL) is usually recognisable by its cytological appearance, even if the type cannot be ascertained. Characteristically, the pattern of spread follows lymphatic pathways, but solitary lesions are occasionally seen. Disseminated NHL in the lung is most likely to be high grade follicle centre lymphoma which has a characteristic cytological appearance: the nucleo/cytoplasmic ratio is usually high, the cytoplasm forms a narrow blue rim on Romanowsky stains and prominent nucleoli often have a punched out appearance or may be attached to the nuclear membrane in alcohol fixed preparations. Hodgkin's disease may spread to the lung and should be considered when there are isolated malignant cells with lobulated

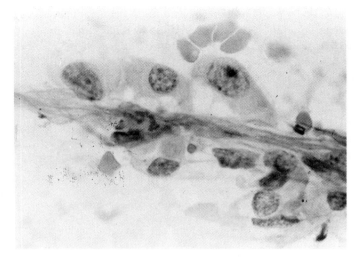

Fig. 6i.4 Pleomorphic cells with pale nuclei and spindle cell cytoplasm loosely attached to a capillary. Bronchial brushings from a man aged 68 years. Direct enquiry elicited a history of resection of angiosarcoma 18 months earlier. Papanicolaou stain.

nuclei with macronucleoli, often associated with eosinophils, histiocytes and lymphocytes. Disseminated lymphoma must be distinguished from primary mucosa-associated lymphoid tissue (MALT) lymphoma, but the latter is most commonly low grade and characterized by monotonous lymphoid cells closely resembling mature lymphocytes (Colby et al 1995).

SARCOMA

Sarcomas frequently spread to lung and may produce malignant cells in brushings, sputum and FNAC (Sterrett et al 1995). The diagnosis is suggested by pleomorphic malignant cells with spindle cell forms, giant cells and vascular cell sheets (Kim et al 1966). The case illustrated in Figure 6i.4 is an FNAC from a bronchial brushing; direct enquiry because of the unusual cytology revealed a recent history of angiosarcoma of the scalp. The diagnosis

Points of best practice

- Cytological diagnosis of disseminated malignancy in the lung is most likely to be achieved if there is a high degree of suspicion when cytological changes are unlike those usually seen in lung cancer.

- Diagnosis may be confirmed by the clinical history, but care must be taken to exclude a second primary or a benign lesion in the lung.

- Clinical probability, radiological pattern of spread, comparison with previous histology or cytology and the occasional use of immunocytochemistry help in the final diagnosis.

can usually be established by cytology correlated with the clinical history, but spindle cell variants of squamous cell lung carcinoma, renal carcinoma and melanoma should be considered in the differential diagnosis. If in doubt, a panel of antibodies may be needed to make the distinction (Colby et al 1995). Not all sarcomas in the lung are metastatic and not all metastases are clinically malignant: for example so called 'benign metastasising leiomyoma' is often hormone responsive and may not be a true neoplasm (Colby et al 1995). Cytological reports of soft tissue lesions should be cautious and must take account of the wide differential diagnosis of such lesions.

References

Askin F B 1993 Something old? Something new? Second primary or pulmonary metastasis in the patient with known extrathoracic carcinoma. Am J Clin Pathol 100: 4–5

Cahan W G, Shah J P, Castro E B 1978 Benign solitary lung lesions in patients with cancer. Ann Surg 187: 241–244

Colby T V, Koss M N, Travis W D 1995 Tumors metastatic to the lung. In: Atlas of tumor pathology: tumours of the lower respiratory tract. Washington DC: Armed Forces Institute of Pathology, 513–546

Johnston W W, Elson C E 1991 Respiratory tract. In: Bibbo M (ed) Comprehensive cytopathology. Philadelphia, Saunders, 325–401

Kim G, Naylor B, Han I H 1986 Fine needle aspiration cytology of sarcomas metastatic to the lung. Acta Cytol 30: 688–694

Linnoila R I, Jensen S M, Steinberg S M et al 1992 Peripheral airway cell marker expression in non-small cell lung carcinoma. Am J Clin Pathol 97: 233–243

Raab S S, Berg L C, Swanson P E, Wick M R 1993 Adenocarcinoma in the lung in patients with breast cancer: a prospective analysis of the discriminatory value of immunohistology. Am J Clin Pathol 100: 27–35

Sterrett G, Frost F, Whitaker D 1995 Tumours of lung and mediastinum. In: Gray W (ed) Diagnostic cytopathology. New York, Churchill Livingstone,69–127

Trott P A 1995 The kidney and retroperitoneal tissues. In: Gray W (ed Diagnostic cytopathology. New York: Churchill Livingstone, 437–454

SECTION ii

Ian D. Buley

Cytology of metastatic neoplasms in lymph nodes

Fine needle aspiration (FNA) is an important tool in making a rapid, relatively non-invasive and cost effective initial diagnosis in lymph nodes containing metastatic malignancy (Orell et al 1992). In known malignancy it is valuable for staging and in monitoring for relapse or the effects of therapy. Imprint cytology can be a useful adjunct to frozen section examination of lymph nodes.

FNA of lymph nodes has pitfalls for the unwary. Particularly in neck masses, the aspirate may incorrectly be identified as being from a lymph node and may even contain lymphoid cells, allowing scope for erroneous diagnosis.

Dr I.D. Buley Department of Cellular Pathology, John Radcliffe Hospital, Headington, Oxford OX3 9DU, UK

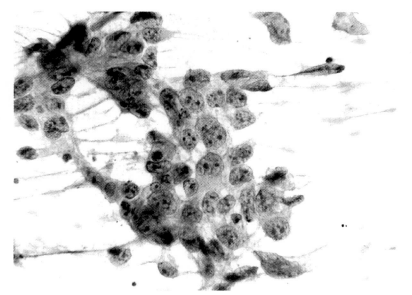

Fig. 6ii.1 This is an FNA of a cervical lymph node from a male aged 41 years. Only after the suggestion of a germ-cell tumour was the history of a painful and slightly swollen left testicle elicited. Subsequent histology confirmed the diagnosis of seminoma, an example of the importance of accurately characterising the nature of this disseminated malignancy which is highly responsive to radiotherapy and chemotherapy.

Pleomorphic adenoma of the parotid can clinically resemble a submandibular lymph node and the unwary, if mislead by the clinical description, may make a misdiagnosis of metastatic mucinous carcinoma particularly where there is the atypia which may be seen in the epithelium of a this adenoma. An aspirate from a Warthin's tumour could lead to misinterpretation of the combination of lymphoid cells, necrotic material and epithelial cells. Equally, peripheral nodules of thyroid tissue involved by autoimmune thyroiditis, with the combination of reactive lymphoid cells and the bizarre cytology seen in Hürthle cells, can be misdiagnosed as metastatic malignancy. The problem of distinguishing degenerative atypia in a branchial cyst aspirate from a necrotic well differentiated squamous carcinoma metastasis is also well known. The risk of misdiagnosis is compounded by poor clinical information and by poor quality specimens.

In true lymph node aspirates, extrinsic cells need not be malignant. They may be cells arising from adjacent normal tissues, non-neoplastic epithelial inclusions (particularly in axillary or parotid lymph nodes) and even benign melanocytic inclusions.

Where there is genuine malignancy broad categorisation into subtype is generally straightforward using conventional cytological criteria. Immuno-cytochemistry is a useful supplementary technique (Buley 1993) enabling refinement of subtyping, particularly in anaplastic malignancy. Consideration needs to be given to specimen collection and preparation to ensure spare material is available: immunocytochemistry on cytological material must be interpreted with caution due to the frequent lack of adequate cytological control material.

The diagnosis of metastatic melanoma may pose particular problems. The cytological appearances in melanoma are very variable. In one study (Nasiell et al 1991) of 81 needle aspirates from metastatic melanoma, 47% were classified as classical in type, 22% as carcinoma-like, 14% as spindle cell type, 6% as lymphoma-like, 6% as undifferentiated, 3% as myxoid and 2% as clear cell type. Overall, melanin pigment was seen in less than two-thirds of the cases; the carcinoma-like, spindle cell and lymphoma-like variants especially were amelanotic in the cytological material available. Immunocytochemistry was necessary to diagnose conclusively more than half of cases.

Increasingly, metastatic malignancy is actively managed and it is important to identify the hormonally responsive, chemotherapy and radiotherapy sensitive tumours (see Fig. 6ii.1). This necessitates cytological expertise, good clinical information and the recognition of the value of biopsy in difficult cases.

References

Buley I D 1993 Update of special techniques in routine cytopathology. J Clin Pathol 46: 881–885

Nasiell K, Tani I, Skoog L 1991 Fine needle aspiration cytology and immunocytochemistry of metastatic melanoma. Cytology 2: 137–147

Orell S R, Sterrett G F, Walters M N-I, Whitaker D 1992 Lymph nodes. Manual and Atlas of Fine Needle Aspiration Cytology. Edinburgh: Churchill Livingstone, 63–95

SECTION iii

Robert P. Hasserjian Thomas Krausz

Diagnosis of primary and secondary lymphomatous effusions

Lymphomatous effusions may be secondary, occurring in patients with nodal lymphoma, or primary, initially occurring and often remaining as an effusion-based malignant lymphoid proliferation (Table 6iii.1). Secondary lymphomatous effusions have been discussed in many texts and we will discuss them only briefly below. We review the diagnosis and pathogenesis of primary effusion lymphomas, including recently described entities.

SECONDARY LYMPHOMATOUS EFFUSIONS

The great majority of lymphomatous effusions are secondary. These effusions can occur in non-Hodgkin's T and B cell lymphomas of various types and grades. They can also occur in Hodgkin's disease, where cytological diagnosis

Dr R.P. Hasserjian, Department of Histopathology, Imperial College School of Medicine, Hammersmith Hospital Campus, Du Cane Road, London W12 0NN, UK
Professor T. Krausz, Department of Histopathology, Imperial College School of Medicine, Hammersmith Hospital Campus, Du Cane Road, London W12 0NN, London, UK

Table 6iii.1 Lymphomas of serous cavities

Secondary
  Non-Hodgkin's lymphoma (T or B)
  Plasmacytoma/multiple myeloma
  Hodgkin's disease
Primary
  Non-Hodgkin's lymphoma (T or B), Burkitt's lymphoma*
  Primary effusion lymphoma*
  Pyothorax-associated lymphoma

*In immunosuppressed patients such as those who are HIV positive.

is difficult. Secondary lymphomatous effusions are usually a late manifestation of systemic lymphoma and often occur in pleural fluid in the setting of a mediastinal or pulmonary mass.

It is important to note that non-lymphomatous reactive effusions may also occur in lymphoma patients. The cytological features of the effusion cells may allow distinction between lymphomatous and reactive lymphocytic effusions (Fig. 6iii.1A); knowing the histological type of the tissue-based lymphoma is important in this regard. Other helpful features include frequent single cell necrosis and the chylous appearance of the fluid in lymphomatous effusions. In difficult cases (especially low-grade lymphomas), immunophenotypic analysis and the demonstration of clonality by immunoperoxidase or gene re-arrangement studies may be essential (Fig 6iii.1B,C).

PRIMARY LYMPHOMATOUS EFFUSIONS

Lymphomas presenting with primary pleural effusions as their initial mani-festation are rare. The most common reported histological types are diffuse large cell lymphoma, follicular lymphoma and small lymphocytic lymphoma; almost

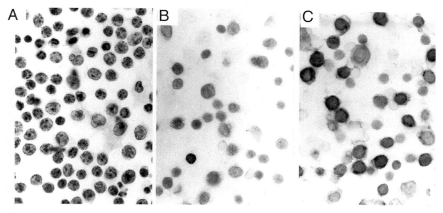

Fig. 6iii.1 Secondary follicular lymphoma in ascitic fluid. Cytospin preparations from ascitic fluid (A, Papanicolaou stain). Numerous small and intermediate sized lymphoid cells are mixed with reactive mesothelial cells. Immunoperoxidase studies on the cytospin preparations showed that nearly all of the lymphoid cells were positive for CD20. The cells were negative for kappa light chain (B) and positive for lambda light chain (C), demonstrating clonality.

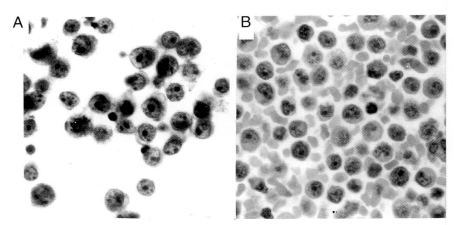

Fig. 6iii.2 Primary effusion lymphoma (PEL). (A, Papanicolaou stain). Cytospin preparations from pleural fluid. (B, H & E stain). Cell-block preparation from pleural fluid. Abundant large immunoblast-like cells with vesicular nuclei, prominent central nucleoli and a moderate amount of cytoplasm are present. (Courtesy of Dr Daniel Jones, Brigham & Women's Hospital, Boston, MA, USA.)

all reported cases are B cell phenotype. Pleural thickening is often present and the diagnosis is usually made on pleural biopsy rather than cytology (Celikoglu et al 1992). Many of these cases have mediastinal lymphadenopathy or a pulmonary mass on radiological studies; classification as primary pleural lymphomas or secondary lymphomas presenting as pleural effusions is, therefore, difficult. However, two primary effusion-based lymphomas appear to represent distinct clinicopathological entities. The cytological features of these effusion-based lymphomas overlap with other non-Hodgkin's lymphomas. Diagnosis of these distinct primary effusion lymphomas may be made on cytological features and ancillary studies in combination with the clinical context. Recent studies have shed light on their pathogenesis.

PRIMARY EFFUSION LYMPHOMA

Primary effusion lymphoma (PEL) is a body cavity based non-Hodgkin's lymphoma that occurs almost exclusively in HIV positive patients, usually in homosexual men (Ansari et al 1996, Jones et al 1996, Nador et al 1996). These tumours present as pleural, pericardial or peritoneal effusions in the absence of solid tumour masses; on biopsy, lymphomatous infiltration of serous membranes may be seen (Table 6iii.2). Throughout their courses these tumours usually remain confined to body cavities. This curious tendency of growth limited to body cavities is intriguing and requires further studies to elucidate its aetiology. Morphologically, the tumour cells have features encompassing large cell, immunoblastic, and anaplastic morphology. The tumour cells are large and pleomorphic with vesicular nuclei, one to several prominent nucleoli and abundant amphophilic or basophilic cytoplasm (Figs 6iii.2). Bizarre cells with irregular nuclei and cells resembling Reed-Sternberg cells are also frequently present. The lymphoma cells show immunoglobulin heavy and light chain gene re-arrangements by molecular methods, but usually fail to

	PEL	PAL	Immuno-suppressed non-PEL
Cytology	Immunoblastic/ anaplastic	Immunoblastic/ anaplastic	Burkitt's
HIV status	Positive	Negative	Often positive
Mass lesion	Absent	Usually present	Absent
Markers			
CD45	+	+	+
pan-B	–	+	–/+
pan-T	–	–	–
CD30	+/–	–	+/–
EMA	+/–	–	+/–
Immunoglobulin genes	Re-arranged	Re-arranged	Re-arranged
T cell receptor genes	Germline	Germline	Germline
EBV	Usually present	Present	Present
HHV-8	Always present	Absent	Absent
c-myc gene	Germline	Germline	Re-arranged

express pan-B cell markers. The cells often co-express CD30, CD38, and EMA and so immunophenotypically resemble activated terminally differentiated B cells. Clonal Epstein-Barr virus (EBV) sequences are detected in almost all cases; unlike Burkitt's lymphoma and most other AIDS-related lymphomas, however, the c-myc gene has been found to be in germline configuration (Karcher et al 1997).

An important characteristic feature of PEL is the presence of human herpes virus 8 (HHV-8, also known as Kaposi's sarcoma-associated herpes virus or KSHV) in the lymphoma cells. HHV-8 viral sequences have been demonstrated by PCR in pleural effusions and this virus has been localised to the tumour cells by *in situ* hybridisation and electron microscopy (Cesarman et al 1995). HHV-8 has also been detected in Kaposi's sarcoma and in multicentric Castleman's disease, both AIDS and non-AIDS associated (Cesarman et al 1997). Many patients who develop PEL have pre-existing Kaposi's sarcoma, and HHV-8 sequence relatedness in both the KS lesions and PEL has been demonstrated in at least one patient. While the role of HHV-8 infection in PEL is not fully understood, production of autocrine factors such as viral IL-6 may contribute to tumour cell proliferation. Interestingly, HHV-8 has also been detected in the neoplastic plasma cells in myelomatous pleural effusions (Tsang et al 1998).

On diagnostic cytology specimens, PEL can be distinguished from secondary body cavity lymphomas by: (i) its almost exclusive involvement of body cavities; (ii) its characteristic pleomorphic morphology; (iii) its 'null-cell' immunophenotype; and (iv) the presence of HHV-8.

In spite of its tendency to remain localised to body cavities, PEL has an extremely poor prognosis, with a median survival of 2–4 months. Causes of death include intractable pleural effusions, respiratory failure, and overwhelming infection.

OTHER PRIMARY EFFUSION LYMPHOMAS IN IMMUNOSUPPRESSED PATIENTS

It is important to note that immunosuppressed patients may develop primary lymphomas in body cavities which are clinicopathologically distinct from PEL. Patients with non-PEL lymphomas presenting in body cavities usually have the morphology of Burkitt's lymphoma rather than immunoblastic lymphoma, are HHV-8 negative and most have have re-arrangements in the *c-myc* gene. These lymphomas are more likely than PEL to disseminate and involve bone marrow.

Recently, cases of PEL occurring in HIV negative patients lacking *c-myc* rearrangements, EBV and HHV8 have also been described (Ichinohasama R et al 1998). The role of other oncogenes and viruses such as hepatitis C in these variant PELs has yet to be elucidated.

PYOTHORAX-ASSOCIATED LYMPHOMA

Pyothorax-associated lymphoma (PAL) was initially observed in Asian patients and has more recently been recognised in Western patients as well. These rare lymphomas occur in the setting of long-standing inflammation of the pleura (Aozasa 1996). The underlying cause of the chronic inflammation is tuberculosis, usually treated with therapeutic pneumothorax. PAL develops after a long latency period of at least 20 years and up to 50 years after the initial pleural injury. Unlike PEL, PAL occurs exclusively in the pleura and usually has an associated pleural or thoracic mass. The incidence does not appear to be increased in immunosuppressed patients.

These neoplasms morphologically resemble PEL, with appearance ranging from immunoblastic to anaplastic and frequent bizarre cells. However, unlike PAL, the tumour cells express pan-B cell markers and do not express the activation marker CD30. EBV viral sequences are detected in most reported cases but HHV-8 positive cases have not been described (Fukayama et al 1993, Martin et al 1994, Molinie et al 1996).

Inflammatory cytokines in long-standing chronic inflammation presumably act in concert with EBV transforming factors in the aetiology of PAL. In particular, IL-6 is produced in some PAL tumour cell lines and appears to enhance their growth in vitro (Kanno et al 1996). As with PEL, autocrine production of IL-6 and/or paracrine production in the setting of chronic inflammation of long duration may contribute to the uncontrolled cell growth in PAL. Like PEL, PAL has a poor prognosis. Most patients die within months of diagnosis, often due to local infiltration of thoracic organs (Molinie et al 1996).

References

Ansari M Q, Dawson D B, Nador R et al 1996 Primary body cavity-based AIDS-related lymphomas. Am J Clin Pathol 105: 221–229

Aozasa K 1996 Pyothorax-associated lymphoma. Int J Hematol 65: 9–16

Celikoglu F, Teirstein A S, Krellenstein D J et al 1992 Pleural effusion in non-Hodgkin's lymphoma. Chest 101: 1357–1360

Cesarman E, Chang Y, Moore P S et al 1995 Kaposi's sarcoma associated herpes virus like DNA sequences in AIDS related body cavity based lymphomas. N Engl J Med 332: 1186–1191

Cesarman E, Knowles D M 1997 Kaposi's sarcoma-associated herpesvirus: a lymphotropic human herpes virus associated with Kaposi's sarcoma, primary effusion lymphoma and multicentric Castleman's disease. Semin Diag Pathol 14: 54–66

Fukayama M, Ibuka T, Hayashi Y et al 1993 Epstein-Barr virus in pyothorax-associated pleural lymphoma. Am J Pathol 143: 1044–1049

Ichinohasama R, Miura I, Kobayashi N et al 1998 Herpes virus type 8-negative primary effusion lyphoma associated with *PAX-5* gene rearrangement and hepatitis C virus. Am J Surg Pathol 22: 1528–1537

Jones D, Weinberg D S, Pinkus G S et al 1996 Cytologic diagnosis of primary serous lymphoma. Am J Clin Pathol 106: 359–364

Kanno H, Yasunaga Y, Iuchi K et al 1996 Interleukin-6-mediated growth enhancement of cell lines derived from pyothorax-associated lymphoma. Lab Invest 75: 167–173

Karcher D S, Alkan S 1997 Human herpes virus-8-associated body cavity-based lymphoma in human immunodeficiency virus-infected patients: a unique B-cell neoplasm. Hum Pathol 28: 801–808

Martin A, Capron F, Liguory-Brunaud M-D et al 1994 Epstein-Barr virus-associated primary malignant lymphomas of the pleural cavity occurring in longstanding pleural chronic inflammation. Hum Pathol 25: 1314–1318

Molinie V, Pouchot J, Navratil E et al 1996 Primary Epstein-Barr virus-related non-Hodgkin's lymphoma of the pleural cavity following long-standing tuberculous empyema. Arch Pathol Lab Med 120: 288–291

Nador R G, Cesarman E, Chadburn A et al 1996 Primary effusion lymphoma: a distinct clinicopathologic entity associated with the Kaposi's sarcoma-associated herpesvirus. Blood 88: 645–656

Tsang P, Flore O, Rafii J et al 1998 Kaposi's sarcoma-associated herpes virus (KSHV/HHV8) in myelomatous effusion. Abstract in the United States and Canadian Academy of Pathology Annual Meeting 1998 141A.

SECTION iv

David MacVicar

New imaging techniques in patients with metastatic neoplasia

Over the past 30 years, medical technology has advanced rapidly but few specialties have experienced such radical change as diagnostic imaging. The mathematical principles of reconstructing the internal composition of a solid object from multiple projections of a thin beam of X-rays through it were worked out in 1917 by the Austrian mathematician Radon. Clinical use of these principles required computing power which was not developed until the late 1960s; this resulted in the introduction of computed tomography (CT) by Hounsfield and Ambrose in 1972. Since that time, the speed and power of CT machines has increased and the space required has reduced. Likewise, the principles of sonography were well understood for many years before computers made ultrasound imaging a clinically viable method. Virtually all recent advances in diagnostic imaging rely to some extent on computers. Magnetic resonance imaging (MRI) is based on a radically different and recently discovered method of generating contrast between body tissues, and advances in isotope imaging have been driven by the development of new radiopharmaceuticals capable of acting as

Dr D MacVicar, Academic Department of Diagnostic Radiology, Royal Marsden NHS Trust, Downs Road, Sutton SM2 5PT, UK

substrates for metabolic mechanisms, thus allowing some demonstration of physiological function.

The capability of modern imaging techniques has led to a drift in clinical practice in oncology. Before the introduction of CT and ultrasound, the diagnosis of metastatic disease was usually made on clinical grounds, sometimes with the assistance of plain radiographs or blood tests. Currently, it is difficult to imagine a diagnosis of metastatic disease being made without the confirmation of at least one computer-based imaging technique and it is, therefore, important for cytopathologists to appreciate the powers and limitations of the common ones.

In the appropriate clinical setting, the radiological diagnosis of metastatic disease rarely poses any problem. Occasionally, atypical imaging features are present, and under such circumstances cytological confirmation may be sought. It is now possible, under imaging control, to place a needle at virtually any site. These minimally invasive techniques are time-consuming and undertaken only if real doubt exists, which should protect cytology and histopathology departments from further increases in workload at least for the time being.

ULTRASOUND

Up-to-date ultrasound equipment is excellent for demonstration of soft tissue lesions in accessible parts of the body. These include the upper abdomen, retroperitoneum, pelvis and the soft tissues of the neck. The chief advantages of ultrasound are its speed and flexibility: solid masses are readily identified and can be approached with a needle under direct vision. Fluid collections in the abdomen, pleural space and pericardium can be aspirated for cytological examination. Its disadvantages are that it has a relatively limited range, lesions deep in the abdomen may be technically difficult to visualise, and pulmonary lesions are inaccessible. However, ultrasound machines continue to develop, giving pictures of astonishing clarity; sophisticated Doppler techniques demonstrate blood flow in large and small vessels and are fuelling research interest into vascularisation of tumours.

COMPUTED TOMOGRAPHY

CT is an ideal screening technique, which makes it the technique of choice in staging asymptomatic patients. The soft tissue contrast available enables all soft tissues, including lung, to be imaged at a single investigation and some information can be gathered about the bones. The technique is versatile and reproducible, and has a high sensitivity for detecting lesions in lymph nodes, liver and other solid abdominal organs, lungs and brain. It is the least technically demanding of methods for guiding biopsy, and generally the most reliable; however, it is relatively time-consuming.

Spiral or helical CT scanning is a recent innovation which requires continuous progress of the patient through the CT gantry while the X-ray tube and detector array spin continually around. This can continue until the heat capacity of the tube is reached. As a result, CT data for the entire body can be acquired in 5–10 min. Computed reformatting of the data can be done at a variety of slice intervals, and in different planes if clinically indicated. In oncology, such subtlety is infrequently required as lumps can usually be detected using axial planes. The chief advantage of spiral CT machines is that they are of relatively recent construction and have high computing capacity, and are, therefore, faster and more reliable.

A further innovation in CT is the electron beam scanner, which functions by fanning an electron beam over a tungsten target, generating an X-ray source without a traditional X-ray tube. They are very expensive.

MAGNETIC RESONANCE IMAGING

MRI first became clinically usable in 1982. The technology is entirely different from CT scanning, though anatomical images may look similar. High power MR scanners rely on a super conducting coil, cooled to close to absolute zero, which induces a powerful magnetic field. The patient is placed within the field; hydrogen ions in the body orientate themselves around the long axis of the magnetic field and oscillate within it, a phenomenon known as precession. In this state, protons are subjected to excitation by a pulse of energy within the radiofrequency range. When allowed to relax between pulses, they emit energy, also within the radiofrequency range, which can be detected by receiving coils and reconstructed into two-dimensional anatomical images. The strength of the returned signal is heavily influenced by physical factors such as the presence of free water in tissues, proximity of biological macromolecules, and contrast agents with paramagnetic or superparamagnetic properties. In addition, the signal information returned can be orientated in any anatomical plane. The variety of pulse sequences and imaging planes is inexhaustible, making MRI the most sensitive and versatile of all imaging techniques. However, the clinical question has to be sharply focused, and the relative lack of easy availability means that MR is not a suitable instrument for routine staging investigations.

The diagnostic accuracy of MR is at its best in detection of bone marrow metastases and in elucidating neurological problems in a patient with cancer. Cord compression, cerebral metastatic disease and meningeal metastatic disease can all be demonstrated using MRI (Fig. 6iv.1). Hepatic metastases are very well visualised by MRI, particularly with the aid of liver-specific contrast agents. Some of the superparamagnetic contrast agents are taken up by macrophages within normal reticulo-endothelial tissue, and it is possible that contrast agents will be developed to discriminate reactive from metastatic causes of lymph node enlargement.

Currently, MRI is not used for detection of pulmonary metastatic disease. However, the capability of MRI is advancing faster than in any other field of imaging, and its uses and indications are subject to constant re-appraisal.

IMAGING WITH RADIOISOTOPES

The principle of cancer-specific imaging in nuclear medicine is to exploit the subtle differences between a cancer cell and a normal cell. A variety of approaches can be used; for example, Technetium-99^M labelled DTPA is an extracellular hydrophilic agent which identifies tumour deposits by a simple diffusion mechanism. Some radiopharmaceuticals depend for their action upon transport protein upregulation in tumours, such as the positron emitter [^{18}F]-fluorodeoxyglucose (^{18}-FDG). ^{123}Iodine labelled meta-iodobenzyl-

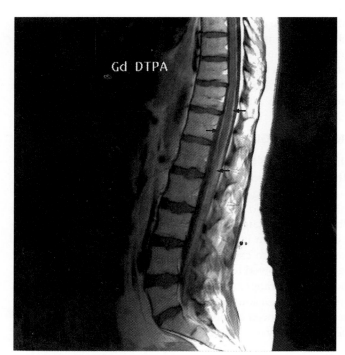

Gd DTPA

Fig. 6iv.1 Metastatic carcinoma of the breast. The patient had mild non-specific headache and backache and a unilateral leg weakness. She was investigated by spinal MR imaging in sagittal plane, using T1-weighted spin-echo sequence following administration of intravenous gadolinium. The scan shows high signal nodularity along the spinal meninges around the conus and cauda equina (arrows). The appearance is typical of seedlings of leptomeningeal metastatic disease from primary breast cancer. The appearance of meningeal disease is similar for most primary tumours.

guanidine (MIBG) attaches to receptors and is stored within cells of the neuroblastoma series. It is also possible to radiolabel antibodies to known tumour-related antigens such as carcino-embryonic antigen.

The principal drawback of nuclear medicine studies is their lack of anatomical detail. However, in the clinical circumstance of a rising tumour marker or a strong suspicion of occult relapse, isotope studies have the advantage that they image the entire body in a single investigation. They can narrow down the area of interest to regions of increased tracer uptake, and the more anatomically precise diagnostic techniques can be concentrated on specific areas, and guide needle biopsy if necessary.

BIOPSY TECHNIQUES

There are very few anatomical sites which are inaccessible to needle biopsy either using cutting needles or cytological aspiration needles. Most radiologists now prefer to use automatic cutting needles rather than manually held Trucut needles. A variety of cytological aspiration needles are also available. The needle used varies with the site of tumour and the preference of the operator. When performing cytological needle aspirations, the radiologist prefers to have a cytologist in the same room, preparing and inspecting slides from specimens retrieved from suspicious lesions until a firm diagnosis of metastatic disease was made or ruled out. Time constraints frequently prevent this, and so training for radiologists in slide preparation would be beneficial.

Further reading

Britton K E, Granowska M 1997 Tumour identification using radiopharmaceuticals. Clin Radiol 52: 731–738
Hoh C K, Schiepers C, Seltzer M A et al 1997 PET in oncology: will it replace the other modalities? Semin Nucl Med 22: 94–106
Husband J E, Reznek R H (eds) 1998 Imaging in oncology. Oxford: ISIS Medical Media
Jones A L, Williams M P, Powles T J et al 1990 Magnetic resonance imaging in the detection of skeletal metastases in patients with breast cancer. Br J C 62: 296–298
Libshitz H I (ed) 1982 Metastatic disease. Radiol Clin North Am 20: 417–605
Thompson W M (ed) 1994 Staging neoplasms. Radiol Clin North Am 32: 1–197

SECTION v

Stephen R. D. Johnston

Cytopathology as a predictive guide to systemic therapy in breast cancer

Our increased understanding of the biology of breast cancer has provided exciting new possibilities for improving systemic anticancer therapy. Biological markers in the tumour can be used to predict the response to conventional therapies, and cytopathological assessment of the primary tumour may allow more appropriate selection of systemic therapies.

RESPONSE PREDICTORS

Expression of oestrogen receptor (ER) has been known strongly to predict response to tamoxifen in metastatic disease (McGuire 1978) and as adjuvant therapy (EBCTCG 1998). Indeed, measurement of change in ER status at relapse during tamoxifen therapy may also guide second-line endocrine therapy (Johnston et al 1995). ER can now be easily measured immunohisto-chemically in paraffin-embedded material or fine needle aspirates, and there is an increasing demand for the routine use of this assay in pathology laboratories to guide clinical decisions about endocrine therapy (Elledge & Osborne 1997). Although endocrine therapy has been thought of as cytostatic, we have shown in pre-operative neo-adjuvant studies that a reduction in the proliferation markers Ki-67 by use of the aromatase inhibitor 4-hydroxy-androstenedione occurs only in ER positive tumours which then respond to treatment (Fig. 6v.1). In addition, we have shown that tamoxifen and the

Dr Stephen R.D. Johnston, Department of Medicine, The Royal Marsden NHS Trust, Fulham Road, London SW3 6JJ, UK

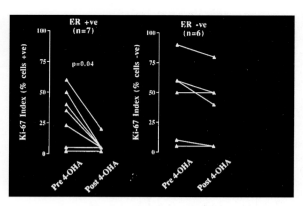

Fig. 6v.1 Change in cell proliferation (Ki-67) in ER positive and ER negative human primary breast carcinomas treated with the aromatase inhibitor 4-hydroxy-androstenedione. A significant fall ($P = 0.04$) in proliferation was seen only in ER positive tumours, which may represent an early cytopathological assessment of response.

steroidal anti-oestrogen ICI 182780 induce apoptosis in the short-term (Ellis et al 1997a). An early change in marker expression during therapy may, therefore, be more predictive of the final response to therapy.

Cytotoxic chemotherapy is being used increasingly as primary medical therapy for patients with large operable breast cancers. The measurement of biological markers in these patients can predict response and guide the use of appropriate systemic treatment. We have studied changes in Ki-67 and apoptosis using *in situ* end-labelling (Fig. 6v.2) after neo-adjuvant infusional chemotherapy in patients with large operable breast cancers. Rapid induction of apoptosis was observed after only 24 h (Ellis et al 1997b), together with a subsequent fall in cell proliferation. We have extended these preliminary observations into a larger randomised clinical trial of neo-adjuvant chemotherapy to see whether early changes in cell growth predict the final clinical response and overall survival. If so, this would allow early selection of patients for whom chemotherapy would be advantageous and identify patients with chemoresistant disease who might benefit from other therapies (see below).

REGULATORY ONCOGENES

There is much interest in the various proto-oncogenes which may regulate the response of a cell to DNA damage induced by specific chemotherapy agents. In particular, *Bcl-2* overexpression may protect many cell types from induction of apoptosis by many different anticancer agents. In an experimental breast cancer model, modulation of *Bcl-2* expression by either hormonal manipulation or antisense oligonucleotides significantly altered the chemosensitivity to doxorubicin (Teixeira et al 1995). It has been postulated, therefore, that Bcl-2 may contribute to drug resistance by preventing an apopotic response. Although there are few clinical data to support this hypothesis, our group has measured Bcl-2 immunohistochemically in primary breast carcinomas before and after therapy (Ellis et al 1998). In tumours that persisted following 4 months of chemotherapy, there was a significant ($P = 0.03$) increase in percentage

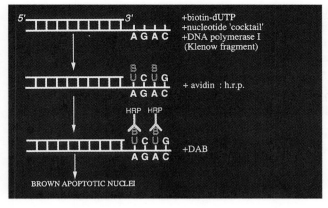

Fig. 6v.2 Methodology for *in situ* end labelling (ISEL) of fragments of DNA in cells undergoing apoptosis by detection of biotinylated nucleotides incorporated into the so-called 'sticky ends'.

expression of *Bcl-2* compared with before chemotherapy. This residual tissue could represent chemoresistant cells in which clonal selection of Bcl-2 expressing cells has occurred. It remains to be seen whether primary and acquired chemoresistance to conventional chemotherapy is associated clinically with overexpression of *Bcl-2*.

The tumour suppressor gene *p53* is mutated in 20–40% of primary breast carcinomas. Critical mutations which disrupt the function of p53 protein may prevent a cell from responding appropriately to DNA damage, either by cell cycle arrest with repair or deletion by apoptosis. Clinical evidence emerged recently from a small study which suggested that p53 may determine chemosensitivity to doxorubicin in primary breast cancer, with resistance being observed in tumours which contain critical mutations in the L2/L3 DNA binding domain (Aas et al 1996). Less clear data are available for the growth factor receptor c-erbB2 which may be a marker for unresponsiveness to chemotherapy. In particular, patients with overexpression of c-erbB2 in the primary tumour may benefit from higher dose CAF adjuvant chemotherapy (Muss et al 1994); other reports have indicated that c-erbB2 is a predictor of poor survival with chemotherapy (Gusterson et al 1992, Wright et al 1992). Although tempting to use these results to tailor conventional drug therapy, it is clear that at present further good quality data on the role of biological markers as primary predictors of response are needed before oncologists can change current practice.

TARGETED THERAPY

Specific abnormalities in some of the above genes are associated with resistance to conventional therapy which may offer new opportunities for targeted therapies. For example, monoclonal antibodies against c-erbB2 demonstrate anticancer activity and may be synergistic when combined with conventional chemotherapy agents (Baselga et al 1996). Direct gene therapy strategies have been developed to restore wild type p53 to tumours in which the gene is mutated; at present, clinical trials are in squamous cell cancers of the lung or head and neck (Roth & Cristiano 1997) and strategies for breast cancer are limited (Ruppert et al 1997). Antisense oligonucleotides against Bcl-2 represent an alternative method for targeting tumour cells, and phase I trials in follicular lymphoma have shown good tolerability and selective modulation of protein expression (Webb et al 1997).

FUTURE OPPORTUNITIES

Advances in automated cytopathological diagnosis using flow cytometry and molecular screening techniques will allow more accurate tumour phenotyping at the time of diagnosis. From studies of primary breast cancer, identification of patients who will, or will not, benefit from conventional endocrine and chemo-therapy treatments may be possible. Oncogene markers which are associated with resistance to these treatments may permit new therapeutic strategies against the malignant cell. To that end, cytopathological analysis of tumour markers could become central to therapeutic decision-making in the clinic.

References

Aas T, Borresen A L, Geisler S et al 1996 Specific p53 mutations are associated with resistance to doxorubicin in breast cancer patients. Nat Med 2; 811–814

Baselga J, Tripathy D, Mendelsohn J et al 1996 Phase II study of weekly intravenous recombinant humanised anti-p185 HER2 monoclonal antibody in patients with HER2/neu overexpressing metastatic breast cancer. J Clin Oncol 14: 737–744

EBCTCG 1998 Tamoxifen for early breast cancer; an overview of the randomized trials. Lancet 351: 1451–1467

Elledge R M, Osborne C K 1997 Oestrogen receptors and breast cancer. BMJ 314: 1843–1844

Ellis P A, Saccani-Joi G, Clarke R et al 1997a Induction of apoptosis by tamoxifen and ICI 182780 in primary breast cancer. Int J Cancer 72: 608–613

Ellis P A, Smith I E, McCarthy K, Detre S, Salter J, Dowsett M 1997b Pre-operative chemotherapy induces apoptosis in early breast cancer. Lancet 349: 849–850

Ellis P A, Smith I E, Detre S et al 1998 Reduced apoptosis and proliferation and increased Bcl-2 in residual breast cancer following pre-operative chemotherapy. Breast Cancer Res Treat 48; 107–116

Gusterson B A, Gelber R D, Goldhirsch A et al 1992 Prognostic importance of c-erbB2 expression in breast cancer. J Clin Oncol 10: 599–605

Johnston S R D, Saccani-Jotti G, Smith I E et al 1995 Changes in estrogen receptor, progesterone receptor and p52 expression in tamoxifen-resistant human breast cancer. Cancer Res 55: 3331–3338

McGuire W L 1978 Hormone receptors; their role in predicting prognosis and response to endocrine therapy. Semin Oncol 5: 428–433

Muss H B, Thor A D, Berry D A et al 1994 c-erbB2 expression and response to adjuvant therapy in women with node positive early breast cancer. N Engl J Med 330: 1260–1266

Roth J A, Cristiano R J 1997 Gene therapy for cancer; what have we done and where are we going? J Natl Cancer Inst 88: 21–39

Ruppert J M, Wrigh M, Rosenfeld M et al 1997 Gene therapy strategies for carcinoma of the breast. Breast Cancer Res Treat 44: 93–114

Teixeira C, Reed J C, Pratt M A C 1995 Estrogen promotes chemotherapeutic drug resistance by a mechanism involving Bcl-2 proto-oncogene expression in human breast cancer cells. Cancer Res 55: 3902–3907

Webb A, Cunningham D, Cotter F et al 1997 BCL-2 antisense therapy in patients with non-Hodgkin lymphoma. Lancet 349: 1137–1141

Wright C, Cairns J, Cantwell B J, Cattan A R, Hall A G, Harris A L 1992 Response to mioxantrone in advanced breast cancer; correlation with expression of c-erbB2 protein and glutathione S-transferases. Br J Cancer 65: 271–274

Peter A. van Dam   Wiebren A.A. Tjalma

Clinical applications of flow cytometry

Flow cytometry has many important research and clinical applications. The most common clinical use of flow cytometry is in the evaluation of circulating blood cells Colvin & Preffer 1987). Progress in defining a role for flow cytometry in the assessment of solid tumours has been slow, partly because of the greater histological complexity of solid tissues, and partly because of practical difficulties in obtaining suitable material. Over the past decade, great advances have been made and flow cytometry is now used more frequently for the measurement of DNA content in solid tumours (Melamed et al 1990).

Recently, the technique has been extended by the development of flow cytometric assays for other cellular components, such as membrane markers, oncoproteins and growth factor receptors (van Dam et al 1992). There can be little doubt that it will become a valuable technique in the study of the biology and treatment of cancer.

PRINCIPLES OF FLOW CYTOMETRY

The principles of flow cytometry have been described in detail in several recent books and review articles (Koss 1987, Melamed et al 1990, Watson 1991). Briefly, flow cytometers measure and record fluorescence and light scatter from cells or other particles, stained with an appropriate fluorochrome, passing an excitation source in a laminar flow jet of liquid suspension medium. The fluorescence of the stained cells is captured by a photomultiplier tube and converted to a digital electronic signal (Steen 1990).

The excitation source can be either a laser or a mercury arc lamp, selected to excite the absorption maxima of the fluorescent dyes used for the analysis of

Prof Dr P.A. van Dam, Department of Obstetrics and Gynaecology, Division of Gynaecological Oncology, Sint Augustinus Hospital, Oosterveldlaan 24, B-2610 Wilrijk, Belgium
Mr Wiebren A.A. Tjalma, Department of Obstetrics and Gynaecology, Division of Gynaecological Oncology, Antwerp University Hospital (UZA), Wilrijkstraat 10, B-2650 Edegem, Belgium

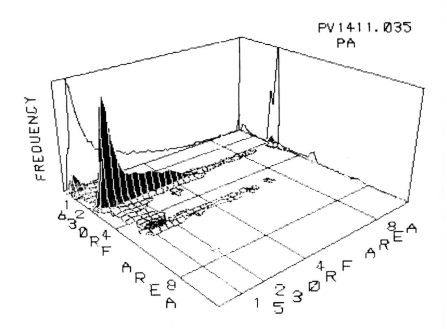

Fig, 7.1 Three dimensional DNA histogram depicting the amount of DNA (630RF AREA) against green oncoprotein fluorescence (530RF AREA) and the cell frequency of an ovarian carcinoma. The tumor is DNA aneuploid and shows heterogenous c-erbB-2 expression. The DNA histogram has a high resolution.

cell components. Some multibeam flow cytometers have combinations of lasers that emit light at different wavelengths, which permits much more versatility in combining fluorochromes for multiparameter analysis (van Dam et al 1995).

Cell sorting, a function associated with flow cytometry, uses electrostatic or mechanical means to divert cells with preselected characteristics from the main stream of the cell suspension. It can be used to isolate populations of cells that are purer than can be obtained by any other means (Shapiro 1988). The sorted cells can be studied directly by microscopy or in cell culture. Cell sorting is, however, a time-consuming and exacting technique that cannot reliably be applied to routine clinical specimens (Koss et al 1989).

Multiparameter flow cytometry permits further characterisation of cell populations without physical separation and isolation of cells. This was achieved first by Kamentsky and coworkers in the 1960s by simultaneous fluorescence and cell size measurements (Kamenstky 1995, Kamenstky et al 1995, Kamentsky & Melamed 1969). At the end of the 1970s, multiparameter flow cytometric assays were developed in which cells were stained with two or more fluorochromes that emitted light at different wavelengths (Koss et al 1989). Dichroic mirrors were used to separate the different wavelengths, which were then recorded by two or more photomultipliers (Watson 1991).

Today, data generated by flow cytometers are either displayed instantaneously on a video screen, or stored in a computer for further analysis, or both. The results of single parameter measurements are usually illustrated as a frequency histogram in which the number of stained cells is plotted as a function of the intensity of fluorescence. Simultaneous measurements of more than one parameter (usually two) are presented as scattergraphs or contour maps showing the relation between the measured features (Fig. 7.1). One type of multiparameter data analysis, in which values of one or more parameters are assessed to determine whether or not to include values of another parameter from the same cell, is referred to as gated analysis (Koss et al 1989).

ADVANTAGES AND LIMITATIONS OF FLOW CYTOMETRY

Conventional biochemical methods used for quantitative measurements of cell constituents are open to errors introduced by dilution of the tumour cell population by necrotic debris and by stromal, inflammatory, and other non-neoplastic cells. Heterogeneity in samples can be masked by taking the averages of measurements. Artefacts can be introduced also from damage to cells caused by the disruption needed in the preparation of cell-free extracts that are used for some of these assays. Immunohistochemistry gives useful qualitative information but is usually subjective, only moderately sensitive, and difficult to standardize. Quantitation is inaccurate if the slides are analyzed without, for example, image densitometry or intensitometry (Baak et al 1988).

Flow technology can overcome some of these problems and is complementary to classical techniques. It can provide objective measurements of a representative sample of cells (10^5 or more) from a large volume of tissue more rapidly and easily than histology, image analysis or spectrometry (van Dam et al 1990). Flow techniques provide statistical accuracy, reproducibility and sensitivity: a detection limit equivalent to 150 molecules of free fluorescein per cell has been achieved (Watson & Walport 1986). As the presence of the compound under investigation is recorded by the cytometer in each individual cell of a sample, small subpopulations of cells can easily be identified.

With multiparameter flow cytometry, necrotic debris and some of the inflammatory and stromal cells can be excluded from the measurements by gating procedures, or by immunostaining the cells for epithelial markers, such as with antibodies to low molecular weight cytokeratins, which allows more accurate analysis of the neoplastic cells of a tumour (Frey 1997). The yield of tumour cells can be enriched for further biochemical analysis by sorting cells or nuclei on the basis of DNA ploidy or other markers (Burmer et al 1989).

Flow cytometry allows simultaneous measurement of several constituents on a cell-to-cell basis by using multicolour staining techniques (van Dam et al 1995). Multivariate analysis of such data yields much information on the relation between the parameters measured. Dynamic events that take from only a few seconds to a few minutes can be studied (Watson 1991).

The main drawback of flow cytometry in comparison with histological, histochemical, immunohistological and image spectrometric studies is the loss of structural information in solid tissues. Careful sampling of tissues and histochemical, immunohistochemical and/or cytochemical controls must be used so that the results can be properly interpreted. In addition, the hardware is very expensive and is not widely available.

SAMPLE PREPARATION

Cells normally in suspension in body fluids, such as blood cells, are prime candidates for analysis by flow cytometry: they need no disaggregation and no spatial information is lost. Mechanical or enzymatic tissue dissociation methods are required to make single cell or single nuclei suspensions from solid tissue samples. Generally, mechanical tissue disaggregation is better for carcinomas than for other tumours, particularly those with large amounts of fibrous tissue in which enzymatic dissociation can produce higher quality single cell suspensions (Slocum 1983, Chassevent et al 1984, Costa et al 1987, Ensley et al 1987a, Ensley et al 1987b, Ensley et al 1987c, Crissman & Steinkamp 1990). Current techniques of solid tissue dissociation remain relatively crude, and more studies are needed to address important questions on the relation between the properties of intercellular junctions, cell loss, and representiveness of the resultant suspensions and of the measurements of the biological substances that are being investigated (Costa et al 1987, Ensley et al 1987c).

Disaggregated single cells or nuclei can be analyzed fresh, or fixed and preserved (Vindolov et al 1982, Vindolov et al 1983a, Vindolov et al 1983b, Alanen et al 1989). Only minimal alterations in the quality of DNA histograms are noted in the latter situation (Coon et al 1988). However, little work has been done on the effect of fixation and storage on measurements of cell components other than DNA (van Dam et al 1995).

The first method for making nuclear suspensions from paraffin blocks was developed by Hedley and colleagues (Hedley et al 1983). The many research and clinical applications of this technique of recovery of DNA have been reviewed recently (Hedley (1989). It allows retrospective DNA analysis by flow cytometry and measurement of nuclear proteins such as oncogene products (Watson et al 1985). Excellent histological controls for the tissue taken for flow cytometry are possible by taking adjacent sections for histology and, if necessary, the cells of interest can be microdissected (Hanselaar et al 1988). Because of the harsh enzymatic digestion required for this tissue dissociation method, however, the quality of these suspensions is usually lower than that of fresh cell suspensions. This is reflected in an inferior resolution of the G_0/G_1 peaks (higher coefficient of variation, CV) and more debris in the former suspensions (Hedley 1989).

An important limitation of the use of paraffin-wax embedded material for flow cytometry is that, at present, only bare nuclei can be analyzed. Cytoplasm, plasma membranes and extracellular material are lost during specimen preparation (van Dam et al 1991). In addition, the handling of the tissue before fixation, the type of fixation, the storage conditions of the paraffin-wax embedded blocks, and the methods of preparing nuclei are all sources of variation and so affect DNA and other nuclear components (Feichter & Goerttler 1986, Alanen et al 1989, Lincoln & Bauer 1990). Despite these drawbacks, the use of paraffin-embedded material has been validated repeatedly by comparison with corresponding fresh tumour material (Camplejohn & Macartney 1985, McIntyre et al 1987, Frierson 1988). Cell and nuclear suspensions prepared from cryopreserved tissue blocks may be less prone to these variables and also permit high quality DNA analysis (Vindolov et al 1982, Dressler et al 1988).

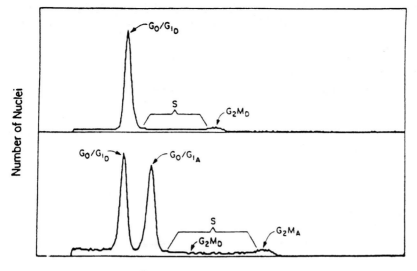

Fig. 7.2 Examples of two DNA histograms. Note that the number of cells is plotted against the relative fluorescence (DNA content). G_0/G_1 peaks are determined by reference to known controls. The upper panel shows a DNA diploid tumour with its G_0/G_1 D peak and S and G_2/M D phase cells. The area under the curves for S and G_2/M phases are estimated via computer. In the lower panel a DNA aneuploid tumour is depicted with a second DNA aneuploid cell population (G_0/G_1 A, S, G_2/M A).

FLOW CYTOMETRIC DNA ANALYSIS

Single parameter measurements of DNA can be accomplished with several established fluorochromes, such as ethidium bromide and propidium iodide, that bind nucleic acids specifically and stoichiometrically (Vindolov et al 1982). RNA is also labelled by these dyes, emphasising the need to incubate the suspensions with ribonuclease to ensure selective DNA staining. As large numbers of cells are analyzed, appropriate statistical methods can be applied to the resulting data to give information on DNA content and cell cycle variables.

DNA histograms are usually interpreted according to guidelines provided by a convention on nomenclature for expressing abnormalities of DNA content (Hiddemann et al 1984). The DNA index (DI) is the mode of the DNA content of the population of cells studied divided by the mode of the DNA content of the corresponding non-neoplastic, normal cells. If the main peak of the DNA histogram centres around the 2C region and the overall DNA distribution is similar to that of normal somatic cells, the tumour is classified as diploid (DI = 1). Populations of cells with a DNA content **not** equal to that of normal cells are referred to as aneuploid (Fig. 7.2) and are further subdivided into hypoploid (DI < 1), hyperploid (DI > 1) and occasionally tetraploid (DI = 2) (Raber & Barlogie 1990). The capacity to resolve subpopulations of cells with minor alterations in DNA content is dependent on technical factors, and is best assessed through the coefficient of variation (CV) of the G_0/G_1 peaks.

Many investigators have reported that an abnormal DNA index is highly specific for malignancy, particularly in solid tumours (Raber & Barlogie 1990). Some normal tissues, however, have tetraploid or haploid cells (such as liver and testis, respectively). There are also a number of premalignant lesions associated with distinctly abnormal DNA cell populations (such as cervical intra-epithelial neoplasia). In addition, artefactual DNA aneuploidy can be detected in autolysed tissue samples (Alanen et al 1989).

Computer software for flow cytometric cell cycle analysis has been developed based on the assumption that the percentage of cells synthesizing DNA (S-phase cells) is a direct reflection of tumour proliferation (Camplejohn & Macartney 1985, Dean 1990). Other authors prefer to report a proliferation index, defined as the percentage of cells in the S and G_2/M phases (Merkel & McGuire 1990). Techniques for estimating S-phase fraction cell populations are numerous and relatively simple when one has 'clean histograms'. In histograms with a high CV, however, when there is a high skew of the modal peak, or large amounts of debris, or aneuploid tumours with several overlapping cycling cell populations, the cell cycle analysis is much more complicated. It then often depends on the judgement of the analyst, and is sometimes impossible (Camplejohn & Macartney 1985, van Dam et al 1992). Delay in fixation of the tissue, suboptimal preservation, archival material, and even intralaboratory and interlaboratory variability are other potential sources of bias (Feichter & Goerrtler 1986, Cross et al 1990).

Some studies have compared flow cytometric cell cycle distribution measurements with other assays of proliferative activity, such as tritiated thymidine labelling index (Roza et al 1985, Walker & Camplejohn 1988). Most of these workers found a moderate or good correlation between those assays and flow cytometric DNA analysis, but there seemed to be a trend towards overestimation of the S-phase fraction by flow cytometry (Raber & Barlogie 1990). This may be because some tumour cells with S-phase DNA content are not cycling (Lacombe et al 1988). Multiparameter flow cytometric assays based on bromodeoxyuridine incorporation in DNA, or assessment of proteins involved in the control of cell proliferation (e.g. Ki67, PCNA/cyclin), have been evaluated and are likely to provide more accurate indices of cell proliferation (Kurki et al 1988, Liu et al 1989).

With the introduction of techniques for the analysis of archival material, it is now possible to correlate flow cytometric DNA analysis with the patient's disease-free interval and overall survival retrospectively (Vindolov et al 1982, Hedley et al 1983). In spite of the pitfalls of DNA analysis, there is clinical evidence for many tumour sites and types that DNA-based measurements of the tumour ploidy and S-phase fraction are useful prognostic factors (van Dam et al 1992).

FLOW CYTOMETRIC QUANTITATION OF NON-DNA CELLULAR COMPONENTS

GENERAL CONSIDERATIONS

The availability of new fluorescent probes and markers provides the potential for new multiparameter flow cytometric investigations. Cell components other than DNA can be labelled with fluorochromes or with antibodies labelled with fluorescent dyes. The introduction of monoclonal antibody technology has started a new era for flow technology, as an almost endless series of highly specific immunological reagents became available for cell classification and the study of cytostructural proteins, cell surface receptors and oncogene products (Kohler & Milstein 1975).

There are several potential problems with using antibodies to quantify cell constituents: tissue disaggregation, cell fixation and subsequent preservation may cause epitope loss or allosteric changes in the conformation of the antigen studied (van Dam et al 1992). Quantitation of cytoplasmic, nuclear and intracellular antigens with antibodies is particularly difficult as it requires cell membrane permeabilisation. Assay of intracellular antigens has been attempted after detergent fixation of fresh cells, in cryopreserved cells and in nuclear suspensions made from paraffin wax blocks (Watson et al 1985, Czerniak et al 1990, Dent et al 1989).

Immunocytological or immunohistological controls and independent biochemical evidence (e.g. immunoprecipitation), together with the use of adequate positive and negative controls and peptide blocking assays, should be used to confirm quantitative data from multiparameter flow cytometry before they are accepted as meaningful. In addition, controls are needed to exclude non-specific binding and trapping of the antibodies.

RNA AND PROTEIN

With the use of different fluorochromes and multiparameter flow cytometry, studies on cell DNA content in relation to total cell protein and RNA have been developed (Darzyniewicz et al 1982, Crissman & Steinkamp 1987). These techniques proved to be useful in detecting abnormalities in the cell cycle (such as uncoupling of transcriptional and translational activity) in experimental conditions as well as elucidating patterns of normal growth and cell cycle patterns (Darzynkiewicz et al 1982, Marrone & Crissman 1988).

CELL SURFACE MARKERS

Multiparameter flow cytometry has become a standard technique for the analysis of surface antigens and proliferation markers in lymphocytes and related cells, and has contributed to the classification of malignant lymphomas and leukaemias. The difficulty of obtaining single cell suspensions from solid tumours has delayed extension of the technique to this field.

Several authors have studied the expression of cell surface markers in cultured cell lines by multiparameter flow cytometry (Nozawa 1989, Bast et al 1990, Berchuck et al 1990, van Dam et al 1990, Acevedo et al 1992a, Acevedo et al 1992b, Meunier et al 1996). Tumour cell subpopulations with high membrane marker expression can be isolated by cell sorting for further detailed study of their behaviour and biochemical characteristics (Paratto & Kimura 1988).

The technique can also be used on cell suspensions, prepared by mechanical or enzymatic disaggregation of solid tissues (Valet & Russmann 1984, Fowler et al 1988, Paratto & Kimura 1988, Baak et al 1990, van Dam et al 1991, Meunier et al 1996). Single and multiparameter flow cytometric assays have been developed to study the expression of membrane markers in cervical smears and biopsy samples of cervical and endometrial tumours (Elias Jones et al 1986, Hendy-Ibbs 1987). It was hoped that these techniques could be used for screening cervical pre-invasive carcinomas. However, no useful applications have been published on the use of flow cytometry for screening of human malignancies.

Durrant et al (1989) used multiparameter flow cytometry to evaluate a panel of cell surface markers that were candidates for antibody-directed therapy on samples of primary ovarian carcinoma. Other groups have used single or multiparameter flow cytometry for identification and quantitation of surface markers in various other tumours (Alam 1990, van Dam et al 1991, Greiner et al 1992).

CYTOKERATINS

A technique has been developed to double-label cells for DNA and keratin which allows the DNA content to be analyzed in epithelial cells alone, with less interference from debris and DNA diploid non-epithelial cells. This approach, improving the accuracy of tumour S-phase fraction calculations, has been applied successfully to endometrial, breast, bladder, colonic, and head and neck carcinomas (Dolbaere et al 1983, Crissman et al 1988, Riccardi et al 1989, Ferrero et al 1990, Rose et al 1996).

PROLIFERATION MARKERS

In vitro and in vivo multiparameter flow cytometric assays that labelled both bromodeoxyuridine (BrdUrd) and DNA are very sensitive, and comparable with the tritiated-thymidine assay for the study of proliferative activity (Dolbaere 1983, Riccardi et al 1989, Sahni et al 1990). Another promising method of assessing cell proliferation consists of simultaneous flow cytometric measurement of proliferating cell nuclear antigen (PCNA/cyclin) or Ki67 and DNA; this has been evaluated in cultured cells (Hall & Levison 1990, Landberg et al 1990, Rosette et al 1990). Attempts are being made to apply the technique in cell suspensions prepared from solid tissues.

ONCOPROTEINS AND GROWTH FACTOR RECEPTORS

Recently, some workers have reported on flow cytometry for measuring oncoproteins in cultured cell lines (Fan 1985, Kelsten et al 1990). Czerniak et al (1990) quantitated the expression of c-myc, c-fos, c-ras and c-erbB-2 oncoproteins in cultured cells by computer-assisted image analysis and flow cytometry. Both techniques gave concordant results.

Very little work has been done to apply flow technology to the study of oncoproteins in solid tumours. Watson et al (1987) assayed the nucleus-associated product of the *c-myc* gene, p62, simultaneously with DNA using flow cytometry on nuclei extracted from archival biopsies of testicular cancer and serous papillary carcinoma of the ovary. Expression of c-myc oncoprotein was significantly higher in the carcinomas compared with normal ovary, and intermediate values were found in borderline ovarian tumours. The same group showed that biopsies of normal cervix had significantly higher c-myc oncoprotein level than carcinomas, but the nuclear content of c-myc oncoprotein did not appear to be a prognostic indicator (Hendy-Ibbs et al 1987). The method has also been successfully used in a variety of other non-gynaecological tumours (Bauer et al 1986, Watson et al 1986, Appley et al 1990, Corver et al 1996). Remvikos et al (1992) studied p53 expression in colorectal tumours with a flow cytometric assay. Kotylo et al (1992) used multiparameter flow cytometry to analyse DNA content and ras p21 oncoprotein expression in ovarian neoplasms. Great care should be taken in the interpretation of this study as nuclear suspensions prepared from paraffin-embedded tissue were used to analyze the expression of a mainly cytoplasmic oncoprotein.

CYTOTOXICITY AND MULTIDRUG RESISTANCE

Flow cytometry has been extensively used in the study of: (i) cytokinetic disturbances in cells incubated in vitro with cytostatic drugs (Edwards et al 1986, Dong et al 1997); (ii) cell cycle phase sensitivity to cytotoxic agents (Kingston et al 1989, Frankfurt et al 1990, Volm & Efferth 1990); (iii) drug resistance in vitro (Lee & Siemann 1989); and (iv) drug resistant cells and their isolation (Sherwood et al 1990).

Measurements of drug influx and efflux using labelled drugs are technically difficult but some drugs commonly used for chemotherapy, such as anthracyclines (e.g. doxorubicin), are intrinsically fluorescent. The intensity of cellular fluorescence can easily be measured by flow cytometry as an indicator of drug uptake and accumulation, which are linked to drug sensitivity (Lee & Siemann 1989, Sherwood et al 1990). Preliminary attempts have been made to apply these techniques to solid tumour samples retrieved from animals or patients treated with cytotoxic agents (Gheuens et al 1991). This should contribute to a better understanding of how these drugs work and might lead to the development of a better in vitro assay for multidrug resistance.

OTHER CELLULAR COMPONENTS

In vitro flow cytometric assays have been used in cultured cells for the study of: (i) steroid receptors (Remvikos et al 1991); (ii) ligand binding (Chatelier & Ashcroft 1987); (iii) dye-permeability (Dive et al 1990); (iv) toxicity (Dallas & Evans 1990); (v) enzyme activity (Robertson et al 1990); (vi) aspects of radiosensitivity and radioresistance (Hodgkiss et al 1991); (vii) the immune response and the cytoskeleton (Giese et al 1990); and (viii) the detection and identification of bacteria, fungi and viruses (Steele-Mortimer et al 1990).

FUTURE APPLICATIONS OF FLOW CYTOMETRY

Many studies suggest that flow cytometric DNA analysis provides useful prognostic information for several tumour types and sites. However, measuring DNA content in neoplasms raises a number of fundamental biological and methodological questions. The molecular basis for DNA

Points of Best Practice

- Good cytological or histological assessment of the samples used for flow cytometry is crucial for the interpretation of the results.•

- Methods of fixation and tissue disaggregation should be optimised.

- Fixation and permeabilisation of single cells is essential for flow cytometric analysis after immunolabelling of intracellular substances.

- Titrate antibodies used and optimise the incubation times.

- Standardise gating and data analysis procedures.

aneuploidy in malignant (and some benign) lesions is unclear. Why DNA aneuploid tumours should behave in a generally more aggressive fashion is also an enigma, but expression of high levels of oncoproteins may account for this, at least in part.

Owing to the limited resolution of current flow cytometric DNA analysis, there remains a grey area between DNA diploidy and aneuploidy. It is, therefore, necessary to establish a more detailed classification of DNA histograms, and to optimise the number of samples needed to allow for tumour heterogeneity.

Flow cytometric DNA analysis should be used with caution to predict the outcome for individual patients. For most tumour types, further prospective studies are needed to establish the precise value of flow cytometric DNA analysis. It has been suggested, however, (Trope & Baak 1995, unpublished data) that one should consider using the technique for stratification of therapeutic regimens for certain tumours, such as borderline carcinoma of the ovary.

Multiparameter flow technology is used widely to study cultured cells in vitro but, at present, there are few clinical applications. As outlined in this chapter, flow cytometry can play an important role in identifying the role of oncogenes, growth factor receptors, and many other substances in the complex carcinogenic process. With a suitable panel of monoclonal antibodies, it may be used for screening, 'biochemical' diagnosis of neoplasia, and rapid drug, hormone, and radiotherapy sensitivity tests. Flow cytometry can also be used to optimise immunotherapy and immunoimaging and, perhaps, to monitor intraperitoneal chemotherapy and/or lymphokine therapy. The combination of flow technology with well-established techniques, such as DNA hybridization, will open further perspectives. The introduction of multiparameter flow cytometry, in particular, should considerably improve the methodology for measurements of tumour cell proliferation. This will increase the prognostic application of flow cytometry in malignant disease and will influence clinical management.

References

Acevedo H F, Krichevsky A, Campbell-Acevedo E A, Galyon J C, Buffo M J, Hartsock R J 1992a Flow cytometry method for the analysis of membrane-associated human chorionic gonadotropin, its subunits, and fragments on human cancer cells. Cancer 69: 1818–1826

Acevedo H F, Krichevsky A, Campbell-Acevedo E A, Galyon J C, Buffo M J, Hartsock R J 1992b Expression of membrane-associated human chorionic gonadotropin, its subunits, and fragments by cultured human cancer cells. Cancer 69: 1829–1842

Alam S M, Whitford P, Cushley W, George W D, Campbell A M 1990 Flow cytometric analysis of cell surface carbohydrates in metastatic human breast cancer. Br J Cancer 62: 238–242

Alanen K A, Joensuu H, Klemi P J 1989 Autolysis is a potential source of false aneuploid peaks in flow cytometric DNA histograms. Cytometry 10: 417–425

Alanen K A, Klemi P J, Joensuu H, Kujari H, Pekkala E 1989 Comparison of fresh, ethanol-preserved, and paraffin-embedded samples in DNA flow cytometry. Cytometry 10: 81–85

Appley A J, Fitzgibbons P L, Chandrasoma P T, Hinton D R, Apuzzo M L 1990 Multiparameter flow cytometric analysis of neoplasms of the central nervous system: correlation of nuclear antigen p105 and DNA content with clinical behaviour. Neurosurgery 27: 83–96

Baak J P, Schipper N W, Wisse-Brekelmans E C et al 1988 The prognostic value of morphometrical features and cellular DNA content in cis-platin treated late ovarian cancer patients. Br J Cancer 57: 503–508

Bast R C, Boyer C M, Olt G J et al 1990 Identification of markers for early detection of epithelial ovarian cancer. In: Sharp, Mason, Leake (eds) Ovarian cancer – biological and therapeutic challenges. London: Chapman and Hall, 265–275

Bauer K D, Clevenger C V, Endow E K, Murad T, Epstein A L, Scarpelli D G 1986 Simultaneous nuclear antigen and DNA content quantitation using paraffin-embedded colonic tissue and multiparameter flow cytometry. Cancer Res 46: 2428–2434

Berchuck A, Olt G J, Soisson A P et al 1990 Heterogeneity of antigen expression in advanced epithelial ovarian cancer. Am J Obstet Gynecol 162: 883–888

Burmer G C, Rabinovitch P S, Loeb L A 1989 Analysis of c-Ki-ras mutations in human colon carcinoma by cell sorting, polymerase chain reaction and DNA sequencing. Cancer Res 49: 2141–2146

Camplejohn R S, Macartney J C 1985 Comparison of DNA flow cytometry from fresh and paraffin embedded samples of non-Hodgkin's lymphoma. J Clin Pathol 38: 1096–1099

Chassevent A, Daver A, Bertrand G et al 1984 Comparative flow DNA analysis of different cell suspensions in breast carcinoma. Cytometry 5: 263–267

Chatelier R C, Ashcroft R G 1987 Calibration of flow cytometric fluorescence standards using isoparametric analysis of ligand binding. Cytometry 8: 632–636

Colvin R B, Preffer F L 1987 New technologies in cell analysis by flow cytometry. Arch Pathol Lab Med 111: 628–632

Coon J S, Deitch A D, DeVere White R W et al 1988 Interinstitutional variability in DNA flow cytometric analysis of tumours. The National Cancer Institute Flow Cytometry Network Experience. Cancer 61: 126–130

Corver W E, Bonsing B A, Abeln E C, Vlak-Theil P M, Cornelisse C J, Fleuren G J 1996 One-tube triple staining method for flow cytometric analysis of DNA ploidy and phenotypic heterogeneity of human solid tumors using single laser excitation. Cytometry 25: 358–366

Costa A, Silvestrini R, Del Bino G, Motta R 1987 Implications of disaggregation procedures on biological representation of human solid tumours. Cell Tissue Kinet 20: 171–180

Crissman H A, Steinkamp J A 1987 A new method for rapid and sensitive detection of bromodeoxyuridine in DNA replicating cells. Exp Cell Res 173: 256–261

Crissman H A, Steinkamp J A 1990 Cytochemical techniques for multivariate analysis of DNA and other cellular constituents. In: Melamed M R, Lindmo T, Mendelsohn M L (eds) Flow cytometry and sorting. New York: Wiley-Liss, 227–247

Crissman J D, Zarbo R J, Niebylski C D, Corbett T, Weaver D 1988 Flow cytometric DNA analysis of colon adenocarcinomas: a comparative study of preparatory techniques. Mod Pathol 1: 198–204

Cross S S, Start R D, Smith J H 1990 Does delay in fixation affect the number of mitotic figures in processed tissue? J Clin Pathol 43: 597–599

Czerniak B, Herz F, Westro R P et al 1990 Quantitation of oncogene products by computer-assisted image analysis and flow cytometry. J Histochem Cytochem 38: 463–466

Dallas C E, Evans D L 1990 Flow cytometry in toxicity analysis. Nature 345: 557–558

Darzynkiewicz Z, Crissman H, Traganos F, Stainkamp J 1982 Cell heterogeneity during the cell cycle. J Cell Physiol 113: 465–474

Dean P N 1990 Data processing. In: Melamed M R, Lindmo T, Mendelsohn M L (eds) Flow cytometry and sorting. New York: Wiley-Liss, 415–444

Dent G A, Leglise M C, Pryzwansky K B, Ross D W 1989 Simultaneous paired analysis by flow cytometry of surface markers, cytoplasmic antigens or oncogene expression with DNA content. Cytometry 10: 192–198

Dive C, Watson J V, Workman P 1990 Multiparametric analysis of cell membrane permeability by two colour flow cytometry with complementary fluorescent probes. Cytometry 11: 244–252

Dolbaere F, Gratzner H G, Pallavicini M G, Gray J W 1983 Flow cytometric measurement of total DNA content and incorporated bromodeoxyuridine. Proc Natl Acad Sci USA 80: 5573-5577

Dong J, Naito M, Tsuruo T 1997 c-myc plays a role in cellular susceptibility to death receptor-mediated and chemotherapy-induced apoptosis in human monocytic leukemia U937 cells. Oncogene 15: 639–647

Dressler L, Clark G, Owens M, Pounds G, Oldaker T, McGuire W L 1988 DNA flow cytometry and prognostic factors in 1331 frozen breast cancer specimens. Cancer 61: 420–427

Durrant L G, Robins A, Baldwin R W 1989 Flow cytometric screening of monoclonal antibodies for drug and toxin targeting to human cancer. J Natl Cancer Inst 81: 688–696

Edwards P G, Nias A H 1986 Cell cycle phase sensitivity to cis-dichloro-bis (isopropylamine) trans-dihydroxyplatinum (IU). Cell Tissue Kinet 19: 419–427

Elias Jones J, Hendy Ibbs P, Cox H, Evan G I, Watson J V 1986 Cervical brush biopsy specimens suitable for DNA and oncoprotein analysis using flow cytometry. J Clin Pathol 39: 577–581

Ensley J F, Maciorowski H, Pietraszkiewicz H et al 1987a Solid tumour preparation for flow cytometry using a standard murine model. Cytometry 8: 479–487

Ensley J F, Maciorowski Z, Pietraszkiewicz H et al 1987b Solid tumor preparation for clinical application of flow cytometry. Cytometry 8: 488–493

Ensley J F, Maciorowski Z, Pietraszkiewicz H, Hassan M, Crissman J, Valdivieso M 1987c Selective and consistent aneuploidal cellular subpopulation losses in enzymatically versus mechanically dissociated human colon specimens analyzed by flow cytometry. Proc Am Assoc Cancer Res 28: 248–251

Fan K 1988 Heterogeneous subpopulations of human prostatic adenocarcinoma cells: potential usefulness of p21 protein as a predictor of bone metastasis. J Urol 139: 318–322

Feichter G E, Goerttler K 1986 Pitfalls in the preparation of nuclear suspensions from paraffin embedded tissue for flow cytometry. Cytometry 7: 616

Ferrero M, Spyratos F, Le Doussal V, Desplaces A, Rouesse J 1990 Flow cytometric analysis of DNA content and keratins by using CK7, CK8, CK19 and KL1 monoclonal antibodies in benign and malignant human breast tumours. Cytometry 11: 716–724

Fowler W C, Maddock M B, Moore D H, Haskill S 1988 Significance of multiparameter flow cytometric analysis of ovarian cancer. Am J Obstet Gynecol 158: 838–845

Frankfurt O S, Seckinger D, Sugarbecker E V 1990 Flow cytometric analysis of DNA damage and repair in the cells resistant to alkylating agents. Cancer Res 50: 4453–4457

Frey T 1997 Correlated flow cytometric analysis of terminal events in apoptosis reveals the absence of some changes in some model systems. Cytometry 28: 253–263

Frierson H F 1988 Flow cytometric analysis of ploidy in solid neoplasms: comparison of fresh tissues with formalin-fixed paraffin-embedded specimens. Hum Pathol 19: 290–294

Gheuens E G, Van Bockstaele D R, van der Kempt I, Tanke H J, van Oosterom A T, De Bruyn E 1991 Flow cytometric double labeling technique for screening of multidrug resistance. Cytometry 12: 636–644

Giese G, Kubbies M, Traub P 1990 Alterations of cell cycle kinetics and vimentin expression in TPA-treated, asynchronous MCP-11 mouse plasmocyte cells. Exp Cell Res; 190: 179–184

Greiner J W, Guadagni V, Goldstein D et al 1992 Intraperitoneal administration of interferon-gamma to carcinoma patients enhances expression of tumor-associated glycoprotein-72 and CEA in malignant ascites cells. J Clin Oncol 10: 735–746

Hall P A, Levison D A 1990 Review: assessment of cell proliferation in histological material. J Clin Pathol 43: 184–192

Hanselaar A G, Vooijs G P, Oud P S, Pahlplatz M M, Beck J L 1988 DNA ploidy patterns in cervical intraepithelial neoplasia grade III, with or without synchronous invasive squamous cell carcinoma. Cancer 62: 2537–2545

Hedley D W 1989 Flow cytometry using paraffin-embedded tissue: five years on. Cytometry 10: 229–241

Hedley D W, Friedlander M L, Taylor I W, Rogg C A, Musgrove E A 1983 Methods for analysis of cellular DNA content of paraffin embedded pathologic material using flow cytometry. J Histochem Cytochem 31: 1333–1335

Hendy-Ibbs P, Cox H, Evan G I, Watson J V 1987 Flow cytometric quantitation of DNA and c-myc oncoprotein in archival biopsies of uterine cervix neoplasia. Br J Cancer 55: 275–282

Hiddemann W, Schumann J, Andreef F M et al 1984 Convention on nomenclature for DNA cytometry. Cytometry 5: 445–446

Hodgkiss R J, Jones G, Long A, Parrick J, Smith K A, Stratford M R 1991 Flow cytometric evaluation of hypoxic cells in solid experimental tumours using fluorescence immunodetection. Br J Cancer 63: 119–125

Kamentsky L A 1965a Rapid biological cell identification by spectroscopic analysis. Proceedings of the 18th Annual Conference on Engineering in Biology and Medicine 7: 178

Kamentsky L A, Melamed M R 1969 Instrumentation for automated examination of cellular specimens. IEEE 57: 2007–2016

Kamentsky L A, Melamed M R, Derman H 1965b Spectrophotometer: new instrument for ultrarapid cell analysis. Science 150: 630–631

Kelsten M L, Berger M S, Maguire H C et al 1990 Analysis of c-erbB-2 protein expression in conjunction with DNA content using multiparameter flow cytometry. Cytometry 11: 522–532

Kingston R E, Sevin B U, Ramos R et al 1989 Synergistic effects of cis-platinum and cytosine arabinoside on ovarian carcinoma cell lines, demonstrated by dual parameter flow cytometry. Gynecol Oncol 32: 282–287

Kohler G, Milstein C 1975 Continuous cultures of fused cells secreting antibody of predefined specificity. Nature 256: 495–497

Koss L G 1987 Automated cytology and histology: a historical perspective. Anal Quant Cytol Histol 9: 369–374

Koss L G, Czerniak B, Herz F, Westro R P 1989 Flow cytometric measurements of DNA and other cell components in human tumours: a critical appraisal. Hum Pathol 20: 528–548

Kotylo P K, Michael H, Fineberg N, Sutton G, Roth L M 1992 Flow cytometric analysis of DNA content and ras p21 oncoprotein expression in ovarian neoplasms. Int J Gynecol Pathol 11: 3

Kurki P, Ogata K, Tan E M 1988 Monoclonal antibodies to proliferating cell nuclear antigen (PCNA)/cyclin as probes for proliferating cells by immunofluorescence microscopy and flow cytometry. J Immunol Methods 109: 49–59

Lacombe F, Belloc F, Benard P et al 1988 Evaluation of four methods of DNA distribution: data analysis based on bromodeoxyuridine/DNA bivariate data. Cytometry 9: 245–253

Landberg G, Tan E M, Roos G 1990 Flow cytometric multiparameter analysis of proliferating cell nuclear antigen/cyclin and Ki-67 antigen: a new view of the cell cycle. Exp Cell Res 187: 111–118

Lee F Y, Siemann D W 1989 Isolation by flow cytometry of a human ovarian tumor cell subpopulation exhibiting a high glutathione content phenotype and increased resistance to adriamycin. Int J Radiat Oncol Biol Phys 16: 1315–1319

Lincoln S T, Bauer K D 1990 Limitations in the measurement of c-myc oncoprotein and other nuclear antigens by flow cytometry. Cytometry 10: 456–462

Liu Y C, Marraccino R L, Keng P C et al 1989 Requirement for proliferating cell nuclear antigen expression during stages of the Chinese hamster ovary cell cycle. Biochemistry 28: 2967–2974

Marrone B L, Crissman H A 1988 Characterization of granulosa cell subpopulations from avian preovulatory follicles by multiparameter flow cytometry. Endocrinology 122: 651–658

McIntire T L, Goldey S H, Benson N A, Braylan R C 1987 Flow cytometric analysis of DNA in cells obtained from deparaffinized formalin-fixed lymphoid tissues. Cytometry 8: 474–478

Melamed M R, Lindmo T, Mendelsohn M L 1990 Flow Cytometry and Sorting, 2nd edn. New York: Wiley-Liss, 1–802

Merkel D E, McGuire W L 1990 Ploidy, proliferative activity and prognosis. DNA flow cytometry of solid tumors. Cancer 65: 1194–1205

Meunier L, Vian L, Langoueyte C et al 1996 Quantification of CD1a, HLA-DR, and HLA class I expression on viable human Langerhans cells and keratinocytes. Cytometry 26: 260–264

Nozawa S, Sakayori M, Ohta K et al 1989 A monoclonal antibody (MSN-1) against a newly established uterine endometrial cancer cell line (SNG-II) and its application to immunohistochemistry and flow cytometry. Am J Obstet Gynecol 161: 1079–1086

Paratto N P, Kimura A K 1988 Isolation and visualisation of Met-72-positive, metastatic variants present in B16 melanoma tumour masses. J Cell Biochem 36: 311–322

Raber M N, Barlogie B 1990 DNA flow cytometry of human solid tumours. In: Melamed M R, Lindmo T, Mendelsohn M L (eds) Flow cytometry and sorting. New York: Wiley-Liss, 745–754

Ramaekers F C, Beck H L, Feitz W F et al 1986 Application of antibodies to intermediate filament proteins as tissue-specific in the flow cytometric analysis of complex tumours. Anal Quant Cytol Histol 8: 271–280

Remvikos Y, Tominaga O, Hammel P et al 1992 Increased p53 protein content of colorectal tumours correlates with poor survival. Br J Cancer 66: 758–764

Remvikos Y, VuHai M T, Laine-Bidron C, Jollivet A, Magdalenat H 1991 Progesterone receptor detection and quantification in breast tumours by bivariate immunofluorescence/DNA flow cytometry. Cytometry 12: 157–166

Riccardi A, Danova M, Dionigi P et al 1989 Cell kinetics in leukaemia and solid tumours with in vivo bromodeoxyuridine and flow cytometry. Br J Cancer 59: 898–903

Robertson F M, Gilmour S K, Beavis A J et al 1990 Flow cytometric detection of ornithine decarboxylase activity in epidermal cell subpopulations. Cytometry 11: 832–836

Rose G S, Tocco L M, Granger G A et al 1996 Development and characterization of a clinically useful animal model of epithelial ovarian cancer in the Fisher 344 rat. Am J Obstet Gynecol 175: 593–539

Rosette C D, DeTeresa P S, Pallavicini M G 1990 Simultaneous flow cytometric detection of cellular c-myc protein incorporated bromodeoxyuridine and DNA. Cytometry 11: 547–551

Roza A, Bhayana R, Ukar K, Kirshnin J, Preisler H 1985 Difference between labelling index and DNA histograms in assessing S-phase cells from a homogeneous group of chronic phase CML patients. Cytometry 6: 445–451

Sahni K, Tribukait B, Einhorn N 1990 Development of ploidy and cell proliferation in serial samples of ascites from patients with ovarian carcinoma. Acta Oncol 29: 193–197

Shapiro H M 1988 Practical flow cytometry, 1st edn. New York: Alan R Liss, 1–45

Sherwood S W, Assaraf Y G, Molina A, Schimke R T 1990 Flow cytometric characterisation of antifolate resistance in cultured mammalian cells using fluoresceinated methotrexate and daunorubicin. Cancer Res 50: 4946–4950

Slocum H, Pavelic Z, Rostum Y et al 1983 Characterization of cells obtained by mechanical and enzymatic means from human melanoma, sarcoma and lung tumor. Cancer Res 41: 1428–1434

Steele-Mortimer O A, Meier-Ewert H, Loser R, Hasmann M J 1990 Flow cytometric analysis of virus-infected cells and its potential use for screening of antiviral agents. J Virol Methods 27: 241–252

Steen H B 1990 Characteristics of flow cytometers. In: Melamed M R, Lindmo T, Mendelsohn M L (eds) Flow cytometry and sorting. New York: Wiley-Liss, 1–10

Valet G, Russmann V 1984 Automated flow cytometric identification of colo-rectal tumour cells by simultaneous DNA, CEA-antibody and cell volume measurements. J Clin Chem Clin Biochem 22: 935–942

van Dam P A, Lowe D G, Watson J V, Chard T, Shepherd J H 1992 Comparative evaluation of fresh, fixed and cryopreserved human solid tumor cells for reliable flow cytometry of fresh DNA and tumour associated antigen. Cytometry 13: 722–729

van Dam P A, Lowe D G, Watson J V, Jobling T, Chard T, Shepherd J H 1991 Multiparameter flow cytometric quantitation of the expression of the tumor associated antigen SM3 in normal and neoplastic ovarian tissues. A comparison with HMFG1 and HMFG2. Cancer 68: 169–177 van Dam P A, Lowe D G, Watson J V, Shepherd J H 1995 Multiparameter flow cytometric measurement of epidermal growth factor receptor and c-erbB-2 oncoprotein in cultured cells and fresh and preserved solid tumor cells. Int J Gynecol Cancer 5: 20–28

van Dam P A, Watson J V, Lowe D G, Cox H, Curling O M, Shepherd J H 1990 Tissue preparation for simultaneous flow cytometric quantitation of tumour associated antigens and DNA in solid tumours. J Clin Pathol 43: 833–839

van Dam P A, Watson J V, Lowe D G, Shepherd J H 1992 Flow cytometric measurement of cell components other then DNA: virtues limitations and applications in gynaecological oncology. Obstet Gynecol 79: 616–621

van Dam P A, Watson J V, Lowe D G, Shepherd J H 1992 Flow cytometric DNA analysis in gynaecological oncology: a review of the literature. Int J Gynecol Cancer 2: 57–65

Vindelov L L, Christensen I J, Nissen N I 1983a A detergent-trypsin method for the preparation of nuclei for flow cytometric DNA analysis. Cytometry 3: 323–327

Vindelov L L, Christensen I J, Jensen G, Nissen N I 1983b Limits of detection of nuclear DNA abnormalities by flow cytometric DNA analysis. Results obtained by a set of methods for sample storage, staining and internal standardization. Cytometry 3: 332–339

Vindolov L L, Cristensen I J, Keiding N, Spang-Thomson M, Nissen N I 1982 Long-term storage of samples for flow cytometric DNA analysis. Cytometry 3: 317–322

Volm M, Efferth T 1990 Relationship of DNA ploidy to chemoresistance of tumours as measured by in vitro tests. Cytometry 11: 406–410

Walker R A, Camplejohn R S 1988 Comparison of monoclonal antibody Ki-67 reactivity with grade and DNA flow cytometry in breast carcinoma. Br J Cancer 57: 281–283

Watson J V 1991 Practical flow cytometry, 1st edn., Oxford: Blackwells

Watson J V, Curling O M, Munn C F, Hudson C N 1987 Oncogene expression in ovarian cancer: a pilot study of c-myc oncoprotein in serous papillary ovarian cancer. Gynecol Oncol 28: 137–150

Watson J V, Sikora K E, Evan G I 1985 A simultaneous flow cytometric assay for c-myc oncoprotein and cellular DNA in nuclei from paraffin embedded material. J Immunol Methods 83: 179–192

Watson J V, Stewart J, Evan G, Ritson A. Sikora K 1986 The clinical significance of flow cytometric c-myc oncoprotein quantitation in testicular cancer. Br J Cancer 53: 331–337

Watson J V, Walport M J 1986 Molecular calibration in flow cytometry with sub-attogram detection limit. J Immunol Methods 93: 171–175

Rodolfo Montironi   Deborah Thompson   Peter H. Bartels

Premalignant lesions of the prostate

For pathologists and urologists there are currently two main issues in prostate pathology. One is the identification of the prognostic factors that predict the outcome of individual patients with prostatic carcinoma (PCa): the goal is to tailor the therapeutic approach to the clinical, morphological and biological features of the case. The other involves the early detection of PCa in the pre-invasive phase; understanding the biology of pre-invasive or precursor lesions has, therefore, become increasingly important. Prostatic intra-epithelial neoplasia is only one of these lesions and is the best known. The role of others, such as atypical adenomatous hyperplasia, is worth exploring (Montironi & Schulman 1996).

PROSTATIC INTRA-EPITHELIAL NEOPLASIA: A PRECURSOR OF ADENOCARCINOMA

Prostatic intra-epithelial neoplasia (PIN) is the precursor of adenocarcinoma originating from the ducts and acini, particularly those of the peripheral zone, of the prostate gland. The morphological continuum that results in early invasive adenocarcinoma is now divided into two grades – low-grade and high-grade – replacing the previous three grade system; PIN1 is considered low grade, and PIN2 and PIN3 are considered high-grade. High-grade PIN has morphological, immunohistochemical, molecular and morphometric features similar to prostatic adenocarcinoma (Bostwick 1996; Fig. 8.1). PIN retains an intact or fragmented basal cell layer, unlike cancer which lacks a basal cell layer. A recent consensus group determined that a small subset of basal cell

Dr Rodolfo Montironi, Institute of Pathological Anatomy and Histopathology, School of Medicine, University of Ancona, Azienda Sanitaria 'Umberto 1º', Via Conca, I-60020 Torrette di Ancona, Italy
Ms Deborah Thompson, Optical Sciences Center, University of Arizona, Tucson, AZ 85721, USA
Prof. Peter H. Bartels, Optical Sciences Center, University of Arizona, Tucson, AZ 85721, USA

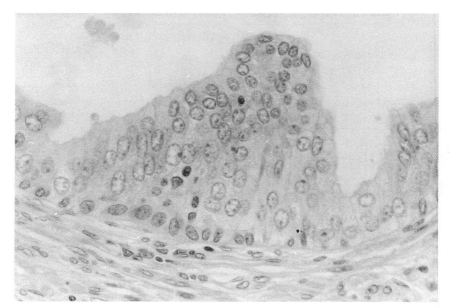

Fig. 8.1 High-grade prostatic intra-epithelial neoplasia.

layer houses the stem cell population. These cells are the presumptive origin of PIN and prostatic adenocarcinoma (Montironi & Schulman 1996).

The clinical importance of recognising PIN is based on its association with prostatic adenocarcinoma. High grade PIN has a high predictive value as a marker for carcinoma, and its identification in biopsy specimens warrants further search for synchronous invasive cancer. The risk of adenocarcinoma in subsequent biopsies is 15 times greater in patients with high-grade PIN. Studies to date have not determined whether PIN remains stable, regresses or progresses, though the implication is that it can progress (Bostwick 1996).

Biopsy is the definitive method for detecting PIN and early invasive cancer, but noninvasive methods are being evaluated. By transrectal ultrasound (TRUS), PIN may be hypo-echoic and, therefore, indistinguishable from carcinoma, though these findings have been disputed. TRUS-directed biopsy permits localisation of the needle and tissue being sampled. Repeat biopsy is indicated if the first attempt is unrevealing. Serum PSA may be elevated in patients with PIN, though this probably results from co-existing cancer. If all procedures fail to identify cancer, close surveillance and follow-up are indicated (Montironi & Schulman 1996).

CELL PROLIFERATION, DEATH AND DIFFERENTIATION IN PIN

The progression from PIN to PCa is a complex process in which the kinetic organisation of the normal prostate epithelium is altered. In fact, the regulation of the stem cells and of the lineages derived from them as well as the homeostatic control between proliferative and non-proliferative behaviour are disrupted, leading to expansion of the cell proliferating compartment due to increased cell proliferation, or decreased cell death, or a combination of both

Table 8.1 Proliferation and apoptotic markers in prostatic intra-epithelial neoplasia

Marker	Method	Results	Reference
PCNA	Immunohistochemistry	Upregulation from NP to PIN and adenocarcinoma	Montironi et al 1993a
Mitotic figures	Microscopic counting	Upregulation from NP to PIN and adenocarcinoma	Giannulis et al 1993
Apoptotic bodies	Microscopic counting	Upregulation from NP to PIN and adenocarcinoma	Montironi et al 1994
bcl-2	Immunohistochemistry	Upregulation from BPH to PIN and adenocarcinoma	Colombel et al 1993

PCNA, proliferating cell nuclear antigen; NP, normal prostate; BPH, benign prostatic hyperplasia; PIN, prostatic intra-epithelial neoplasia.

(Colombel et al 1993, Montironi et al 1993a; Table 8.1). This depends on several factors, including hormonal status and growth factor milieu.

Cell proliferation

In some studies, cell proliferation has been determined in prostate tissue by evaluating the frequency and location of proliferating cell nuclear antigen (PCNA) (Montironi et al 1993a). Results similar to those observed with PCNA have been obtained with other proliferation markers such as MIB-1 and Ki-67 and with DNA static cytometry as well as by analyses of mitoses and silver-stained nucleolar organiser regions (AgNORs) (Bostwick et al 1996).

The frequency of PCNA-positive nuclei in PIN lesions is higher than in normal prostate and close to the values in PCa, revealing that the epithelial proliferating fractions are progressively greater from normal prostate through PIN to PCa (Montironi et al 1993a). In normal prostate, only the nuclei in the basal position express PCNA. In fact, the basal cell layer of prostate ducts and acini, which contains cells able to divide or dividing, includes the proliferative compartment. The luminal layer, which is unable to proliferate because it contains post-mitotic maturing and mature cells, is the differentiated compartment. PIN lesions show PCNA-positive nuclei in all the cell layers, though the proportion of positive nuclei decreases towards the lumen because the cells acquire some degree of differentiation. This indicates that cells able to proliferate appear in all cell layers of PIN and PCa, thus resulting in the expansion of the proliferative compartment (Montironi et al 1994).

Cell death (apoptosis)

The frequency of apoptotic bodies (ABs) increases from normal prostate through PIN to PCa. The increased frequency of apoptotic bodies from normal prostate to PCa parallels that observed with PCNA immunostaining (Montironi et al 1993c, Montironi et al 1994). However, the apoptotic body-related values are approximately an eighth to a tenth of those obtained in the PCNA study. In PIN, apoptotic bodies are present in all cell layers, including

Table 8.2 Differentiation markers in prostatic intra-epithelial neoplasia

Marker	Method	Results (% positive)	Reference
Neuroendocrine cells	Immunohisto-chemistry	Downregulation in high-grade PIN and adenocarcinoma	Bostwick et al 1994
PSA	Immunohisto-chemistry	Downregulation in high-grade PIN	McNeal et al 1991
Telomerase	PCR	Upregulation in high-grade PIN and adenocarcinoma	Kim et al 1994
AR gene	PCR	Upregulation in mets	Taplin et al 1995
AR	Immunohisto-chemistry	No AR gene mutations in hormone-refractory adenocarcinoma	Ruizeveld et al 1994
Type IV collagenase	mmunohisto-Ichemistry/ISH	Upregulation from BPH to high-grade PIN and adenocarcinoma	Boag et al 1993
C-CAM	Immunohisto-chemistry	Decreased in BPH and PIN; absent in adenocarcinoma	Kleinerman et al 1995
Cathepsin B	Immunohisto-chemistry	Upregulation in adeno-carcinoma; correlation with grade	Sinha et al 1995
Cathepsin D	Immunohisto-chemistry	Benign usually negative; upregulation with adenocarcinoma	Makar et al 1994
Cathepsin D	Immunohisto-chemistry	Benign usually negative; upregulation in high-grade PIN and adenocarcinoma	Maygarden et al 1994
Cathepsin D	Immunohisto-chemistry	Correlates with cancer grade and DNA ploidy, but not stage	Ross et al 1995
Lewis Y antigen	Immunohisto-chemistry	Benign usually negative; PIN 88%; adenocarcinoma 100%	Myers et al 1995
GST-Pi	Immunohisto-chemistry/blot	Benign 100%; PIN and adenocarcinoma much lower	Lee et al 1994
E-Cadherin	Immunohisto-chemistry	Downregulated in mets	Umbas et al 1994
E-Cadherin	Northern and Southern blot analysis	Downregulated in high-grade adenocarcinoma	Morton et al 1993
MMP-9	Zymography	Expression in 64% with bone mets	Hamdy et al 1994

PSA, prostate-specific antigen; AR androgen receptor; PCR, polymerase chain reaction; ISH, in situ hybridization; blot, blotting; BPH, benign prostatic hyperplasia; PIN, prostatic intra-epithelial neoplasia; mets, metastases; GST, glutatione-S-transferase; CAM, cell adhesion molecule.

the luminal, the frequency decreasing progressively towards the lumen. The results of the location of the apoptotic bodies parallel those related to PCNA. This means that the location of apoptotic bodies basically corresponds to the extension of the proliferative compartment, which may be the main site of apoptotic body production and/or accumulation.

Histologically, some apoptotic bodies are seen in intercellular spaces, some in the cytoplasm of epithelial cells and some in the lumen where the apoptotic bodies appear in the cytoplasm of macrophages. The relation of apoptotic bodies with viable cells may indicate how apoptotic bodies are eliminated: ABs are dispersed from their site of origin along intercellular spaces; some of those arising in epithelia are extruded into the lumen, but most are phagocytosed and degraded by the adjoining cells; epithelial cells as well as cells of the mononuclear phagocytic system participate in this disposal.

Apoptosis has also been investigated with other techniques such as the terminal deoxynucleotide transferase-mediated dUTP-digoxigenin (or dUTP-biotin) nick end-labelling (or TUNEL) procedure which detects *in situ* DNA strand breaks in cells undergoing apoptosis. The results are comparable to those obtained with the evaluation of the apoptotic bodies by light microscopy.

The increasing occurrence of apoptosis in PIN and PCa may depend on intrinsic mechanisms of growth control, abnormal cell division and abnormalities in DNA content. The apoptotic phenomenon may in part be linked to abnormally dividing epithelial cells in PIN and PCa, thus resulting in the formation of apoptotic bodies (El-Labban et al 1986). Colombel et al (1992) identified a defective cell cycle leading to apoptosis in the prostate gland experimentally. Alternatively, the apoptotic phenomenon could also be one way to eliminate genetically aberrant cells or cells with serious abnormalities in DNA content, resulting from either abnormal mitotic division or genotoxicity due to an unknown agent (Falkvoll 1990).

Cell differentiation

The differentiated compartment is partly obscured in PIN because the cells show a defective expression of differentiation markers (Bostwick et al 1996; Table 8.2). Virtually all studies of differentiation markers indicate that high-grade PIN is more closely related to carcinoma than to benign epithelium. Many markers are downregulated with increasing grades of PIN and cancer, including markers of secretory differentiation, such as prostatic acid phosphatase and prostate-specific antigen (PSA). Reduction of some cytoplasmic differentiation markers during the pre-invasive phase may be followed by abrupt re-expression at the site of invasion. Other secretory products are upregulated in PIN and adenocarcinoma, including estramustine binding protein, oestrogen-inducible protein pS2, glycoprotein A-80, fatty acid synthase, and Lewis X and Lewis Y antigens (Brawer et al 1994, Myers et al 1995).

MOLECULAR PATHOLOGY OF PIN

Peptide growth factors appear to control development of normal and neoplastic prostatic epithelium by acting as autocrine or paracrine mediators of epithelial-stromal interaction and growth (Table 8.3). Most studies to date have focused on the families of peptides associated with epidermal growth factor (EGF) and transforming growth factor (TGF) (for review see Bostwick et al 1996). The EGF family of peptides and associated oncoproteins includes EGF, TGF-α and other factors that influence mitogenesis through the same transmembrane glycoprotein receptor and tyrosine kinase. EGF is expressed weakly in benign epithelium and PIN and may be upregulated in cancer, although results are contradictory (Myers et al 1993). Conversely, EGF receptor

Table 8.3 Growth factors and related receptors in prostatic intra-epithelial neoplasia

Marker	Method	Results (% positive)	Reference
EGF	Immunohisto-chemistry/ISH	Upregulation from BPH to high-grade PIN and adenocarcinoma	Turkeri et al 1994
EGFR	Immunohisto-chemistry	Downregulation from BPH to high-grade PIN and adenocarcinoma	Robertson et al 1994
EGFR	ISH	Downregulation from BPH to high-grade PIN and adenocarcinoma	Montone et al 1993
EGFR	Immunohisto-chemistry/ISH	Downregulation from BPH to high-grade PIN and adenocarcinoma	Turkeri et al 1994
EGFR	Immunohisto-chemistry	Downregulation from BPH to high-grade PIN and adenocarcinoma	Maygarden et al 1994
EGFR	Immunohisto-chemistry	Downregulation from BPH to high-grade PIN and adenocarcinoma	Ibrahim et al 1993
TGF-α	Immunohisto-chemistry/ISH	Upregulation from BPH to high-grade PIN and adenocarcinoma	Turkeri et al 1994
TGF-α	Immunohisto-chemistry	Downregulation from BPH to high-grade PIN and adenocarcinoma	Robertson et al 1994
TGF-α	Immunohisto-chemistry	Upregulation from BPH to high-grade PIN and adenocarcinoma	Myers et al 1995
c-erbβ-2/B-3	Immunohisto-chemistry	Upregulation from BPH to high-grade PIN and adenocarcinoma	Myers et al 1994
c-erbβ-2	Immunohisto-chemistry	Upregulation from PIN to adenocarcinoma	Ibrahim et al 1992

EGF, epidermal growth factor; EGFR, epidermal growth factor receptor; TGF, transforming growth factor; PCR, polymerase chain reaction; ISH, in situ hybridization; BPH, benign prostatic hyperplasia; PIN, prostatic intra-epithelial neoplasia.

is downregulated in PIN and cancer (Maddy et al 1989). Overexpression of p160[erbB-3] and p185[erbB-3] reflects an increase in cellular proliferative activity (Myers et al 1994). The transforming growth factor-β (TGF-β) family of peptides, including TGF-β1 and TGF-β2, appears to regulate cell proliferation and differentiation. Expression of the TGF-β receptor appears to be under negative androgen regulation, suggesting that it plays a role in cell death as a consequence of androgen deprivation (Thompson et al 1985).

Mitogen-activated protein (MAP) kinases are key elements of the signalling systems that transduce different extracellular messages into cellular responses. At least three parallel MAP kinase pathways have been identified (Loda et al 1996). One, stimulated by serum and growth factors to activate extracellular signal-regulated protein kinases (ERKs) by dual tyrosine and threonine phosphorylation, triggers cell proliferation or differentiation; the other two, induced by a variety of cellular stresses to activate c-jun N-terminal kinases (JNKs) and re-activating kinase (p38/RK), result in growth arrest and induction of apoptosis. Mitogen-activated protein kinase phosphatases (MKPs) inactivate MAP kinases through dephosphorylation and so can modulate the MAP kinase pathways.

Overexpression of three MAP kinases (JNK-1, ERK-1 and p38/RK) and MKP-1 mRNA has been found in all cases of high-grade PIN compared with normal prostate. Immunoreactivity for MKP-1 protein has been found to be as intense as in normal glands or weaker in 30% and 56% of the PIN cases, respectively. Of PIN cases, 14% do not stain with MKP-1 antibody. The proportion of apoptosis is significantly higher in PIN lesions which do not express MKP-1 protein than in those that do express this protein. According to Magi-Galluzzi et al (1998), these data support the contention that MKP-1, even in PIN, may shift the balance between cell proliferation and death by inhibiting pathways leading to apoptosis.

Unlike other oncogenes that influence cell proliferation rates or differentiation, the *bcl-2* gene suppresses apoptosis and increases the length of survival of cells. Overexpression of *bcl-2* is observed in PIN and cancer compared with normal prostatic tissue. Colombel et al (1993) speculated that *bcl-2* expression might play a role in the progression of PIN and low-grade cancer by interfering with apoptosis, thus resulting in accumulation of genetic abnormalities.

The *p53* gene and its protein products play a critical role in cell cycle check points that control cell growth and differentiation. Mutations of the suppressor gene *p53* have been found only in a minority of cases of early prostate cancer and apparently participate in later stages of prostatic carcinogenesis (Batsakis et al 1995). According to most reports, the retinoblastoma gene and its protein products do not appear to participate in the early stages of prostatic carcinogenesis (Brooks et al 1995).

Recent studies reveal consistent downregulation of epithelial cell adhesion molecules and transmembrane proteins in prostatic carcinogenesis (Bostwick et al 1996). The expression of C-CAM, a cell adhesion molecule from the immunoglobulin gene family, is decreased in PIN and cancer, suggesting that it is a tumour suppressor gene (Kleinerman et al 1995). Similarly, the calcium-dependent cell–cell adhesion molecule E-cadherin is downregulated in prostate cancer. Loss of expression of this transmembrane glycoprotein reflects loss of epithelial integrity. The function of E-cadherin is regulated by a group of protein called catenins, which couple the cadherin molecule to the microfilament cytoskeleton (Morton et al 1993, Umbas et al 1994). Mutational inactivation or deletion of the α-catenin gene is another mechanism that results in loss of normal cell–cell adhesion in prostate carcinogenesis. A variety of hemidesmosomal proteins and related proteins are present in PIN, and not in PCa, including integrin α4β6, laminin γ2 and type VII collagen. These findings indicate that the composition and cellular attachments of the basement membrane in prostate cancer are abnormal. Downregulation of epithelial cell adhesion molecules in PIN and cancer is accompanied by upregulation of many of the enzymes for degradation of the extracellular matrix, including matrix metalloproteinases and type IV collagenases (Boag & Young 1993).

QUANTITATIVE MORPHOLOGY OF PIN

McNeal and Bostwick (1986) observed that PIN is characterised by proliferation and anaplasia of the secretory cells of pre-existing ducts and acini. The changes are based on the subjective evaluation of cytological, architectural and associated features.

Premalignant lesions of the prostate

Secretory cell changes in PIN

There are several studies in which the features above are quantitatively evaluated in histological sections (Montironi et al 1992, Petein et al 1991). The data reported show that quantitation analyses help to define some traditional morphological features better. These can be defined objectively because the changes are represented by numbers and not by the subjective evaluation of morphological clues. Second, quantitation analyses help to identify subtle abnormalities. Take, for example, nucleoli. The nucleolar size and frequency are objectively defined in numerical terms. Moreover, the degree of nucleolar margination is a new diagnostic feature, easily evaluated as the proportion of nucleoli touching the nuclear membrane. Even though not included in the original list of features identified by McNeal & Bostwick (1986), marginated nucleoli have already been marked in the original diagram by Bostwick and Brawer (1987). Thirdly, quantitation analyses provide useful insights into the understanding of some of the morphological changes, such as nuclear enlargement. The changes in nuclear DNA content and in chromatin distribution and pattern (see also below under 'Malignancy-associated changes') could contribute to the explanation of nuclear enlargement. In particular, the incidence of aneuploidy in high-grade PIN varies from 32–68%, somewhat lower than in carcinoma, which shows aneuploidy in 55–63% of cases (Amin et al 1993, Berner et al 1993, Crissman et al 1993, Montironi et al 1990, Weinberg & Weidner 1993). About 70% of aneuploid cases of high-grade PIN are associated with aneuploid carcinoma, but only 29% of cases of aneuploid cancer are associated with aneuploid PIN (Baretton et al 1994).

The changes in the DNA content and chromatin texture can be related to chromosomal changes such as loss of heterozygosity and chromosome gains (Alers et al 1995, Emmert-Buck et al 1995, Qian et al 1995, Takahashi et al 1994; Table 8.4). Allelic loss is common in high-grade PIN and prostate cancer. Using novel microdissection techniques, Emmert-Buck et al (1995) described loss of heterozygosity for 8p12-21 in 64% of foci of high-grade PIN and 91% of carcinomas, compared with 0% in normal prostate. Sakr and colleagues (1994) have found allelic loss of 8p, 10q, and 16q in 29% of cases of high-grade PIN and 42% of primary cancers. Qian et al (1995), using centromere-specific probes for fluorescence *in situ* hybridisation (FISH) directed against chromosomes 7, 8, 10, 12 and Y, have found an equal overall frequency of numeric chromosomal anomalies in foci of high-grade PIN and prostate cancer (50% and 51%, respectively), suggesting that these foci are pathogenetically linked. Gain on chromosome 8 is the most frequent numerical anomaly in high-grade PIN and PCa. Gain on the chromosome 8 centromere has been shown by FISH, and loss of portions of the 8 p-arm by PCR in specimens of high-grade PIN and carcinoma, suggesting that alterations of this chromosome may be important for the initiation or early progression of prostate cancer (Emmert-Buck et al 1995). The frequency of trisomy 7 is higher in carcinoma than in high-grade PIN, suggesting that gain of chromosome 7 may play a role in the progression of PIN to PCa (Greene et al 1994).

Architectural changes of the ducts and acini with PIN

PIN is associated with changes in the basal cell layer, as shown immuno-histochemically with a basal cell-specific monoclonal antibody directed against

Table 8.4 Loss of heterozygosity and other chromosomal changes in prostatic intra-epithelial neoplasia

Chromosome	Method	Results (% positive)	Reference
8p, 10q, 12p, 16q	PCR	*8p22:* benign, 0%; high-grade PIN, 29%; primary adenocarcinoma, 29%; *10q11.2-qter:* benign, 0%; high-grade PIN, 25%; primary adenocarcinoma, 18%; *12pter-p12:* benign, 0%; high-grade PIN, 20%; primary adenocarcinoma, 42%; *16q22.1:* benign, 0%; high-grade PIN, 0%; primary adenocarcinoma, 0%	Sakr et al 1994
8p12-21	PCR	*Benign,* LOH in 0%; high-grade PIN, LOH in 64%; adenocarcinoma, LOH in 91%	Emmert-Buck et al 1995
Y	ISH	*High-grade PIN,* LOH in 8%; adenocarcinoma, LOH in 8%	Alers et al 1995
7q31.1	Multiplex PCR	*Adenocarcinoma,* LOH in 28%, gain in 2%	Takahashi et al 1994
7, 8, 10, 12, Y	FISH	*High-grade PIN:* gain of chromosome 8 in 32%, 10 in 13%, 7 in 10%, 12 in 4% and Y in 4% *Adenocarcinoma:* gain of chromosome 8 in 30%, 7 in 28%, 12 in 9% and Y in 9%	Qian et al 1995

PCR, polymerase chain reaction; ISH, in situ hybridization; FISH, fluorescence in situ hybridization; LOH, loss of heterozygosity; PIN, prostatic intra-epithelial neoplasia.

high molecular weight keratin (34βE12 antikeratin monoclonal antibody). Morphologically, basal cell layer disruption is present in 56% of cases of high-grade PIN (Bostwick & Brawer 1987), and is more common in glands adjacent to PCa than in distant glands. The amount of disruption increases with increasing grades of PIN, with abnormality of more than one-third of the basal cell layer in 52% of foci of high-grade PIN. Early invasive PCa occurs at sites of glandular outpouching and basal cell loss. Tumour cells consistently fail to find this antibody whereas normal prostatic epithelium is invariably stained with a continuous and intact circumferential basal cell layer.

Morphological observation alone does not permit accurate measurement of the distance between basal cells and, therefore, quantitation of the amount of basal cell layer disruption. This problem has been addressed by the Machine Vision in Pathology project under development at the Optical Sciences Center, University of Arizona. The scope of the project is to bring objective assessment to conventional diagnostic criteria and concepts in premalignant and malignant prostatic lesions.

Images of whole glands of normal prostate, low-grade PIN and high-grade PIN have been digitised. The images have been processed by a Machine Vision system, automatically segmented and a number of histometric characteristics of the deterioration of the basal cell layer have been derived (Bartels et al 1998b): (i) degree of enclosure expressed as a percentage, i.e. how much of the duct is represented by the basal cell layer; (ii) number and length of gaps in the basal cell layer; (iii) basal cell layer thickness and variance; (iv) epithelial lining thickness and variance; (v) ratio of the secretory cell area to the basal cell layer

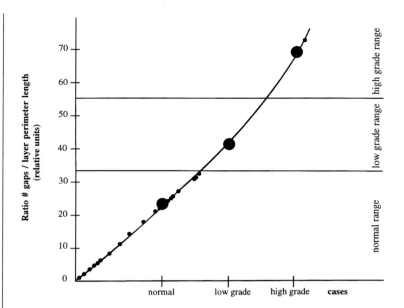

Fig. 8.2 Trend in the histometric variable 'proportion of gland perimeter covered by basal cell layer' as a function of PIN lesion progression.

component area (this feature together with the previous represents the degree of stratification of the epithelial lining, and, in particular, of the secretory cell component); and (vi) crowding index of the secretory cell component.

The histometric characterisation of the deterioration of the basal cell layer has shown changes related to the progression of PIN. In particular, Figure 8.2 shows the results derived from the number of gaps in the basal cell layer relative to the gland perimeter length, plotted over the progression of PIN lesions. There is an almost linear relation. This histometric index could serve as a measure of lesion progression, or regression following intervention. In the same project, high resolution images of nuclei still facing, or no longer facing intact segments of the basal cell layer have been recorded and karyometrically analysed. The degree of deterioration of the basal cell layer is accompanied by statistically highly significant changes in the chromatin texture and spatial distribution in secretory cell nuclei no longer facing an intact segment of that layer.

Stromal changes associated with PIN

The interaction of the stroma and epithelium probably plays a critical role in prostate carcinogenesis. Substantial changes occur in the stroma around ducts and acini with PIN and PCa, including angiogenesis.

Angiogenesis, a prerequisite for normal growth and development (Montironi et al 1996b), is a complex process involving interactions between endothelial cells, tumour cells, tumour infiltrating leukocytes and extracellular matrix. In particular, the background biology of angiogenesis is represented by five main stages (Folkman & Shing 1992): (i) activation of endothelium; (ii) destruction of stroma and capillary basement membrane by proteolytic enzymes, including type IV collagenase; (iii) endothelial cell proliferation; (iv) migration of endothelial cells towards the angiogenic stimulus; and (v) formation of patent capillaries. Abnormal angiogenesis is a critical feature of many diseases including malignant tumours and their precursors, such as prostate cancer and PIN (Folkman 1992, Montironi et al 1993c).

The expression of type IV collagenase (72 kDa metalloproteinase, MMP-2) is seen as cytoplasmic staining in epithelial cells and to a lesser extent in stromal cells, which showed weak to moderate immunoreactivity. MMP-2 immunostaining increases progressively from normal prostate, through PIN, to invasive adenocarcinoma (Montironi et al 1996c; Weidner et al 1993). In some areas, endothelial cells lining capillaries are weakly to moderately immunopositive indicating that this type of cell can also express MMP-2. This finding is in keeping with studies in colorectal neoplasia (Poulson et al 1992) and breast cancer and gives further support to the concept that destruction of stroma and capillary basement membrane are needed to permit the migration of capillary endothelial cells. In their study on proliferation, basement membrane changes, metastasis and vascularisation patterns in human breast cancer, Verhoeven and Van Marck (1993) came to a similar conclusion.

The percentage of PCNA-stained nuclei in endothelial cells is much lower than in epithelial cells in the prostate. The lowest values are seen in prostatic atrophic ducts and acini and in normal prostate. The highest values are seen in invasive PCa. The percentage of PCNA-stained nuclei in the stroma is lower than in the epithelial component but slightly higher than in the endothelium (Montironi et al 1996c). The PCNA-related data obtained in the capillary endothelial cells indicate that endothelial cell proliferation in the precursors of adenocarcinoma is as high as in capillary endothelium in invasive malignancy.

The quantitative investigation of the capillary architecture shows that, going from normal prostate through PIN to invasive PCa, an increasing proportion of capillaries becomes shorter, with open lumina and undulating contours and with a greater number of endothelial cells. The highest proportion of touching capillaries is seen in the normal prostate, while the lowest is in invasive PCa, being intermediate in PIN (Table 8.5). When the PIN samples are divided into low-grade and high-grade, the feature values in the low-grade approaches those in normal prostate, whereas in the high-grade they are close to invasive adenocarcinoma.

These studies show that the preneoplastic and neoplastic lesions of the human prostate are associated with increasing qualitative and quantitative changes in the capillary architecture (Montironi et al 1993b). Vascularisation may be an essential requirement for the development of PIN, such as is true for invasive adenocarcinoma, or may be a consequence of factors arising in PIN. Understanding the events controlling angiogenesis could enable new therapeutic approaches to prevent neoplastic progression as well as to induce regression of cancers and their precursors.

STATISTICAL CLASSIFICATION OF PIN

PIN comprises a continuum of nuclear and cytoplasmic abnormalities in the cells lining prostatic ducts and acini (Bostwick 1996). In its most severe expression, dysplasia produces cells which are individually indistinguishable

Table 8.5 Microvessel density in prostatic intra-epithelial neoplasia

Marker	Method	Results	Reference
Microvessels	Lectin binding	Upregulation from NP to PIN and adenocarcinoma	Montironi et al 1996b
Microvessels	Immunohisto-chemistry	Upregulation from BPH to PIN and adenocarcinoma	Sinha et al 1995
Microvessels	Immunohisto-chemistry	Upregulation from NP to PIN and adenocarcinoma	Bigler et al 1993

NP, normal prostate; BPH, benign prostatic hyperplasia; PIN, prostatic intra-epithelial neoplasia.

from those of invasive carcinoma. Do classifications based on statistical analyses of quantitative data support the concept of the continuity of morphological abnormalities? Linear discriminant analysis, a procedure used to assign objects to categories, has been applied to quantitative data. This is based on analysis of cases assigned to agreed categories and gives rise to a rule (the canonical discriminant function, CDF) that serves as the basis for classifying further cases into one of the categories. One of the advantages of linear discriminant analysis is that only a small selection of features that best represents the lesions is included in the calculation of the CDF scores. Each PIN lesion is represented by only two CDF values or scores which summarise the information on quantitation (Montironi et al 1991).

The plot of the two CDFs shows the separation achieved between the diagnostic categories and gives an idea of the spatial distribution of the samples (Fig. 8.3). CDF1 shows that normal prostate, PIN and invasive PCa appear as contiguous categories, with some overlap, mainly between PIN and PCa. On the other hand, CDF2 shows that from normal prostate through PIN to PCa the samples become more scattered. This could be interpreted as an increasing variability among the samples in the higher categories. Moreover, the area occupied by the PIN samples in the scatterplot of Figure 8.3 can be divided into two parts (indicated by the interrupted line) separating the low grade PIN samples (closer to the normal prostate samples) from high grade PIN (closer to PCa samples). Therefore, quantitation analyses, when associated with advanced statistics, graphically confirm the concept of the continuum of abnormalities (Montironi et al 1990).

From the practical point of view, histological grading of PIN is important. Originally three grades were adopted, though Helpap suggested four (1980). A two-grade system was always preferred, on the basis of cluster analysis. This multivariate method can be used when the number of categories and criteria for membership of each category are unknown for all cases, and may identify homogeneous categories on the basis of their similarities.

Hierarchical and non-hierarchical clustering methods give similar results: cases of low-grade PIN are clustered with normal prostate cases, whereas high-grade PIN clusters with PCa (Montironi et al 1991). This corresponds to the morphological observation that low-grade PIN is closer to normal prostate whereas high-grade PIN is closer to PCa. The results obtained with cluster

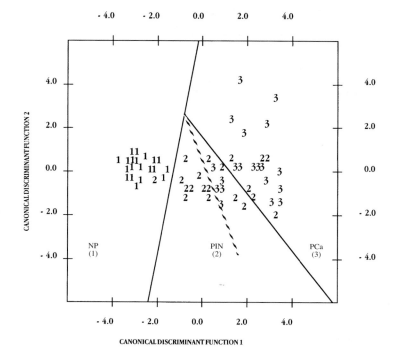

Fig. 8.3 Scatterplot of the spatial distribution of the cases of normal prostate (NP), prostatic intra-epithelial neoplasia (PIN) and invasive adenocarcinoma (PCa). The cases appear as continuous categories with overlap mainly between PIN and PCa. The two lines divide the scatterplot into the three categories. The part corresponding to PIN can be subdivided into two parts (interrupted line), separating the low-grade PIN (close to the NP) from high-grade PIN (close to PCa). Reproduced with permission from Montironi et al, 1990.

analysis confirm the report by Drago et al (1989) in which the Bethesda Workshop Investigators agreed on a grading system that described low and high-grade PIN by incorporating the previous grades 2 and 3 into the high-grade. The two-grade system is probably preferable to three or four grades because the two PIN grades reflect the current understanding of premalignant or pre-invasive malignant lesions in different organs where two contiguous grades are identified.

It has been argued that diagnostic pathology is based on identification rather than classification (Bartels et al 1997). Statistical classification is constrained by the fact that it operates in a closed system: classification is based only on a limited number of features. In contrast, diagnostic identification functions in an open system in which many features can be assessed simultaneously and lack of data on one feature might stimulate a search for information on other features.

In prostatic pathology, the weighting of individual features is allowed to vary depending on available information. This approach can be readily applied to **descriptive** data through the use of methods such as Bayesian belief networks, but could be difficult to model mathematically for the assessment of **quantitative** data.

DIAGNOSTIC DECISION SUPPORT SYSTEMS

Diagnostic decision support systems (DDSSs) can be applied to prostate histopathology to provide guidance in situations involving complex decision sequences. DDSSs are designed to result in a systematic, ordered, and exhaustive evaluation of evidence and to weight individual items of evidence as they are gathered to form the basis for a final decision. Most DDSSs provide a numeric measure of confidence in the final decision or diagnostic recommendation (Bartels et al 1995a). The decisive advantage of diagnostic DDSSs is the ability to process symbolic information, in contrast to systems limited to numerical information only, for which extensive analytical procedures are already well established. As much of the human knowledge and insight required for diagnostic and prognostic evaluations is in symbolic form – as concepts and linguistic terms – the new methodology opens the way for a systematic evaluation of evidence to provide diagnostic and prognostic support (Bartels et al 1995b). DDSSs may be implemented as inference networks (Bayesian belief networks) for assessment of uncertainty in PIN diagnosis and grading.

Bayesian belief network

The diagnosis and grading of PIN is difficult because its morphological appearances form a continuum of changes, ranging from lesions devoid of architectural and cytological atypia bordering on normal prostate to degrees of atypia that are typical of invasive carcinoma. As guidelines for the identification of PIN are established and the prognosis of patients with PIN becomes clear, accurate recognition and reporting of PIN will become essential.

Montironi et al (1995) attempted to standardise the morphological criteria for identification and grading of PIN through the use of a Bayesian belief network. This network is designed to distinguish between normal prostate, low-grade PIN, high-grade PIN, cribriform adenocarcinoma (i.e. Gleason primary grade 3C) and large acinar adenocarcinoma (i.e. Gleason primary grade 3A). The network consists of a single layer of evidence nodes supplying a single decision node. The relation among each feature and the diagnostic decision node is quantified as a conditional probability matrix.

Initially, the numeric response of this network was tested with prototype likelihood ratio vectors for each diagnostic. This variable has shown that not one of the diagnostic clues is capable by itself of identifying all five diagnostic alternatives. Normal prostate, low-grade PIN, high-grade PIN and cribriform adenocarcinoma are identified more than once by different diagnostic variables and all of the clues are useful in recognising large acinar adenocarcinoma. For all five diagnostic categories to be identified, at least two diagnostic variables must be assessed; secretory cell stratification and basal cell nuclear recognition are the strongest.

The network has recently been tested on a series of prostate lesions comprising normal prostate, PIN and adenocarcinoma. For the benign and malignant categories, the network has given high belief values, in general > 0.8, in favour of the respective groups. When considering lesions showing PIN, the network classified most of the cases with high certainty though there were some cases which showed equivocal belief values among the diagnostic groups (Fig. 8.4). This reflects the difficulties that pathologists face when

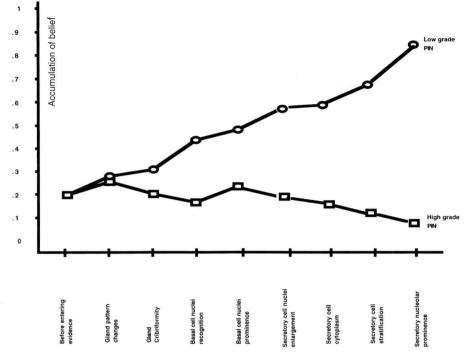

Fig. 8.4 The Bayesian belief network provides a useful quantitative measure of certainty in the diagnostic alternatives. The accumulation of belief for the low-grade PIN category (PINlow) and for high-grade PIN (PINhigh) is shown.

attempting to grade such lesions. However, the belief network provides a useful quantitative measure of certainty in the diagnostic alternatives.

The Bayesian belief network approach reported here reflects the way the pathologist behaves when making a diagnosis and applying a grading system. Several features are evaluated, selected and combined to support one of the alternatives. However, the belief in the alternatives cannot be quantitated. In contrast, the network provides a numeric value for the belief in the most appropriate diagnostic alternative (Hamilton et al 1995).

PIN AND CHEMOPREVENTION

The most desirable way of reducing the impact of cancer is prevention, provided this can be done with minimal risk or inconvenience. It follows that if PIN is indeed a precursor to invasive cancer then the elimination, retardation, or reduction of PIN would lead to a parallel reduction in cancer incidence. The chemoprevention of premalignant prostatic lesions such as PIN is a strategy designed to inhibit or reverse the process of carcinogenesis by administering one or more non-cytotoxic drugs.

A major pathway of chemoprevention unique to the prostate is the inhibition of androgen-induced effects on prostate growth. In fact, overwhelming evidence suggests that androgens play an important role in the development and progression of prostate cancer. Moreover, to control PIN progression, total androgen ablation might not be necessary and a monotherapy with single agent androgen deprivation, such as with bicalutamide or flutamide, might be more than sufficient. On the other hand, a patient at high risk of developing a morphological precursor of PCa and subsequently cancer might have some kind of genetic susceptibility. In this situation, finasteride (a 5-α-reductase inhibitor) may be of use as it reduces the level of a testosterone metabolite, dehydrotestosterone, which promotes tumour growth (Brawer & Ellis 1995).

Androgen ablation in relation to cell proliferation and death

There is a lower prevalence and extent of high-grade PIN in prostates of patients receiving androgen deprivation therapy than in untreated patients (Ferguson et al 1994). These findings indicate that the dysplastic prostatic epithelium is hormone dependent. The lower prevalence and extent of high-grade PIN is accompanied by cytoplasmic clearing and extensive glandular atrophy with a decreased ratio of glands to stroma. The two main effects of androgen ablation on prostate epithelial cells consist of reducing proliferation and enhancing apoptosis. The number of PCNA-stained nuclei in treated cases is lower than in untreated (PCNA location is unaffected). The low PCNA values and absence of mitoses in PIN, normal prostate and PCa indicates suppressed proliferation activity as a consequence of androgen deprivation therapy (Magi-Galluzzi et al 1993, Montironi et al 1994). Oomens et al (1991) assessed the proliferative cell fraction of human prostatic carcinoma using Ki-67 and found that the percentage of positive nuclei decreased significantly after androgen deprivation, dropping to 7% of the initial values after 3 months. Armas et al (1993) reported decreased PCNA expression due to pre-operative androgen deprivation therapy on prostatic carcinoma.

Apoptotic bodies are more frequent in treated PIN and PCa (and in the adjacent normal prostate) than in untreated cases and are found in all cell layers as well as in the lumina. This suggests that androgen ablation induces a certain degree of epithelial regression by enhancing apoptosis. The findings are in agreement with the experimental study of Szende et al (1990), who investigated the effects of LHRH agonists and somatostatin on cancer in hamsters. This observation probably corresponds to the finding of 'progressive nuclear pyknosis' observed by Helpap (1985) in patients on hormone therapy. Apoptosis was evaluated by Stiens et al (1981) in patients with prostatic carcinoma before and after oestrogen and radiation therapy. They found that the apoptosis index can increase 10-fold in the first 10 days of therapy.

Inhibition of angiogenesis in prostate cancer and its precursors

Anti-angiogenic agents could be of use in inducing regression of PIN and PCa. The rationale for this is that angiogenesis is necessary, but is not alone sufficient, for progression and expansion of a tumour population, but the absence of angiogenesis or its inhibition can severely restrict tumour growth (Folkman & Ingber 1992). If a tumour-bearing animal could be successfully treated with a specific angiogenesis inhibitor, this would strengthen the hypothesis that human tumour growth is also angiogenesis-dependent. Many well-characterised inhibitors are now being studied (Folkman & Ingber 1992, Rak et al 1995).

The expression of PCNA and type IV collagenase in prostate cancer and PIN specimens from patients treated pre-operatively with total androgen ablation has been recently investigated (Montironi et al 1996b). There was no PCNA expression in endothelial cell nuclei, but type IV collagenase positivity in the endothelial, stromal and epithelial cells was decreased when compared with untreated lesions. Capillaries were reduced in frequency.

These observations suggest that angiogenesis is inhibited in the prostate by total androgen ablation, which induces cell regression and activation of apoptosis. Consequently, prostate cells are prevented from expressing, producing or exporting angiogenic molecules. The reduced expression of type IV collagenase is in agreement with experimental studies, in which the anti-angiogenic effect of collagenase inhibitors affected basement membrane synthesis and degradation which are critical steps in the formation of new capillary blood vessels. Marshall and Narayan (1993) speculated that suppression of angiogenesis may be achieved through any hormonal manipulation that caused androgen deprivation.

ATYPICAL ADENOMATOUS HYPERPLASIA

A precursor of prostatic adenocarcinoma or a simple proliferative lesion?

Atypical adenomatous hyperplasia (AAH), also referred to as adenosis, is a localised proliferation of small acini in the prostate that may be mistaken for PCa (Gleason primary grade 1 or 2; Fig. 8.5). AAH can be distinguished from well-differentiated carcinomas by having a fragmented basal cell layer, infrequent crystalloid and inconspicuous nucleoli (Parkinson 1995). Despite these morphological features, diagnosis of AAH and its distinction from well-

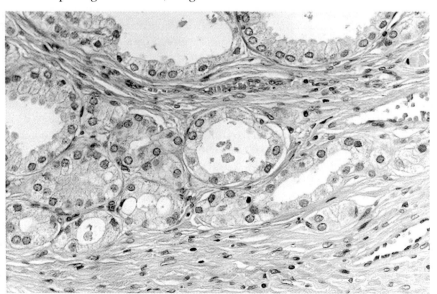

Fig. 8.5 Atypical adenomatous hyperplasia (adenosis). Localised proliferation of small acini.

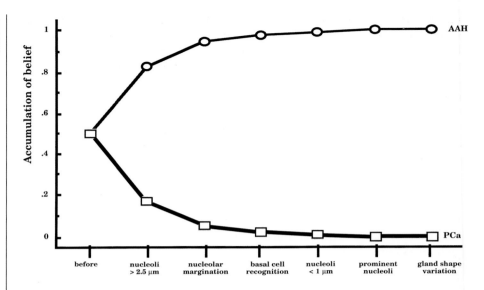

Fig. 8.6 Bayesian belief network for the identification of atypical adenomatous hyperplasia. When evidence for six features is entered, the accumulation of belief is progressive and monotonic towards 1.0.

differentiated prostatic adenocarcinoma with small acinar pattern can be difficult because of terms and concepts.

A Bayesian belief network has been used to reduce the problem of uncertainty in diagnostic assessment. A network has been developed with a node of two diagnostic alternatives (e.g. AAH versus PCa), and 12 descendant nodes for the diagnostic features (Montironi et al 1996a). Eight of these nodes were based on cell features, three on the type of gland lumen contents and one on the gland shape. The results showed that the diagnostic alternatives were reliable and that the network could differentiate AAH from PCa with certainty.

The features which best contributed to the highest level of diagnostic certainty were nucleolar size, frequency and location. In particular, after analysis of five nucleolar features (prominent nucleoli, inconspicuous nucleoli, multiple nucleoli, nucleoli with diameter >2.5 μm, and nucleolar margination), the result for AAH was 1.0, and was very close to 1.0 when the three features were evaluated. The contribution of gland lumen contents (mucinous material, corpora amylacea and crystalloids) is such that the final result did not exceed 0.8. Results with the remaining features (basal cell presence or absence, variation in gland shape, cytoplasm appearance, variation in nuclear size) were slightly better. These features allow a substantial accumulation of belief which is already greater than 0.9 when only three are polled. However, the maximum belief value is never obtained. Therefore, a Bayesian belief network for AAH diagnosis offers a descriptive classifier which allows the use of linguistic, fuzzy variables and the accumulation of evidence presented by diagnostic clues (Fig. 8.6).

AAH has been proposed as a precursor of prostatic adenocarcinoma in the transition zone because of the following: (i) age peak that precedes that of PCa; (ii) increased incidence in association with PCa; (iii) topographic relationship with small acinar PCa; (iv) increased nuclear area and diameter; (v) a proliferative index similar to that of small acinar PCa; (vi) and occasional cases with some genetic alterations. However, the data are insufficient to conclude that AAH is a premalignant lesion and its link to PCa has not yet been proven. For this reason, the term 'adenosis' was suggested to replace 'atypical adenomatous hyperplasia'. This has not been accepted as yet and 'atypical' has been retained to indicate the unusual pattern of small acinar formations that characterise AAH (Montironi & Schulman 1996).

Atypical adenomatous hyperplasia is a particular pattern of microglandular proliferation present in the transition zone. This may possibly be a transition between normal prostate epithelium and the well-differentiated adeno-carcinomas usually seen in the transition zone.

MALIGNANCY-ASSOCIATED CHANGES

A precursor of prostate adenocarcinoma?

Malignancy-associated changes (MACs) have been described by Nieburgs (Montironi & Schueman 1996) as subtle changes in normal cells near premalignant and malignant lesions. Most studies have been made on colonic mucosa and uterine cervix (for review see Montironi et al 1997). In two recent studies, MACs have been described in association with PIN and PCa.

MACs were first identified in a paper on the usefulness of PIN-related Bayesian belief networks for the assessment of non-neoplastic prostatic tissue either associated or not with inflammation or adjacent to PCa and PIN (Montironi et al 1997). The investigation included a series of prostatectomy specimens subdivided as follows: prostatic tissue not associated with neoplasia or other diseases; and tissues associated with acute or chronic inflammation and adjacent to accidentally discovered PCa or PIN. For specimens found to have PCa or PIN, the Bayesian results for normal prostate were intermediate between those from normal prostatic tissue associated with inflammation and those not associated with inflammation. Moreover, it was found that subtle changes were present at a distance from the tumour or PIN lesions. It was concluded that the network can be used to differentiate with certainty non-neoplastic prostate adjacent to PCa or PIN from non-neoplastic prostatic tissue associated with inflammation or not.

Bartels et al (1998a) documented the changes in chromatin pattern in secretory cell nuclei from prostates with PIN and PCa. High resolution images of nuclei provided a set of features descriptive of the chromatin texture and spatial distribution. From these data, features with a monotonic trend of progression were selected and plotted to reveal trends of lesion progression. Sets of images were recorded in prostates with PIN lesions or PCa at defined distances from the margins of cancer to explore the spatial extension of the malignancy-associated changes.

The nuclear chromatin in secretory cells in prostates with either PIN or PCa underwent distinct and statistically significant changes in its texture and distribution. Two trends of progressive change were documented. The values of a number of features descriptive of the degree of clumping of the chromatin increase: values found in normal prostate were lower than those recorded in nuclei in histologically otherwise normal prostate with PIN or malignant

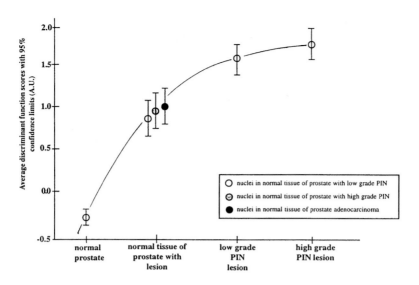

Fig. 8.7 Malignancy associated changes. Mean discriminant function scores for the progression trend from normal prostate to high grade PIN lesions. Note the ranking of secretory cell nuclei recorded in the normal appearing tissue of glands with a high grade PIN lesion, between normal tissue, and low grade PIN lesions.

adenocarcinoma. There is a further increase in clumping for nuclei in low-grade PIN to high-grade PIN lesions (Fig. 8.7).

The second trend is a decrease in the values of the same features from those found in nuclei in high-grade PIN lesions that still have an intact basal cell layer, to those without a basal cell layer, which may be the first step in progression towards development of a malignant lesion; there is a further decrease in size of nuclei from glands immediately adjacent to a malignant lesion, and in adenocarcinoma itself. The described changes appear to be widespread and detectable in the histologically normal appearing tissue of prostates with PIN or a malignant lesion.

There are four possible interpretations for MACs: (i) it is possible that this change is entirely a non-specific response of the prostate epithelium to any irritant factor; (ii) this change might reflect the spread of prostate cancer; (iii) this change could be a preneoplastic response to carcinogenic stimuli, leading to prostate carcinoma; (iv) this could be a specific response to the presence of carcinoma, i.e. a change induced by the adjacent neoplasm. The third or fourth possibility could be applicable to the prostate. There is no agreement among MAC-related reports on interpretation. For example, in studies on morphologically normal colons from patients with colon cancer, the interpretation was that people with colon cancer may have morphologically normal colonic tissue that is genetically abnormal. In the cervix, the MAC finding may represent an influence of the neoplasm on the adjacent mucosa; however, it cannot excluded that these changes reflected a subtle premalignant condition in apparently normal mucosa adjacent to a cervical neoplasm.

Whatever the explanation, it may be possible to use MACs as an important tool in the management of patients with PIN or PCa. In particular, the possibility of detecting MACs in the prostate may be applicable to many clinical situations, such as the detection of malignancy in the prostate when only non-neoplastic changes are found in a biopsy.

DO OTHER PRECURSOR LESIONS EXIST IN THE PROSTATE?

There are some variants of PCa in which the existence of precursors is speculative or unknown. For example, basaloid carcinoma is one of the prostate basaloid lesions. There is no proof that some forms of basaloid lesions, for instance atypical basal cell hyperplasia, might represent a precursor of this variant of prostate carcinoma, so the problem remains unsolved (Devaraj & Bostwick 1993). The answer could be found in the basal cell layer, which is, therefore, worth investigating for its precise composition and function. Is it composed exclusively of stem cells? Does the basal cell layer also include some kind of differentiated cells the function of which is different from that of the secretory cells? Studies addressing these questions have been undertaken by Bonkhoff and colleagues. They showed that cells in the basal layer have the capacity of multi-directional differentiation, including a neuroendocrine pathway (Bonkhoff et al 1994, di Sant'Agnese 1995).

Prostatic duct carcinoma has been well characterised from the morphologically and clinically and shown to have features in common with the acinar variants of PCa. Intraductal papillae and a cribriform pattern are seldom observed in the adjacent parenchyma: these components have been interpreted as the result of intraductal spreading of malignant cells. However, a similar feature present in other organs and tissues adjacent to carcinoma has been considered as an intra-epithelial or non-invasive component, such as in *in situ* ductal carcinoma of breast and salivary carcinoma (Luna et al 1987).

CONCLUSIONS

The several precursors of prostate cancer reflect the multiplicity of patterns and variants of PCa. A big step forward in understanding some basic aspects has already been made, especially in relation to PIN. Quantitation analysis was used accurately to compare PIN and PCa, contributing to the detection of subtle changes that characterise the wide morphological spectrum of PIN and the similarities between PIN and PCa.

Quantitation was applied to evaluate the degree of cell renewal changes in PIN by cell proliferation and cell death markers. Recently, better quantitation techniques have become available, so that the automated detection and analysis of prostate gland structure and components are now possible. Molecular pathology permits identification of subtle changes at the chromosomal level and detection of an abnormal expression of oncogenes. The results have contributed to our understanding of the changes in the proliferation and differentiation processes reported in earlier studies.

Research in the fields of quantitation and molecular pathology is now directed towards the identification and clarification of those PIN subsets that have already acquired the genotypic and phenotypic features of PCa and so can progress to invasive cancer.

Points of Best Practice

- Prostatic intra-epithelial neoplasia is the most likely precursor of adenocarcinoma originating from ducts and acini, particularly those in the peripheral zone of the prostate gland.

- High-grade prostatic intra-epithelial neoplasia has a high predictive value as a marker for carcinoma and its identification in biopsy specimens warrants further search for concurrent invasive cancer.

- Progression from prostatic intra-epithelial neoplasia to prostate cancer is a complex process in which the kinetic organisation of the normal prostate epithelium is altered. This depends on several factors including hormonal status and growth factors.

- Molecular pathology has allowed the identification of subtle changes at the chromosomal level and detection of abnormal expression of oncogenes. The results obtained have contributed to our understanding of the changes in proliferation and differentiation processes.

- Quantitation analysis was originally used to compare accurately prostatic intra-epithelial neoplasia and prostate cancer and to contribute to the detection of the subtle changes that characterise the morphological spectrum of prostatic intra-epithelial neoplasia and the similarities between prostatic intra-epithelial neoplasia and prostate cancer. Recently, quantitation techniques have become available that permit automated detection and analysis of prostate gland structures and lesions.

- Diagnostic decision support systems can be applied to prostate histopathology to provide guidance when complex decisions must be made. The advantage of diagnostic decision support systems is the ability to process symbolic information.

- There is a great decrease in the prevalence and extent of high-grade prostatic intra-epithelial neoplasia in prostates after androgen deprivation therapy compared to untreated prostates. The two basic effects of androgen ablation on epithelial cells consist of reducing proliferation and enhancing apoptosis.

- Atypical adenomatous hyperplasia has been proposed as a possible precursor of prostatic adenocarcinoma in the transition zone. The data are insufficient to conclude that atypical adenomatous hyperplasia is a premalignant lesion and its link to prostate cancer has not yet been established.

- It may be possible to use malignancy associated changes as important variables in the management of patients with prostatic intra-epithelial neoplasia or prostate cancer. Detection of malignancy associated changes in the prostate may be useful in many clinical situations, such as detection of malignancy in the prostate when only non-neoplastic changes are found in a biopsy because of sampling problems.

- Some variants of prostate cancer have unknown precursors.

References

Alers C A, Krijtenburg P J, Vissers K J et al 1995 Interphase cytogenetics of prostatic adenocarcinoma and precursor lesions: analysis of 25 radical prostatectomies and 17 adjacent prostatic intraepithelial neoplasias. Genes Chromosom Cancer 12: 241–250

Amin M B, Schultz D S, Zarbo R J et al 1993 Computerized static DNA ploidy analysis of prostatic intraepithelial neoplasia. Arch Pathol Lab Med 117: 794–798

Armas O A, Melamed A, Aprikian A et al 1993 Effect of preoperative androgen deprivation therapy in prostatic carcinoma. Lab Invest 68: 55A

Baretton G B, Vogt T, Blasenbreu S et al 1994 Comparison of DNA ploidy in prostatic intraepithelial neoplasia and invasive carcinoma of the prostate: an image cytometric study. Hum Pathol 25: 506–513

Bartels P H, Montironi R, Hamilton P W et al 1998a Nuclear chromatin texture in prostate. PIN and malignancy associated changes. Analyt Quant Cytol Histol 20: 397–406

Bartels P H, Montironi R, Thompson D et al 1998b Statistical histometry of the basal cell/ secretory cell bilayer in prostatic intraepithelial neoplasia. Anal Quant Cytol Histol 20: 381–388

Bartels P H, Thompson D, Montironi R et al 1995a Diagnostic decision support for prostate lesions. Pathol Res Pract 191: 945–957

Bartels P H, Thompson D, Weber J E 1995b Diagnostic and prognostic decision support systems. Pathologica 87: 221–236

Bartels P H, Wied G 1997 Automated screening for cervical cancer: diagnostic decision procedures. Acta Cytol 41: 6–10

Batsakis J G, El-Naggar A K 1995 p53: fifteen years after discovery. Adv Anat Pathol 2: 71–88

Berner A, Danielsen H E, Pettersen E O et al 1993 DNA distribution in the prostate. Normal gland, benign and premalignant lesions, and subsequent adenocarcinomas. Anal Quant Cytol Histol 15: 247–252

Bigler S A, Deering R E, Brawer M K 1993 Comparison of microscopic vascularity in benign and malignant prostate tissue. Hum Pathol 24: 220–226

Boag A H, Young I D 1993 Immunohistochemical analysis of type IV collagenase expression in prostatic hyperplasia and adenocarcinoma. Mod Pathol 6: 65–68

Bonkhoff H, Stein V, Remberger K 1994 Multidirectional differentiation in the normal, hyperplastic, and neoplastic human prostate: simultaneous demonstration of cell-specific epithelial markers. Hum Pathol 25: 42–46

Bostwick D G 1996 Progression of prostatic intraepithelial neoplasia to early invasive adenocarcinoma. Eur Urol 30: 145–152

Bostwick D G, Brawer M K 1987 Prostatic intra-epithelial neoplasia and early invasion in prostate cancer. Cancer 59: 788–794

Bostwick D G, Dousa M K, Crawford B G et al 1994 Neuroendocrine differentiation in prostatic intraepithelial neoplasia and adenocarcinoma. Am J Surg Pathol 18: 1240–1246

Bostwick D G, Pacelli A, Lopez-Beltran A 1996 Molecular biology of prostatic intraepithelial neoplasia. Prostate 29: 117–134

Brawer M, Deering R, Brown M et al 1994 Predictors of pathological stage in prostatic cancer. The role of neovascularity. Cancer 73: 678–687

Brawer M K, Ellis W J 1995 Chemoprevention for prostate cancer. Cancer 75: 1783–1789

Brooks J D, Bova G S, Isaacs W B 1995 Allelic loss of the retinoblastoma gene in primary human prostatic adenocarcinoma. Prostate 26: 35–39

Colombel M, Olsson C A, Ng P-Y et al 1992 Hormone-regulated apotosis results from reentry of differentiated prostate cells into a defective cell cycle. Cancer Res 52: 4313–4319

Colombel M, Symmans F, Gil S et al 1993 Detection of the apoptosis-suppressing oncoprotein bcl-2 in hormone-refractory human prostate cancers. Am J Pathol 143: 390–400

Crissman J D, Sakr W A, Hussein M E et al 1993 DNA quantitation of intraepithelial neoplasia and invasive carcinoma of the prostate. Prostate 22: 155–162

Devaraj L T, Bostwick D G 1993 Atypical basal cell hyperplasia of the prostate. Immunophenotypic profile and proposed classification of basal cell proliferations. Am J Surg Pathol 17: 645–659

di Sant'Agnese A 1995 Neuroendocrine differentiation in prostatic carcinoma. Recent findings and new concepts. Cancer 75: 1859–1859

Drago J R, Mostofi F K, Lee F 1989 Introductory remarks and workshop summary. Urology 34 (Suppl.): 2–3

El-Labban NG, Osorio-Herrera E 1986 Apoptotic bodies and abnormally dividing epithelial cells in squamous cell carcinoma. Histopathology 10: 921–931

Emmert-Buck M R, Vocke C D, Pozzati R O et al 1995 Allelic loss on chromosome 8p12-21 in microdissected prostatic intraepithelial neoplasia (PIN). Cancer Res 55: 2959–2962

Falkvoll K H 1990 The occurrence of apoptosis, abnormal mitoses, cells dying in mitosis and micronuclei in a human melanoma xenograft exposed to single dose irradiation. Strahlenther Onkol 166: 487–492

Ferguson J, Zincke H, Ellison E et al 1994 Decrease of prostatic intraepithelial neoplasia (PIN) following androgen deprivation therapy in patients with stage T3 carcinoma treated by radial prostatectomy. Urology 44: 91–95

Folkman J 1992 The role of angiogenesis in tumor growth. Semin Cancer Biol 3: 65–71

Folkman J, Ingber D 1992 Inhibition of angiogenesis. Semin Cancer Biol 3: 89–96

Folkman J, Shing Y 1992 Angiogenesis. J Biol Chem 267: 10931–10934

Giannulis I, Montironi R, Magi Galluzzi C et al 1993 Frequency and location of mitoses in prostatic intraepithelial neoplasia (PIN). Anticancer Res 13: 2447–2452

Greene D R, Rogers E, Wessels E C et al 1994 Some small prostate cancers are nondiploid by nuclear image analysis: correlation of deoxyribonucleic acid ploidy status and pathological features. J Urol 151: 1301–1307

Hamdy F C, Fadlon E J, Cottam D et al 1994 Matrix metalloproteinase 9 expression in primary human prostatic adenocarcinoma and benign prostatic hyperplasia. Br J Cancer 69: 177–182

Hamilton P W, Bartels P H, Montironi R 1995 Improved diagnostic decision making in pathology: do inference networks hold the key? J Pathol 175: 1–5

Helpap B 1980 The biological significance of atypical hyperplasia of the prostate. Virchows Archiv A Pathol Anat 387: 307–317

Helpap B 1985 Treated prostatic carcinoma. Histological, immunohistochemical and cell kinetic studies. Appl Pathol 3: 320–341

Ibrahim G K, Kerns B J M, MacDonald J A et al 1993 Differential immunoreactivity of epidermal growth factor receptor in benign, dysplastic and malignant prostatic tissue. J Urol 149: 170–173

Ibrahim G K, MacDonald J A, Kerns B J M et al 1992 Differential immunoreactivity of herb-2/neu oncoprotein in prostatic tissues. Surg Oncol 1: 151–155

Kim N W, Piatyszek M A, Prowse K R et al 1994 Specific association of human telomerase activity with immortal cells and cancer. Science 266: 2011–2015

Kleinerman D I, Troncoso P, Lin S et al 1995 Consistent expression of an epithelial cell adhesion molecule (C-CAM) during human prostate development and loss of expression in prostate cancer: implication as a tumor suppressor. Cancer Res 55: 1215–1220

Lee W K, Morton R A, Epstein J I et al 1994 Cytidine methylation of regulatory sequences near the p-class glutathione S-transferase gene accompanies human prostatic carcinogenesis. Proc Natl Acad Sci USA 91: 11733–11737

Loda M, Capodieci P, Mishra R et al 1996 Expression of MAP kinase phosphatase-1 (MKP-1) in the early phases of human epithelial carcinogenesis. Am J Pathol 149: 1553–1564

Luna M A, Batsakis J G, Ordonez N G et al 1987 Salivary gland adenocarcinoma: a clinicopathologic analysis of three distinctive types. Semin Diagn Pathol 4: 117–135

Maddy S Q, Chisholm G D, Busuttil A et al 1989 Epidermal growth factor receptors in human prostate cancer: correlation with histological differentiation of the tumour. Br J Cancer 60: 41–44

Magi-Galluzzi C, Montironi R, Cangi M G et al 1998 Mitogen-activated protein kinases and apoptosis in PIN. Virchows Arch 432: 407–413

Magi-Galluzzi C, Montironi R, Giannulis I et al 1993 Prostatic invasive adenocarcinoma. Effect of combination endocrine therapy (LHRH agonist and flutamide) on the expression and location of Proliferating Cell Nuclear Antigen (PCNA). Pathol Res Pract 189: 1154–1160

Makar R, Mason A, Kittelson J M et al 1994 Immunohistochemical analysis of cathepsin D in prostate carcinoma. Mod Pathol 7: 747–751

Marshall S, Narayan P 1993 Treatment of prostatic bleeding: suppression of angiogenesis by androgen deprivation. J Urol 149: 1553–1554

Maygarden S J, Novotny D B, Moul J W et al 1994 Evaluation of cathepsin D and epidermal growth factor receptor in prostate carcinoma. Mod Pathol 7: 930–936

McNeal J E, Bostwick D G 1986 Intraductal dysplasia: a premalignant lesion of the prostate. Hum Pathol 17: 64–71

McNeal J E, Villers A, Redwyne E A et al 1991 Microcarcinoma in the prostate: its association with duct-acinar dysplasia. Hum Pathol 22: 644–652

Montironi R, Bartels P H, Hamilton P W et al 1996a Atypical adenomatous hyperplasia (adenosis) of the prostate. Development of a Bayesian belief network for its distinction from well-differentiated adenocarcinoma. Hum Pathol 27: 396–407

Montironi R, Bartels P H, Thompson D et al 1995 Prostatic intraepithelial neoplasia (PIN). Performance of Bayesian belief network for diagnosis and grading. J Pathol 177: 153–162

Montironi R, Diamanti R, Pomante R et al 1997 Subtle changes in benign tissue adjacent to prostate neoplasia detected with a Bayesian belief network. J Pathol 182: 442–449

Montironi R, Diamanti L, Thompson D et al 1996b Analysis of the capillary architecture in the precursor of prostate cancer: recent findings and new concepts. Eur Urol 30: 191–200

Montironi R, Lucarini G, Castaldini C et al 1996c Immunohistochemical evaluation of type IV collagenase (72-kd metalloproteinase) in prostatic intraepithelial neoplasia. Anticancer Res 16: 2057–2062

Montironi R, Magi-Galluzzi C, Diamanti L et al 1993a Prostatic intra-epithelial neoplasia. Expression and location of proliferating cell nuclear antigen (PCNA) in epithelial, endothelial and stromal nuclei. Virchows Archiv A Pathol Anat 422: 185–192

Montironi R, Magi-Galluzzi C, Diamanti L et al 1993b Prostatic intra-epithelial neoplasia. Qualitative and quantitative analyses of the blood capillary architecture on thin tissue sections. Pathol Res Pract 189: 542–548

Montironi R, Magi-Galluzzi C, Scarpelli M et al 1993c Occurrence of cell death (apoptosis) in prostatic intra-epithelial neoplasia. Virchows Archiv A (Pathol Anat) 423: 351–357

Montironi R, Magi-Galluzzi C, Scarpelli M et al 1994 Quantitative characterisation of the frequency and location of cell proliferation and death in prostate pathology. J Cell Biochem 19 (Suppl): 238–245

Montironi R, Scarpelli M, Magi-Galluzzi C et al 1991 Diagnostic quantitative pathology: classification by multiple variables and multivariate analyses. Arch Pathol 23: 29–48

Montironi R, Scarpelli M, Magi-Galluzzi C et al 1992 Aneuploidy and nuclear features of prostatic intraepithelial neoplasia (PIN). J Cell Biochem (Suppl): 47–53

Montironi R, Scarpelli M, Sisti S et al 1990 Quantitative analysis of prostatic intraepithelial neoplasia on tissue sections. Anal Quant Cytol Histol 12: 366–372

Montironi R, Schulmann C C 1996 Precursors of prostatic cancer: progression, regression and chemoprevention. Eur Urol 30: 133–137

Montone K T, Tomaszewsky J E 1993 In situ hybridization for epidermal growth factor receptor (EGFR) external domain transcripts in prostatic adenocarcinoma. J Clin Lab Anal 7: 188–195

Morton R A, Ewing C M, Nagafuchi A et al 1993 Reduction of E-cadherin levels and deletion of the alpha-catenin gene in human prostate cancer cells. Cancer Res 53: 3585–3590

Myers R B, Kudlow J E, Grizzle W E 1993 Expression of transforming growth factor-alpha, epidermal growth factor and the epidermal growth factor receptor in adenocarcinoma of the prostate and benign prostatic hyperplasia. Mod Pathol 6: 733–737

Myers R B, Srivastava S, Grizzle W E 1995 Lewis Y antigen as detected by the monoclonal antibody BR96 is expressed strongly in prostatic adenocarcinoma. J Urol 153: 1572–1574

Myers R B, Srivastava S, Oelschlager D K et al 1994 Expression of p160^{erbB-3} and p185^{erbB-3} in prostatic intraepithelial neoplasia and prostatic adenocarcinoma. J Natl Cancer Inst 86: 1140–1145

Oomens E H G M, van Steenbrugge G J, van Der Kwast T H et al 1991 Application of the monoclonal antibody Ki-67 on prostate biopsies to assess the proliferative cell fraction of human prostatic carcinoma. J Urol 145: 81–85

Parkinson M C 1995 Pre-neoplastic lesions of the prostate. Histopathology 27: 301–311

Petein M, Michel P, Van Velthoven R et al 1991 Morphonuclear relationship between prostatic intraepithelial neoplasia and cancer as assessed by digital cell image analysis. Am J Clin Pathol 96: 628–634

Poulsom R, Pignatelli M, Stetler-Stevenson W G et al 1992 Stromal expression of 72 kDa type IV collagenase (MMP-2) and TIMP-2 mRNAs in colorectal neoplasia. Am J Pathol 141: 389–396

Qian J, Bostwick D G, Takahashi S et al 1995 Chromosomal anomalies in prostatic
intraepithelial neoplasia and carcinoma detected by fluorescence in situ hybridization.
Cancer Res 55: 5408–5414

Rak J W, St Croix B D, Kerbel R S 1995 Consequences of angiogenesis for tumor progression,
metastasis and cancer therapy. Anti-Cancer Drugs 6: 3–18

Robertson C N, Roberson K M, Herzberg A J et al 1994 Differential immunoreactivity of
transforming growth factor alpha in benign, dysplastic and malignant prostatic tissues.
Surg Oncol 3: 237–242

Ross J S, Nazeer T, Figge H L et al 1995 Quantitative immunohistochemical quantitation of
cathepsin D levels in prostatic carcinoma biopsies. Correlation with tumor grade, stage,
PSA level, and DNA ploidy status. Am J Clin Pathol 104: 36–41

Ruizeveld de Winter J A, Janssen P J A, Sleddens H M A B et al 1994 Androgen receptor status
in localized and locally progressive hormone refractory human prostate cancer. Am J
Pathol 144: 735–746

Sakr W A, Macoska J A, Benson P et al 1994 Allelic loss in locally metastatic multisampled
prostate cancer. Cancer Res 54: 3273–3277

Sinha A A, Gleason D F, Staley N A et al 1995 Cathepsin B in angiogenesis of human prostate:
an immunohistochemical and immunoelectron microscopic analysis. Anat Rec 241:
353–362

Sinha A A, Wilson M J, Gleason D F et al 1995 Immunohistochemical localization of cathepsin
B in neoplastic human prostate. Prostate 26: 171–178

Stiens R, Helpap B, Weissbach L 1981 Quantitative untersuchungen zum zellverlust in
prostatakarzinomen. Klinisch-morphologische aspekte. Verh Dtsch Ges Urol 32: 73–74

Szende B, Srkalovic G, Schally A V et al 1990 Inhibitory effects of analogs of luteinizing
hormone-releasing hormone and somatostatin on pancreatic cancers in hamsters. Cancer
65: 2279–2290

Takahashi S, Qian J, Brown J A et al 1994 Potential markers of prostate cancer aggressiveness
detected by fluorescence in situ hybridization. Cancer Res 54: 3574–3579

Taplin M-E, Bubley G J, Shuster T D et al 1995 Mutation of the androgen-receptor gene in
metastatic androgen-independent prostate cancer. N Engl J Med 332: 1393–1398

Thompson D M, Gill G N 1985 The EGF receptor, structure, regulation, and potential role in
malignancy. Cancer Surv 4: 767–788

Turkeri L N, Sakr W A, Wykes S M et al 1994 Comparative analysis of epidermal growth
factor receptor gene expression and protein product in benign, premalignant, and
malignant prostate tissue. Prostate 25: 199–205

Umbas R, Isaacs W B, Bringuier P P et al 1994 Decreased E-cadherin expression is associated
with poor prognosis in patients with prostate cancer. Cancer Res 54: 3929–3933

Verhoeven D, Van Marck E 1993 Proliferation, basement membrane changes, metastasis and
vascularization patterns in human breast cancer. Pathol Res Pract 189: 851–861

Weidner N, Carrol P R, Flax J et al 1993 Tumor angiogenesis correlates with metastasis in
invasive prostate carcinoma. Am J Pathol 143: 401–409

Weinberg D S, Weidner N 1993 Concordance of DNA content between prostatic intraepithelial
neoplasia and concomitant carcinoma. Evidence that prostatic intraepithelial neoplasia is a
precursor of invasive prostatic carcinoma. Arch Pathol Lab Med 117: 1132–1137

Richard G. A. Faragher David Kipling

CHAPTER 9

Detection and significance of senescent cells in tissue

IMPORTANCE OF THE MEASUREMENT OF CELL SENESCENCE

Ageing is of serious concern to governments, scientists and clinicians. Recent interest in ageing research has highlighted both the scale of the problem and the lack of data integrating the ageing of individual cells and that of intact tissue. The potential impact of the ageing process on medical services is enormous. By the year 2030, people over the age of 60 will constitute one-fifth of the British population (Greengross et al 1997). Similar demographic trends exist in both developed and less developed nations (Lutz W et al 1997). Elderly patients account for one-quarter of hospital beds and more than half of all prescriptions (Davies 1983). To deal with a problem of this magnitude, basic research into the ageing process was recommended as a priority area by the Technology Foresight Panel on Health and Life Sciences (1995) instigated by the British government. This article aims to provide basic information on one potential cause of the ageing of tissue – the senescence of the cells which compose it. Biochemical markers of the senescent state are also reviewed.

The term senescence describes the finite capacity of normal human cells to divide in culture. Senescence was first conclusively demonstrated in a series of experiments carried out by Hayflick and Moorehead in the 1960s (Hayflick & Moorehead 1961, Hayflick 1965). They showed that a culture of normal human fibroblasts could not be propagated indefinitely: after a finite number of passages, the culture would enter a static phase and fail to expand further. Subsequent experiments demonstrated that the failure of such cultures to grow continually was not due to cell death (Macieira-Coelho et al 1966). More recent experiments have shown that senescence is also distinct from apoptosis

Dr R. G. A. Faragher, Ocular Research Group, Department of Pharmacy, University of Brighton, Cockcroft Building, Moulsecomb, Brighton BN2 4GJ, UK
Dr D. Kipling, Department of Pathology, University of Wales College of Medicine, Heath Park, Cardiff CF4 4XN, UK

Table 9.1 Evidence linking cell senescence and whole organism ageing

Observation	Reference
Human cell cultures show a decline in growth potential with advancing donor age	Martin et al 1970, Schneider & Mitsui 1976, Gilchrest 1983, Lipman & Taylor 1987, Perillo et al 1987, Bermach et al 1991, Blake et al 1997
The proliferative lifespan of fibroblasts in culture correlates strongly with the lifespan of the species from which they were taken	Rohme 1981
Calorie restriction extends the lifespan of whole organisms and leads to a reduced number of senescent cells in lens epithelium in vivo	Li et al 1997
Cultures of vascular endothelial cells derived from arteriosclerotic arteries show a greatly reduced lifespan compared to autologous cultures derived from veins	Van Hinsburgh 1992
Organ cultured corneae show a strongly age-linked increase in the number of senescent cells in the endothelial layer	Hoppenreijs et al 1994
The pattern of gene expression in senescent cells in vitro is consistent with the development of age-related degenerative disease in vivo	Gray & Norwood 1995, Linskens et al 1995
The number of senescent cells observed within dermal tissue sections increases in a strongly age-dependent manner	Dimri et al 1995
The proliferative lifespan of fibroblasts from donors with progeroid syndromes is significantly reduced	Brown et al 1984, Faragher & Kipling 1997, Vazari 1997

(Norsgaard et al 1996) and, in culture systems where the processes can be distinguished, from terminal differentiation (Hornsby & Gill 1980, Norsgaard et al 1996). The 'senescence' of cells in culture is a process distinct from the 'senescence' of organisms in the environment. The mechanism controlling the entry of cells into senescence is not a 'clock' which controls the ageing of mammals. Indeed it is unlikely that any such central clock exists at all (Kirkwood 1996).

Cell senescence is implicated in the pathogenesis of the normal ageing process. A series of experiments summarised in Table 9.1 demonstrated that the proliferative potential of cells in culture correlates inversely with the age of the donor in a wide range of normal human cell types. The mean maximum lifespan of many animal species correlates well with the growth potential of their fibroblasts in culture. Recent studies on a range of breeds of the domestic dog support this observation and show that both lifespan and cell growth potential are susceptible to the influence of selective breeding (Li et al 1996). Patients with accelerated ageing diseases, such as Werner's syndrome, show both extremely poor fibroblast growth and a wide range of age-related

Table 9.2 Selected alterations in cell phenotype with the onset of senescence

Phenotypic alteration in senescence	Cell type	Reference
Repression of c-fos	Fibroblasts, T lymphocytes	Sheshadri & Campisi 1990, Sikora et al 1992
Repression of cyclin A and B	Fibroblasts	Stein & Dulic 1995
G_2 arrest on restimulation without division	Fibroblasts, T lymphocytes	Kill & Shall 1990, Perillo et al 1993
Elevated collagenase	Fibroblasts	Millis et al 1989
Elevated stromelysin	Fibroblasts	Zeng & Millis 1996
Elevated PAI-2	Fibroblasts	Kumar et al 1992
Elevated ceramide	Fibroblasts	Venable et al 1995
Transcriptional represssion of IGF-1 gene	Fibroblasts	Ferber et al 1993
Reduced active TGFβ-1	Fibroblasts	Zeng et al 1996
Elevated IL-1α expression	Fibroblasts	Zeng & Millis 1996
Senescence associated β-galactosidase activity	Fibroblasts, keratinocytes, mammary epithelial cells, endothelial cells, neonatal melanocytes	Dimri et al 1995
Altered regulation of intracellular Ca^{2+}	Fibroblasts	Brooks-Frederich et al 1993
Elevation of cytochrome b and NADH 4/4L subunit	Fibroblasts	Kodama et al 1995

disorders suggesting that cell senescence and tissue ageing are related (Faragher & Kipling 1997). Experimental studies have also demonstrated that when the lifespan of mice is extended by calorie restriction the accumulation of senescent lens cells is reduced (Li et al 1997). Taken together these observations suggest that the progressive accumulation of senescent cells may contribute to the development of age-related diseases in tissues largely composed of renewing or conditionally renewing cell types.

STRUCTURAL AND BIOCHEMICAL CHANGES ASSOCIATED WITH CELL SENESCENCE

A wide range of changes occur in normal cells which enter senescence (Campisi 1997). These comprise a permanent and active repression of DNA synthesis and a series of changes in gene expression which alter the phenotype of the growth-arrested cell. These changes have been described mostly in human fibroblasts in culture; similar changes have been reported in other tissues (Table 9.2).

In fibroblasts, senescence is associated with a series of structural changes that are clearly visible in culture (see Fig. 9.1). At the ultrastructural level, these

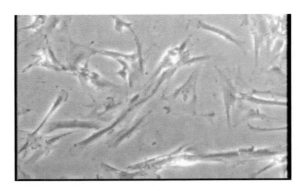

Fig. 9.1 Senescent culture of normal human corneal fibroblasts (Strain EK1.BR). See text for description of senescent phenotype.

changes include an increase in cell size, an increase in nuclear size and enlarged lysosomes (Stanulis-Praeger 1987). This increase in lysosomal size is associated with increases in activity of lysosomal enzymes (Stanulis-Praeger 1987, Dimri et al 1995). Mitochondrial mass increases (Goldstein & Korczack 1981) though respiratory efficiency appears to decline. Senescent fibroblasts generally have a more rigid cytoskeleton than their growing counterparts which is associated with decreased filamin expression (Kelly et al 1985). These changes may be associated with a decline in migration rate (Schneider & Mitsui 1976). Human fibroblasts also show a decline in invasiveness and a decreased ability to contract collagen lattices (Bell et al 1979). Though production of several growth factors is severely curtailed (Goldstein 1990, Ferber et al 1993), growth factor receptor numbers and affinity are generally unaffected by the onset of senescence (Goldstein 1990, Norwood et al 1990). However, downstream components of the normal signal transduction pathway are affected by irreversible growth arrest: the *c-fos* gene is transcriptionally repressed in senescent cells (Sheshadri & Campisi 1990, Campisi 1997) and endogenous levels of ceramide are also greatly increased, probably due to elevated sphingomyelinase activity (Obeid & Venable 1997). Addition of artificial ceramide to growing cells has recently been shown to mimic many of the effects of senescence (Venable et al 1995, Obeid & Venable 1997). Ceramide appears to function as an effector of cell senescence rather than the primary trigger, so it is appropriate to consider the nature of this trigger mechanism with an explanation of the kinetics of the senescence process.

THE KINETICS OF SENESCENCE

Early work on the senescence of fibroblasts assumed that the cell cultures studied were homogeneous populations of cells which all divided a roughly identical number of times before entering senescence in relative synchrony (Hayflick 1965, Shall 1987). However, long pulse labelling experiments in the 1970s using tritiated thymidine at every passage throughout the lifespan of fibroblast cultures demonstrated that cells which never incorporated label were present in the cultures from the very first passage and smoothly increased in number until they became the predominant cell type (Cristofalo & Scharf 1973). These experiments have been confirmed using cloning

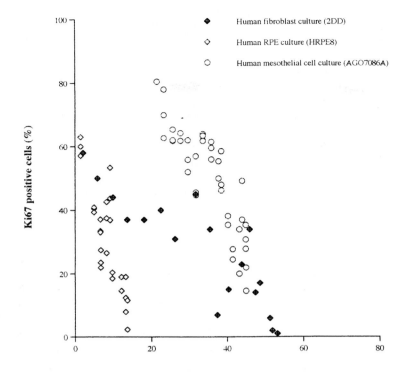

Fig. 9.2 Kinetics of senescence in a variety of cultured human primary cells. Rates of senescence vary depending on cell type. Data reproduced from Thomas et al 1997 and Rawes et al 1997 with permission.

techniques and endogenous proliferation markers (Smith & Whitney 1980, Faragher et al 1993) and show that primary cell cultures are mixtures of growing and senescent cells, the proportions of which alter as the cells are serially passaged. This behaviour is consistent with a counting mechanism that operates at each cell division (Shall 1987). The cloning experiments also demonstrated that this mechanism contains has a strong stochastic element (Smith & Whitney 1980). At each cell cycle, each individual fibroblast has a chance of entering senescence or continuing to divide. This chance is not fixed but increases with the number of times the cell has divided before. Conversely, a fibroblast which has divided only once or twice can be 'unlucky' and enter senescence when its probability of doing so is extremely low. It is important to stress that complete exhaustion of the proliferative capacity of a cell population is not required before the impact of senescence is felt.

Historically, the kinetics of cell senescence were extensively studied only in fibroblasts, with the evaluation of senescence in other cell types confined to confirmation of a limited culture lifespan and measurement of its extent (quoted as population doublings) (Stanulis-Praeger 1987). Recently, formal comparative studies of the kinetics of senescence in several cell types have been performed. These involved human mesothelial and retinal pigmented epithelial cells and were conducted to determine whether the rate of entry into senescence was fixed across a range of tissues (Thomas et al 1997, Rawes et al 1997). Mesothelial cells have a lifespan similar to human fibroblasts and thus provided a useful theoretical comparator, whilst retinal pigmented epithelial cells are the primary tissue affected in age-related macular degeneration and so of consequent clinical interest. These experiments suggest that the kinetics of senescence differ considerably between cell types (Fig. 9.2). Extrapolating from these data to the clinical situation, any process or insult that triggers cell turnover in vivo may shift the proportions of growing and senescent cells to a greater extent in a retinal or peritoneal layer than in a corresponding layer of dermal fibroblasts. Such experiments also have a purely theoretical value as they provide multiple sets of kinetic criteria with which any theory seeking to explain the control of normal cell senescence must be compatible. The most plausible current theory for the constitutive mechanism of senescence – the loss of telomeric DNA – is discussed below.

TELOMERE SHORTENING AS A HUMAN CELL DIVISION COUNTING CLOCK

Human chromosomes have telomeres as the specialised structures at their ends. Telomeres distinguish these natural chromosome ends from double-strand breaks which can lead to fusion and recombination between chromosomes and the activation of genome damage-monitoring systems (Kipling 1995a). Telomeres enable the ends of human chromosomes to behave differently because of the presence of a specific terminal DNA sequence (arrays of the hexamer TTAGGG) which, in turn, binds proteins such as hTRF1 and hTRF2 (Broccoli et al 1997, Smith & de Lange 1997, van Steensel et al 1998).

Telomeres facilitate the replication of the ends of chromosomes. Conventional DNA replication faces a major problem with the ends of a DNA molecule – the so-called end replication problem (Kipling 1995a). The consequence of this is that a small amount of terminal DNA is not duplicated in each S-phase, resulting in an inexorable loss of terminal DNA with repeated cell division. In addition to the end replication problem, there is also evidence of terminal sequence loss by a separate mechanism (Makarov et al 1997, McElligott & Wellinger 1997). Human cells can compensate for terminal sequence losses by *de novo* synthesis of telomeric sequences by the enzyme telomerase (Kipling 1995a). Telomerase activity is present in human germ-line cells and immortal human cell lines (Harley & Villeponteau 1995, Kipling 1995b). By contrast, in virtually all normal somatic cells telomerase activity cannot be detected. Telomere shortening might, therefore, act as a 'clock' to count cell division (Harley 1991, Holt et al E 1996, Olovnikov 1996).

Cultured human fibroblasts and many other cell types show a decrease in telomere length with cell division (Harley et al 1990, Allsopp et al 1995, Henderson et al 1996), and residual telomere length is a good predictor of replicative lifespan in fibroblasts (Allsopp et al 1992). Very recent data (Bodnar et al 1998) have for the first time provided direct, experimental evidence consistent with telomere shortening being a necessary part of normal human cell senescence. Forced expression of telomerase via expression with hTRT – the catalytic subunit of human telomerase (Kilian et al 1997, Meyerson et al 1997, Nakamura et al 1997) – halts telomere shortening sufficient to prevent senescence in three human cell types (fibroblasts, vascular endothelial cells and retinal pigmented epithelial cells), conferring an extended lifespan of at least 20 population doublings (Bodnar et al 1998).

In the following section we ask two related questions: can telomere loss in telomerase-negative somatic cells (Harley & Villeponteau 1995) provide a useful and informative marker for the replicative history of a cell; and will recent data (Bodnar et al 1998) on preventing the senescent phenotype provide new therapies?

TELOMERE SHORTENING WITH AGE – a biomarker of replicative history

In telomerase-negative cells, ongoing cell proliferation will lead to inexorable terminal sequence loss. For this reason, several studies have used telomere length as a marker of differential replicative history in human cells in vivo (Allsopp et al 1995). To date, all of these have used terminal restriction length analysis. This involves digestion of genomic DNA with a combination of restriction enzymes that cleave the genome (but do not cut within the $(TTAGGG)_n$ arrays at the telomeres), followed by agarose gel electrophoresis, Southern blotting and finally detection of the $(TTAGGG)_n$-containing terminal restriction fragments with an appropriate hybridisation probe. Variants of this protocol have been developed to use gel hybridisation (which avoids technical problems related to Southern transfer of large fragments), and radioactive and non-isotopic probe detection systems have been successfully used. A commercial kit (TeloQuant™, PharMingen) for terminal restriction length analysis is now available which uses non-isotopic detection and includes a detailed protocol for signal quantitation.

The main drawback of terminal restriction length analysis is the large number (10^5-10^6) of cells that are required. This is not a protocol that can be applied to single cells or in an *in situ* format. Although telomere shortening with in vitro cell division has been detected by fluorescence *in situ* hybridisation (Henderson et al 1996), there is no information on whether this protocol can be adapted to tissue sections to provide meaningful data. One technological development that may help in the future is the use of peptide nucleic acid probes for telomere *in situ* hybridisation (Lansdorp et al 1996). This is an accurate method of determining telomere length on metaphase human chromosomes and may be a route to single-cell quantitation of total telomere length in interphase cells. Such a development would permit study of the cell hypothesis of ageing to move from the study of fully senescent cells (see below) to the analysis of the division capacity of individual cells in aged tissues. This is important as there are several situations where reduced potential to proliferate (cells having fewer divisions 'left on the clock') may be clinically relevant, such as tissues in which high levels of cell division are normal, or where a burst of cell proliferation is required during tissue repair.

TELOMERE LENGTH IN RELATION TO AGE IN THE PROLIFERATIVE COMPARTMENT

At least two processes lead to terminal sequence loss in cell division, and this can be assessed using terminal restriction length analysis. Such telomere shortening dependent on cell division is well documented in cultured primary human cells, such as fibroblasts (Allsopp et al 1995). A similar loss with division would be expected in vivo and, indeed, this is the case. Telomere length decreases with age in human fibroblasts (Harley et al 1990, Henderson et al 1996), peripheral blood leukocytes (Hastie et al 1990), skin dermal and epidermal cells (Lindsey et al 1991), colon epithelial cells (Hastie et al 1990) and T cells (Weng et al 1995). Telomere shortening with age has also been described for candidate human stem cells (CD34$^+$ CD38^{lo}; Vaziri et al 1994) and stem cell proliferation following bone marrow transplantation produces similar telomere shortening (Notaro et al 1997). Vascular endothelial cells show not only telomere shortening with age: areas with high haemodynamic stress and thus increased cell turnover (e.g. iliac artery versus iliac vein) show a faster rate of telomere shortening with age (Chang & Harley 1995). In contrast, cells which are telomerase-positive (or recently derived from telomerase-positive precursors, such as spermatozoa; Allsopp et al 1992) or which do not divide during adult life (such as mature neurones in the brain; Harley & Villeponteau 1995) show no decline in telomere length with donor age. These data are all consistent with the premise that telomere length provides a useful biomarker of proliferative history.

One problem with such analyses is genetic polymorphism in terminal restriction length (Slagboom et al 1994); there is considerable scatter on graphs of terminal restriction length with donor age in cross-sectional studies (Allsopp et al 1992). However, if in vitro replicative capacity is measured for fibroblasts from a range of donors and compared to initial terminal restriction length there is a good correlation between the two (Allsopp et al 1992). These and other data (Allsopp & Harley 1995) indicate that terminal restriction length is a good predictor of replicative capacity in vitro (Allsopp & Harley 1995). Therefore, though it may be a poor indicator of chronological time, telomere length is a far better criterion of the biologically relevant variable with respect to ageing, namely replicative history.

A second problem can occur if rates of telomere shortening are altered. Telomere dynamics have been investigated in a variety of human diseases which show features consistent with premature ageing (Faragher & Kipling 1997, Martin 1997). These include ataxia telangiectasia, Hutchinson-Gilford progeria and Down's syndrome. Telomere lengths in all three disorders are shorter than equivalent age-matched normal controls (Allsopp et al 1992, Broccoli & Cooke 1993, Vaziri et al 1993, Metcalfe et al 1996). However, though this may reflect accelerated cell turnover in these cases, data for both ataxia telangiectasia and Werner's syndrome reveal altered rates of telomere loss with cell division in vitro (Schulz et al 1996, Vaziri et al 1997), and it is difficult in this case to use telomere data to determine the in vivo cell kinetics.

The cell numbers required for terminal restriction length analysis limits studies to those instances where sufficient cells are available. Many of the studies described above can be categorised as 'proof of principle'. However, there have been several attempts to use terminal restriction length analysis as a biomarker for proliferative history in the haematopoietic system to yield new data on cell turnover.

TELOMERE DYNAMICS IN THE HAEMATOPOIETIC SYSTEM

Although cells from peripheral blood are easy to obtain, ironically this is one system where interpreting terminal restriction length data is fraught with difficulties; many of the cells studied are either telomerase-positive, or recently derived from telomerase-positive precursors. The presence of telomerase makes it possible for cell division to occur with no telomere shortening, breaking the link between cell division and telomere length. This can be illustrated by attempts to use terminal restriction length analysis to determine cell kinetics following HIV-1 infection.

One of the prominent features of HIV-1 infection and AIDS is a progressive decrease in the number of CD4$^+$ T-cells, which correlates well with disease progression. Work using other techniques has suggested a very high rate of turnover of CD4$^+$ T-cells during HIV-1 infection, raising the possibility that AIDS might result, at least in part, from exhaustion of the capacity to generate CD4$^+$ T-cells (Ho et al 1995, Wei et al 1995). There have been several attempts to investigate the cell kinetics in HIV-1 infection using telomere length as a biomarker.

Terminal restriction lengths of both naive and memory T-cells decrease with in vitro culture and with donor age (Weng et al 1995). However, a decrease in CD4$^+$ terminal restriction length in HIV-1 infection is not observed (Wolthers et al 1996). Indeed, when using monozygotic twins of whom only one is HIV-positive, the TRF lengths of CD4$^+$ T-cells were actually **longer** in the HIV-positive sibling (Palmer et al 1997). These observations appear at odds with data (Ho et al 1995, Wei et al 1995) supportive of a higher rate of CD4$^+$ T cell turnover in HIV-1 infection, as this should lead to decreased rather than increased telomere lengths.

How are we to interpret these data? The answer may come from the observation that many of the cells under study are telomerase positive; substantial amounts of the enzyme are found in CD4$^+$ CD8$^+$ thymocytes, and also in activated CD4$^+$ T-cells in peripheral blood (Palmer et al 1997). Since the presence of telomerase has the potential to stop, or even reverse, telomere shortening, it is far from simple to determine cell kinetics in HIV-1 infection using TRF data (Weng et al 1997).

One illustration of the potential for a strongly telomerase-positive cell compartment to produce unexpected terminal restriction length data is provided by the example of B lymphocyte differentiation (from antigen-naive cells, through to being germinal centre B cells, and finally to memory B cells in the peripheral blood). During this differentiation process, telomere length actually increases in the germinal centre (Weng et al 1997), which correlates with very high levels of telomerase at this point in B lymphocyte development. This illustrates well the capacity for telomerase to distort the link between telomere length and replicative history. It should be stressed, therefore, that terminal restriction length analyses should ideally be used as a biomarker only for the replicative history of cells that are fully telomerase-negative. As already indicated, the presence of telomerase in various cell types in the haematopoietic system can cause the data to be difficult or impossible to interpret. Other cell types that should perhaps be avoided are epithelial cells. Although *ex vivo* these cells are usually telomerase-negative, when stimulated to divide in culture many become telomerase-positive. This has now been demonstrated for human uroepithelial, prostate and mammary epithelial cells (Belair et al 1997), oral keratinocytes (Chang & Harley 1995), epidermal and ectocervical keratinocytes, and simple endocervical epithelial cells (Harlebachor & Boukamp 1996, Yasumoto et al 1996).

TELOMERASE AS 'GENE THERAPY FOR AGEING'

Human telomerase has now been cloned (Kipling 1997). Telomerase is a ribonuclear protein consisting of a small essential RNA molecule (hTR) (Hastie et al 1990) which provides the template for TTAGGG synthesis, together with a catalytic protein subunit (hTRT). hTRT has been cloned by several groups (Harrington et al 1997, Kilian et al 1997, Meyerson et al 1997, Nakamura et al 1997). As expected from its biochemical function of synthesising DNA complementary to a RNA template, the amino acid sequence of hTRT contains regions which show similarity to motifs found in reverse transcriptases. In vitro reconstitution experiments indicate that hTR and hTRT are sufficient to form active telomerase (Weinrich et al 1997). Transfection of hTRT expression constructs into primary human cells is sufficient to restore telomerase activity (Weinrich et al 1997, Bodnar et al 1998, Nakayama et al 1998), demonstrating that the reason that such cells are normally telomerase-negative is because they lack hTRT. This provides encouragement for the use of antibodies against hTRT as a non-enzymatic marker for telomerase, an enzyme widely expressed in human malignancy.

The recent observation that cellular lifespan can be extended by forced expression of telomerase (Bodnar et al 1998) raises interesting practical implications. In the long-term this might provide a route to delay some of the age-related changes ascribable to replicative senescence. Indeed, it may even be possible to reverse the senescent phenotype, as opposed to delaying its occurrence. This possibility is raised by the observation that in certain situations replicative senescence can indeed be reversed. The first situation occurs upon the experimental addition of vascular endothelium growth factor to fully senescent human dermal microvascular cells (Watanabe et al 1997). This causes them to re-enter division, revert to a 'young' appearance and continue to proliferate for many generations. Secondly, micro-injection of p53-neutralising antibodies into senescent human fibroblasts leads to resumption of cell division and reversion to a 'young' appearance (Gire & Wynford-Thomas 1998).

Now, the key experiment is to determine whether extending telomeres in a senescent cell to a length found in young cells will reverse senescence. As an anti-ageing therapy, it would be illogical to reverse the in vivo senescent phenotype by use of vectors expressing viral oncoproteins because of their tumorigenic potential, despite the cellular lifespan extension and phenotype reversal this would confer. Such a system would allow only cell division and maintenance of a 'young' phenotype in the continued presence of the onco-protein. However, assuming short telomeres are necessary for senescence and that the state can be reversed, a potentially safer approach might be transient expression of telomerase (e.g. transient delivery of an hTRT-expression construct) leading to telomere elongation. Not only would the senescent state be reversed, but crucially once telomerase was removed (hence the require-ment for transient delivery) the cells would continue to be young and have the potential to divide. A more prosaic but potentially more tractable system would be to use transient telomerase expression to give some extra division potential to growing cells; this could well find application in developing gene therapy modalities where limited cellular lifespan restricts the ability of the manipulated cells to repopulate in vivo (Decary et al 1997).

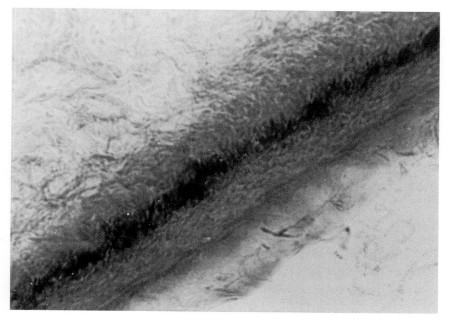

Fig. 9.3 Senescent cells stained using the senescence associated β-galactosidase technique (*see* Table 9.3) in a dermal section from an elderly donor. Note intense dark area of staining (blue). Photograph reproduced with kind permission of Dr Judy Campisi.

POTENTIAL MARKERS OF THE SENESCENT STATE

Histochemical markers

Regardless of the mechanism by which they arise, the central tenet of the cell hypothesis of ageing is that senescent cells progressively accumulate during the ageing of regenerative tissue in vivo. A crucial test of the hypothesis is, thus, the demonstration of senescent cells in tissue sections. However, until recently, progress in this area was hampered by the lack of a marker for senescence which did not also recognise quiescent cells. Support for the hypothesis was thus largely based on extrapolation from in vitro systems and was necessarily derivative (Martin et al 1970, Schneider & Mitsui 1976; Gray & Norwood 1995). Attempts to identify senescent cells in tissue based upon subtle aspects of their phenotype were inconclusive (Macieira-Coelho 1995).

However, senescence is reported to be associated with elevated β-galactosidase activity in many cell types (Dimri et al 1995). The practical advantage of this observation was that it became possible to modify a standard histochemical assay for β-galactosidase activity such that it functioned equally efficiently in vivo and in vitro. When this assay was applied to dermal sections from donors of increasing age a sustained increase in senescence associated β-galactosidase positive cells was observed (Fig. 9.3).

The mechanistic basis of senescence associated β-galactosidase is currently unknown and may be related to the over-expression of the enzyme at senescence or to a simple increase in cell size correlating with entry into the permanently non-dividing state (Dimri et al 1995, Thomas et al 1997). As the

Table 9.3 Protocol for detection of senescence associated endogenous β-galactosidase activity (reproduced with kind permission of Dr Judy Campisi)

Required reagents

Citric acid/sodium phosphate buffer (100 ml)
  36.85 ml 0.1 M citric acid solution
  63.15 ml 0.2 M sodium phosphate (dibasic) solution
  Verify that pH is 6.0
Citric acid solution (0.1 M)
  2.1 g citric acid monohydrate in 100 ml distilled water
Sodium phosphate solution
  2.84 g per 100 ml sodium dibasic phosphate or
  3.56 g per 100 ml sodium dibasic phosphate dihydrate
X-gal powder (stored in dark at –20°C)
Sodium chloride (5 M)
Dimethylformamide (DMF)
Potassium ferrocyanide
Potassium ferricyanide
Magnesium chloride (1 M)

These reagents are combined to make the **staining solution** below:

Component	Volume	Final conc.
Citric acid/sodium phosphate buffer	4 ml	40 mM
X-gal (20 mg in DMF)		1 mg/ml
[Few drops of DMF only since this inhibits the β-galactosidase]		
100 mM potassium ferrocyanide	1 ml	5 mM
100 mM potassium ferricyanide	1 ml	5 mM
5 M sodium chloride	0.6 ml	150 mM
1 M magnesium chloride	40 µl	2 mM
Water	13.4 ml	
Total volume	20 ml	

Fixative
  2% formaldehyde/0.2% glutaraldehyde in PBS:
  β-galactosidase staining is also compatible with 3% formaldehyde

Protocol (adherent cells/tissue)

1. Wash material twice in PBS

2. Fix for 3–5 min at room temperature, prolonged fixation will inactivate the enzyme

3. Repeat washes in PBS

4. Add staining solution (1–2 ml per 35 mm diameter dish)

5. Incubate at 37°C. Blue colour is detectable in some cells within 2 h, staining is usually maximal after 12–16 h

7. Material can be mounted in aqueous mountants (e.g. Apathy's syrup) and can be counterstained with fast green or similar colour compatible stain

Combined detection of activity and proliferation.

Staining is compatible with [³H]-thymidine labelling (10 mCi/ml for 72 h). Label. carry our β-galactosidase staining, allow colour to develop, wash twice with PBS, twice with methanol, air dry, coat with NTB2 emulsion, expose and develop

The authors own laboratory have had success with combining β-galactosidase with bromodeoxyuridine labelling (72 h) and antisera to pKi67 (Mib rabbit polyclonal). β-galactosidase staining also supports cell permeabilisation with 0.2% Triton X-100.

technique itself is relatively simple and potentially useful it is reproduced in Table 9.3. Dimri et al (1995) list a series of cell types on which the assay has been validated. Variants of the technique have also been employed with essentially similar results (Thomas et al 1997).

Also of potential use to pathologists interested in the objective quantification of senescent cells is lipofuscin. Lipofuscin is sometimes also termed 'age-pigment'. Lipofuscin emits a distinct yellow-orange fluorescence when excited with UV light, it is also readily detectable by several methods (Ohtani & Kawashima 1983, Ivy et al 1984, Faragher et al 1993, Katz et al 1993). In cultured cells, lipofuscin accumulation correlates with senescence in normal and Werner's syndrome fibroblasts (Poot et al 1985), retinal pigmented epithelial cells (Faragher et al 1993) and tumour cells forced into growth arrest by genetic manipulation (Sugrue et al 1997). Whilst potentially useful, lipofuscin accumulation also occurs in irreversibly post-mitotic cells from static populations such as neurons (Ohtani & Kawashima 1983). Evaluation should, thus, be conducted with care.

Molecular markers

The ideal marker for senescent cells in tissue would be a gene which is expressed only by senescent cells, is expressed heavily, and is induced by the onset of senescence in as wide a range of cell types as possible. As gene techniques designed to identify differentially expressed sequences have been available for over a decade and have recently improved in sensitivity and sophistication with the advent of differential display PCR and suppression subtractive hybridisation, it would appear to be relatively simple to identify such an ideal marker. However, historically, identification of genes expressed only by senescent cells has been hampered by two distinct problems:

1. There is a tendency for many growth arrest specific sequences to be common to both the quiescent and senescent states (Wang 1987) though this is not always the case (Cowled et al 1994). Quiescence (G_0Q) is a transient growth-arrested state which can be induced by the removal of serum from the medium of primary or immortal cells or through contact inhibition. Quiescence can be reversed by serial passage or by the re-addition of serum. Unfortunately, most cells in normal regenerative tissue are quiescent until called upon to divide and thus genes common to quiescence and senescence offer limited potential as ex vivo markers of tissue composition.

2. There are technical difficulties of library construction and screening using primary cell cultures. As such cultures are mixtures of growing and senescent cells, both senescent and growing RNA is present in the pools of RNA which are compared. This leads to differences which appear to be relative (over or under expression) rather than unique; expression ratios of greater than 4 between the senescent and growing RNA pools represent significant differences to date. Though gene sequences have been identified using various differential display/ subtractive hybridisation techniques (Table 9.4), none has been formally validated on tissue sections though many may have the potential to serve as useful markers

Table 9.4 A selection of genes found to be overexpressed with the onset of cell senescence

Gene	Function	Cell type	Senescence specific	How identified	Reference
Ws3.10	Suppression of Ca^{2+}-dependent membrane currents	Fibroblasts	Possible	cDNA library screen	Thweatt et al 1992
Fibronectin	Extracellular matrix protein	Fibroblasts, endothelial cells	No, **	Multiple methods	Gray & Norwood 1995
α1-procollagen	Extracellular matrix protein	Fibroblasts	No, **	Multiple methods	Gray & Norwood 1995
IGFBP-3	Binding protein for insulin-like growth factor 3	Fibroblasts	No, **	cDNA library screen	Wang et al 1996
PAI-1	Control of haemostasis	Fibroblasts, endothelial cells	No, **	Enhanced DD	Linskens et al 1995
SPARC	Extracellular matrix proteins	Fibroblasts	No, **	cDNA library screen	Wang et al 1996
LPC-1, LPC-14	?	Fibroblasts	Possible	cDNA library screen (phagemid)	Doggett et al 1992
LPC-16X, LPC-20	?	Fibroblasts	Possible	As above	Doggett et al 1992
LPC-24, LPC-26	?	Fibroblasts	Possible	As above	Doggett et al 1992
Cytochrome b	Component of electron transport chain	Fibroblasts	No, **	Multiple methods	Doggett et al 1992, Kodama et al 1995
ND4	Subunit 4 mitochondrial NADH dehydrogenase	Fibroblasts	No, **	Multiple methods	Doggett et al 1992, Kodama et al 1995
SAG	Transcription factor	Fibroblasts-	Possible	Library screen (cDNA λZAP)	Wistrom & Villeponteau 1992
Endothelin 1	Vaso-constrictor	Endothelial cells	No, **	Multiple methods	Kumazaki et al 1997
p21wdf/SDf	Inhibitor of CDKs	Multiple types	No, **	Plasmid expression screen	Noda et al 1994, Gray & Norwood 1995
TIMP-2	Tissue inhibitor of MMP	Fibroblasts	No, **	Enhanced DD	Linskens et al 1995
IGFBP-5	Binding protein for insulin-like growth factor 3	Fibroblasts	No, **	Enhanced DD	Linskens et al 1995
HSCDN7	?	Fibroblasts	No, **	Enhanced DD	Linskens et al 1995
EST00718	?	Fibroblasts	No, **	Enhanced DD	Linskens et al 1995
MnSOD	Free radical scavenger	Fibroblasts	No, **	Enhanced DD	Linskens et al 1995
Heregulin	EGF-like growth factor	Fibroblasts	No, **	Enhanced DD	Linskens et al 1995
CD44	Hyaluronic acid receptor	Fibroblasts	No, **	Enhanced DD	Linskens et al 1995

**A gene expressed in growing cells which is upregulated at senescence; ? indicates that the function of the sequence is unknown; DD indicates use of differential display PCR.

The concept that the progressive accumulation of senescent cells may contribute to the development of age related disorders in tissues composed largely of renewing or conditionally renewing cell types has found support within a range of medical disciplines (Eldred 1993, Buckwalter 1995).

Musculoskeletal and dermatological systems

As the main characteristic of senescent cells is their simple failure to divide, the wound healing response of aged patients has been an area of basic interest to those seeking a link between cell senescence and tissue ageing. Although the age of a patient is often quoted anecdotally as a cause in the delay of wound healing, it has been recently shown that the evidence for this is lacking (Goodson & Hunt 1979, Ashcroft et al 1995). However, this appears to be due to a failure to conduct systematic experiments in appropriate model systems. Given these caveats, it is perhaps encouraging that the evidence for age-related alterations in wound healing is as robust as it is. With appropriate caution, it is pertinent to examine the effect cell senescence may have on the wound healing process, with particular attention to the healing of dermal wounds.

The dermis is the only tissue in which senescent cells have been shown to accumulate in an age-dependent manner (Dimri et al 1995). There is also a well characterised change in the extracellular matrix of elderly people. In particular, the proportions of collagen, elastin and glycosaminoglycans alter in a manner resembling the changes in extracellular matrix production seen between senescent and growing fibroblasts in vitro (Ashcroft et al 1995, Passi et al 1997). A number of in vitro features of senescent fibroblasts – including decreased migration rate, ability to contract collagen and over-production of a range of extracellular matrix degrading enzymes – also have the potential to affect adversely wound healing. However, these studies have mostly been conducted using dermal fibroblasts; fibroblastoid cells from other areas of the body may show differences in functional capacity when examined in detail (Solmi et al 1996).

Age-related degeneration of the intervertebral discs is frequently identified as a common cause of back pain and stiffness (Buckwalter 1995). Such problems are common among middle aged and old people and represent a major impairment to their quality of life. Intervertebral discs are essentially discrete bodies of connective tissue maintained by a relatively sparse population of fibrocytic cells. The ability of this macromolecular network to allow diffusion of nutrients into the disc appears central to its structural integrity and senescence of the intervertebral cell population has been specifically proposed as a mechanism by which the function of the matrix may be compromised (Buckwalter et al 1993). Quantitative studies on intervertebral disc cell senescence (either in vitro or ex vivo) remain to be conducted.

Cardiovascular system

Atheroma is one of the major killers in old age. About 60% of men surviving to the sixth decade show 75–100% stenosis of at least one coronary artery

(Lakatta 1980). A wide range of aetiological factors have been implicated which have been generically described as the repeated induction of tissue 'repair' responses which eventually become fatal (Van Hinsburgh 1992). The disease is age-linked and currently irreversible. A major cell type involved is the vascular endothelium, which regulates haemostasis. Senescent endothelial cells have been shown to upregulate urokinase-type plasminogen activator (u-PA) and plasminogen activator inhibitor-1 (PAI-1) more than 50-fold relative to non-senescent controls (West et al 1996). Elevated PAI levels in vivo are a major risk factor for myocardial infarction and deep vein thrombosis and, in transgenic studies, PAI-1 overexpression leads to thrombotic disease (Auwerx et al 1988, Erickson et al 1990). The implication that senescent endothelium has reduced fibrinolytic activity is thus strong. Endothelial cells also relax contracted smooth muscle cells via the production of nitric oxide. However, senescent endothelial cells in culture lack the ability to produce nitric oxide, suggesting the inability of senescent endothelial cells to modulate vascular tone in vivo (Sato et al 1993). Unfortunately no evidence is available to date on the distribution of senescent endothelial cells within the vasculature.

The eye

In developed countries, ageing is the single most important risk factor for vision loss. Ageing research in the eye has tended to focus on cataracts and related problems, such as presbyopia. The ageing of lens fibre cells is clearly a post-mitotic phenomenon and will not be discussed here, though cultures of the fibre precursor cells (the lens epithelium) have been shown to demonstrate a clear age-related reduction in growth potential (Lipman & Taylor 1987). Lens epithelial cells synthesise the G0 marker statin on induction of terminal differentiation but, unlike many other cell types, do not do so while quiescent (Muggleton Harris & Wang 1989). This difference underlines the need to study senescence in a range of different cell types and it is perhaps regrettable that senescent lens epithelial cells have not been characterised in more detail.

A common feature of some age-related ocular problems is the need for surgical intervention to correct them. This usually involves incision surgery into the cornea, a three layered avascular structure. Compromised wound healing by corneal fibroblasts (keratocytes) has been documented in Werner's syndrome (Jonas et al 1987) and normal ageing (Faragher et al 1997).

The commonest cause of age-related blindness is macular degeneration, essentially a failure of the retinal pigmented epithelial cell layer to break down the tips of the rod cell effectively (Silvestri 1997), a process associated with an increase in lipofuscin. Similar changes occur in retinal pigmented epithelial cells undergoing senescence in culture (Rawes et al 1997). The potential for a link between macular degeneration and retinal pigmented epithelial senescence is thus provocative and is strengthened by the observation that calorie restriction slows the rate of accumulation of lipofuscin (Katz et al 1993).

The immune system

Immunosenescence comprised a subtle remodelling of the immune system rather than a simple deterioration (Franceschi et al 1995) of every component.

Although some aspects of the immune system (such as NK cell activity) appear unaffected by ageing (Krishnaraj 1992) and the propensity of aged granulocytes to induce an oxidative burst in response to stimuli appears to increase with age, significant deficits do occur, particularly in the T-cell compartment (Effros & Pawelec 1997). The relation between ageing and immunity has interested the biomedical community for over 30 years, but the cell hypothesis of ageing received scant attention until T-cell senescence was formally demonstrated in the late 1980s (Burnet 1971, Perillo et al 1987, Perillo et al 1993). A decline in T-cell proliferative response in vivo has been reported with ageing and correlated with flow cytometry studies which suggest that there is an increasing fraction of non-mitogen responsive cells and a fraction of G_2 arrested cells with similar characteristics to those seen in restimulated cultures of senescent T-cells (Perillo et al 1993). Theoretical calculations by Pawelec predict that, if the proliferative potential of T-cells is the same in the body as it is ex vivo then the number of divisions which a particular cell clone can undergo in response to antigen stimulation is not indefinite and is probably less than ten (Adibzadeh et al 1996). Reports have also indicated that, in addition to a non-responsive population and a responsive population with increased cell cycle transit times, there is a population of 'presenescent' T-cells, with reduced division potential in aged people (Fillit 1994). An extremely rare accelerated ageing disease (Mulvihill-Smith syndrome) shows both poor fibroblast growth and compromised T cell proliferation in vitro (Ohashi 1993). Unfortunately, at the moment, a good marker for the senescent state in T lymphocytes is not available, so direct tests of the cell hypothesis of ageing in the immune system are currently difficult. Identification of such a marker is clearly a key goal in the study of immunosenescence and cell senescence generally.

Points of best practice

- The ageing of the population will pose a growing challenge to health care.

- Strong circumstantial evidence links cell senescence to the ageing of regenerative tissue.

- Histopathologists are well qualified to provide quantitative data on the effects of senescence on tissue structure and to relate these effects to cellular changes identified in vitro.

- Senescence is not cell death.

- An ideal marker for senescent cells in vivo is currently not available. However simple histochemical staining for β-galactosidase works well in tissue sections.

- A wide range of senescence-associated genes are currently being identified which may provide useful markers in the near future.

- The mechanism of cell senescence appears to be closely linked to telomere shortening. *In situ* determination of telomere length has the potential to identify senescent and presenescent cells.

Detection and significance of senescent cells in tissue

ACKNOWLEDGEMENT

The authors thank Dr E. Ostler for critical reading and assistance in drafting this manuscript.

References

Adibzadeh M, Mariani E, Bartoloni C et al 1996 Lifespans of T lymphocytes. Mech Age Dev 91: 145–154

Allsopp R C, Vaziri H, Patterson C et al 1992 Telomere length predicts replicative capacity of human fibroblasts. Proc Natl Acad Sci USA 89: 10114–10118

Allsopp R C, Harley C B 1995 Evidence for a critical telomere length in senescent human fibroblasts. Exp Cell Res 219: 130–136

Allsopp R C, Chang E, Kashefi-Aazam M et al 1995 Telomere shortening is associated with cell division in vitro and in vivo. Exp Cell Res 220: 194–200

Ashcroft G S, Horan M A, Ferguson P 1995 The effects of ageing in cutaneous wound healing in mammals. J Anat 187: 1–26

Auwerx J, Bouillon R, Collen D, Gebeors J 1988 Induction of tissue-type plasminogen activator and plasminogen activator inhibitor in diabetes mellitus. Arteriosclerosis 8: 68–72

Belair C D, Yeager T R, Lopez P M, Reznikoff C A 1997 Telomerase activity: a biomarker of cell proliferation, not malignant transformation. Proc Natl Acad Sci USA 94: 13677–13682

Bell E, Ivarsson B, Merrill C 1979 Production of tissue-like structure by contraction of collagen lattices by human fibroblasts of different proliferative potential in vitro. Proc Natl Acad Sci USA 76: 1274–1278

Bermach G, Mayer U, Naumann G O H 1991 Human lens epithelial cells in culture. Exp Eye Res 52: 113–119

Blake D A, Yu H, Young D L, Caldwell D R 1997 Matrix stimulates the proliferation of human corneal endothelial cells in culture. Invest Ophthalmol Vis Sci 38: 1119–1129

Bodnar A G, Ouellette M, Frolkis M et al 1998 Extension of life-span by introduction of telomerase into normal human cells. Science 279: 349–352

Broccoli D, Cooke H 1993 Aging, healing, and the metabolism of telomeres. Am J Hum Genet 52: 657–660

Broccoli D, Smogorzewska A, Chong L et al 1997 Human telomeres contain two distinct myb-related proteins, TRF1 and TRF2. Nature Genet 17: 231–235

Brooks-Frederich K M, Cianciarulo F L, Rittling S R, Cristofalo V J 1993 Cell cycle dependent regulation of Ca^{2+} in young and senescent WI-38 cells. Exp Cell Res 205: 412–415

Brown W T, Zebrower M, Kieras F 1984 Progeria: a model disease for the study of accelerated ageing. Basic Life Sci 375: 396

Buckwalter J A 1995 Aging and degeneration of the human intervertebral disc. Spine 20: 1307–1314

Buckwalter J A, Woo S L, Goldberg V M et al 1993 Soft tissue aging and musculoskeletal function. J Bone Joint Surg [Am] 75: 1533–1548

Burnet M 1971 Genes, dreams and realities. London: Pelican, 163–184

Campisi J 1997 The biology of replicative senescence. Eur J Cancer 33: 703–710

Chang E, Harley C B 1995 Telomere length and replicative ageing in human vascular tissues. Proc Natl Acad Sci USA 92: 11190–11194

Cowled P A, Ciccarelli C, Coccia E, Philipson L, Sorrentino V 1994 Expression of growth arrest specific (gas) genes in senescent murine cells. Exp Cell Res 211: 197–202

Cristofalo V J, Scharf B B 1973 Cellular senescence and DNA synthesis; Exp Cell Res 76 :419–427

Davies I 1983 Ageing. London: Edward Arnold, 1–2

Decary S, Mouly V, Ben Hamida C, Sautet A, Barbet J P, Butler-Brown G S 1997 Replicative potential and telomere length in human skeletal muscle: implications for satellite cell-mediated gene therapy. Hum Gene Ther 8: 1429–1438

Dimri G, Lee X, Basile B et al 1995 A biomarker that identifies senescent human cells in culture and in aging skin in vivo. Proc Natl Acad Sci USA 92: 9362–9367

Doggett D L, Rotenburg M O, Pignolo R J, Phillips P D, Cristofallo V J 1992 Differential gene expression between young and quiescent, senescent WI-38 cells. Mech Age Dev 65: 239–255

Effros R B, Pawelec G 1997 Replicative senescence of T cells: Does the Hayflick Limit lead to immune exhaustion? Immunol Today 18: 450–454

Eldred G E 1993 Biochemical ageing in the retina and RPE. Prog Retinal Res 12: 101–121

Erickson L A, Fici G J, Lund J E, Boyle T P, Polites G, Marrotti K R 1990 Development of venous occlusions in mice transgenic for plasminogen activator inhibitor. Nature 346: 74–76

Faragher R G A, Kill I R, Tannock T C A et al 1993 Is the Werner's syndrome gene a 'clock' gene which counts cell division? Proc Natl Acad Sci USA 90: 12030–12034

Faragher R G A, Kipling D 1997 Progeroid syndromes: probing the molecular basis of aging? Mol Pathol 50: 234–241

Faragher R G A, Mulholland B, Tuft S J, Sandeman S, Khaw P T 1997 Aging and the cornea. Br J Ophthalmol 81: 814–817

Ferber A, Chang C, Sell C et al 1993 Failure of senescent human fibroblasts to express the insulin-like growth factor 1 gene. J Biol Chem 268: 17883–17888

Fillit H 1994 Clinical immunology of aging. Rev Clin Gerontol 4: 187–197

Franceschi C, Monti D, Sansoni P, Cossarizza A 1995 The immunology of exceptional individuals: the lesson of centenarians. Immunol Today 16: 12–16

Gilchrest B A 1983 Relationship between actinic damage and chronologic aging in keratinocyte cultures in human skin. J Invest Dermatol 81: 184s–189s

Gire V, Wynford-Thomas D 1998 Reinitiation of DNA synthesis and cell division in senescent human fibroblasts by microinjection of anti-p53 antibodies. Mol Cell Biol In press

Goldstein S 1990 Replicative senescence: the human fibroblast comes of age. Science 249: 1129–1133

Goldstein S, Korczack L B 1981 Status of mitochondria in living human fibroblasts during growth and senescence in vitro. J Cell Biol 91: 392–398

Goodson H, Hunt T K 1979 Wound healing and aging. J Invest Dermatol 73: 88–91

Gray M D, Norwood T H 1995 Cellular aging in vitro. Rev Clin Gerontol 5: 369–381

Greengross S, Murphy E, Quam L et al 1997 Aging: a subject that must be top of world agendas. BMJ 315: 1029–1030

Harlebachor C, Boukamp P 1996 Telomerase activity in the regenerative basal layer of the epidermis in human skin and in immortal and carcinoma-derived skin keratinocytes. Proc Natl Acad Sci USA 93: 6476–6481

Harley C B 1991 Telomere loss: mitotic clock or genetic time bomb? Mutat Res; 256: 271–282

Harley C B, Futcher A B, Greider C W 1990 Telomere shorten during ageing of human fibroblasts. Nature 345: 458–460

Harley C B, Villeponteau B 1995 Telomeres and telomerase in aging and cancer. Curr Opin Genet Dev 5: 249–255

Harrington L, Zhou W, McPhail T et al 1997 Human telomerase contains evolutionarily conserved catalytic and structural subunits. Genes Dev 11: 3109–3115

Hastie N D, Demptster M, Dunlop M G, Thompson A M, Green D K, Allshire R C 1990 Telomere reduction in human colorectal carcinoma and with ageing. Nature 346: 866–868

Hayflick L 1965 The limited in vitro lifespan of human diploid cell strains. Exp Cell Res 37: 614–636

Hayflick L, Moorehead P S 1961 The serial cultivation of human diploid cell strains. Exp Cell Res 25: 585–621

Henderson S, Allsopp R, Spector D, Wang S S, Harley C 1996 In situ analysis of changes in telomere size during replicative ageing and cell-transformation. J Cell Biol 134: 1–12

Ho D D, Neumann A U, Perelson A S et al 1995 Rapid turnover of plasma virions and CD4 lymphocytes in HIV-1 infection. Nature 373: 123–126

Holt S E, Shay J W, Wright W E 1996 Refining the telomere–telomerase hypothesis of aging and cancer. Nat Biotech 14: 836–839

Hoppenreijs V P T, Pels E, Vrensen G F J M, Treffers W F 1994 Effects of platelet derived growth factor on endothelial wound healing of human corneas. Invest Ophthalmol Vis Sci 35: 150–161

Hornsby P J, Gill G N 1980 Loss of division potential in culture: aging or differentiation? Science 208: 1482–1483

Ivy G O, Schottler F, Wenzel J, Baudry M, Lynch G 1984 Inhibition of lysosomal enzymes: accumulation of lipofuscin-like dense bodies in the brain. Science 226: 985–987

Jonas J B, Ruprect K W, Schmitzvalckenberg P et al 1987 Ophthalmic surgical complications in Werner's syndrome: report of 18 eyes of nine patients. Ophthalmol Surg 18: 760–764

Katz M L, White H A, Gao C L, Roth G S, Knapka J J, Ingram D K 1993 Dietary restriction slows age pigment accumulation in the retinal pigment epithelium. Invest Ophthalmol Vis Sci 34: 3297–3302

Kelly R O, Mann P L, Perdue B D, Marek L F 1985 Reduction of filamin in late passage human diploid fibroblasts (IMR90). Mech Age Dev 30: 79–98

Kilian A, Bowtell D D L, Abud H E et al 1997 Isolation of a candidate human telomerase catalytic subunit gene, which reveals complex splicing patterns in different cell types. Hum Mol Genet 6: 2011–2019

Kill I R, Shall S 1990 Senescent human diploid fibroblasts are able to support DNA synthesis and to express markers associated with proliferation. J Cell Sci 97: 473–478

Kipling D 1995a The telomere. Oxford: OUP

Kipling D 1995b. Telomerase: immortality enzyme or oncogene? Nat Genet 9: 104–106

Kipling D 1997 Mammalian telomerase: catalytic subunit and knockout mice. Hum Mol Genet 6: 1999–2004

Kirkwood T B L 1996 Human senescence. Bioessays 18: 1009–1016

Kodama S, Yamada H, Annab L, Barrett J C 1995 Elevated expression of mitochondrial cytochrome b and NADH dehydrogenase subunit 4/4L in senescent human cells. Exp Cell Res 219: 82–86

Krishnaraj R 1992 Immunosenescence of human NK cells: effects on tumor target recognition, lethal hit and interferon sensitivity. Immunol Lett 34: 79–84

Kumar S, Millis A J T, Baglioni C 1992 Expression of interleukin-1-inducible genes and production of interleukin-1 by ageing human fibroblasts. Proc Natl Acad Sci USA 89: 4683–4687

Kumazaki T, Wadhwa R, Kaul S C, Mitsui Y 1997 Expression of endothelin, fibronectin and mortalin as aging and mortality markers. Exp Gerontol 32: 95–103

Lakatta E G 1980 Health in an older society. Institute of Medicine and National Research Council: Committee on Aging Society. Washington DC. National Academic Press, 73–104

Lansdorp P M, Verwoerd N P, van de Rijke F M et al 1996 Heterogeneity in telomere length of human chromosomes. Hum Mol Genet 5: 685–691

Li Y, Deeb B, Pendergrass W, Wolf N 1996 Cellular proliferative capacity and life span in small and large dogs. J Gerentol 51A: B403–B408

Li Y, Yan Q, Wolf N S 1997 Long-term calorie restriction delays age-related decline in proliferation capacity of murine lens epithelial cells in vitro and in vivo. Invest Ophthalmol Vis Sci 38: 100–108

Lindsey J, McGill N I, Lindsey L E et al 1991 In vivo loss of telomeric repeats with age in humans. Mutat Res 256: 45–48

Linskens M H K, Feng J, Andrews W H et al 1995 Cataloging altered gene expression in young and senescent cells using enhanced differential display. Nucleic Acid Res 23: 3244–3251

Lipman R D, Taylor A 1987 The in vitro replicative potential and cellular morphology of human lens epithelial cells derived from different aged donors. Curr Eye Res 6: 1453–1457

Lutz W, Sanderson W, Scherbov S 1997 Doubling of world population unlikely. Nature 387: 803–805

Macieira-Coelho A 1995 The last mitoses of the human fibroblast proliferative lifespan, physiopathologic implications. Mech Age Dev 82: 91–104

Macieira-Coelho A, Ponten J, Philipson L 1966 The division cycle and RNA synthesis in diploid human cells at different passage levels in vitro. Exp Cell Res 42: 673–684

Makarov V L, Hirose Y, Langmore J P 1997 Long G tails at both ends of human chromosomes suggest a C strand degradation mechanism for telomere shortening. Cell 88: 657–666

Martin G M 1997 The genetics of aging. Hosp Pract 32: 47–75

Martin G M, Sprague C A, Epstein C J 1970 Replicative lifespan of cultivated human cells. Effects of donor's age, tissue and genotype. Lab Invest 73: 3584–3588

McElligott R, Wellinger R J 1997 The terminal DNA structure of mammalian chromosomes. EMBO J 16: 3705–3714

Metcalfe J A, Parkhill J, Campbell L et al 1996 Accelerated telomere shortening in ataxia telangiectasia. Nat Genet 13: 350–353

Meyerson M, Counter C M, Eaton E N et al 1997 hEST2, the putative human telomerase catalytic subunit gene, is up-regulated in tumor cells and during immortalization. Cell 90: 785–795

Millis A J T, Sottile J, Hoyle M, Mann D M, Diemer V 1989 Collagenase production by early and late passage cultures of human fibroblasts. Exp Gerontol 24: 559–575

Muggleton Harris A L, Wang E 1989 Statin expression associated with terminally differentiating and post replicative lens epithelial cells. Exp Cell Res 182: 152–159

Nakamura T M, Morin G B, Chapman K B et al 1997 Telomerase catalytic subunit homologs from fission yeast and human. Science 277: 955–959

Nakayama J I, Tahara H, Tahara E et al 1998 Telomerase activation by hTRT in human normal fibroblasts and hepatocellular carcinoma. Nat Genet 18: 65–68

Noda A, Ning Y, Venable SF et al 1994 Cloning of senescent cell-derived inhibitors of DNA synthesis using an expression screen. Exp Cell Res 211: 90–98

Norsgaard H, Clark B F C, Rattan S I S 1996 Distinction between differentiation and senescence and the absence of increased apoptosis in human keratinocytes undergoing cellular aging in vitro. Exp Gerontol 31: 563–570

Norwood T H, Smith J R, Stein G H 1990 Aging at the cellular level: the human fibroblast-like cell model. In: Schneider E L, Rowe J W (eds) Handbook of the biology of aging. San Diego: Academic Press, 131–154

Notaro R, Cimmino A, Tabarini D et al 1997 In vivo telomere dynamics of human hematopoietic stem cells. Proc Natl Acad Sci USA 94: 13782–13785

Obeid L M, Venable M E 1997 Signal transduction in cellular senescence. J Am Geriatr Soc 45: 361–366

Ohashi H, Tasukahara M, Murano I et al 1993 Premature aging and immunodeficiency: Mulvihill-Smith syndrome? Am J Med Genet 45: 597–600

Ohtani R, Kawashima S 1983 Reduction of lipofuscin by centrophenoxine and chlorpromazine in the neurons of rat cerebral hemisphere in primary culture. Exp Gerontol 18: 105–112

Olovnikov A M 1996 Telomeres, telomerase, and ageing – origin of the theory. Exp Gerontol 31: 443–448

Palmer L D, Weng N P, Levine B L, June C H, Lane H C, Hodes R J 1997 Telomere length, telomerase activity, and replicative potential in HIV infection: analysis of CD4(+) and CD8(+) T cells from HIV-discordant monozygotic twins. J Exp Med 185: 1381–1386

Passi A, Albertini R, Campagnari F, De Luca G 1997 Modifications of proteoglycans secreted into the growth medium by young and senescent human fibroblasts. FEBS Lett 402: 286–290

Perillo N L, Naeim F, Walford R L, Effros R B 1993 In vitro aging in T lymphocyte cultures: analysis of DNA content and cell size. Exp Cell Res 207: 131–135

Perillo N L, Walford R L, Newman M A, Effros R B 1987 Human T lymphocytes possess a limited in vitro lifespan. Exp Gerontol 24: 177–178

Poot M, Visser W J, Verkerk A, Jongkind J F 1985 Autofluorescence of human skin fibroblasts during growth inhibition and in vitro ageing. Gerontology 31: 158–165

Rawes V, Kipling D, Kill I R, Faragher R G A 1997 The kinetics of senescence in retinal pigmented epithelial cells: a test for the telomere hypothesis of ageing? Biochemistry (Moscow) 62: 1291–1296

Rohme D 1981 Evidence for a relationship between longevity of mammalian species and life spans of normal fibroblasts in vitro and erythrocytes in vivo. Proc Natl Acad Sci USA 78: 5009–5013

Sato I, Morita I, Kaji K, Ikeda M, Nagao M, Murota S 1993 Reduction of nitric oxide producing activity associated with in vitro aging in cultured human umbilical vein endothelial cell. Biochem Biophys Res Commun 195: 1070–1076

Schneider E L, Mitsui Y 1976 The relationship between in vitro cellular aging and in vivo human age. Proc Natl Acad Sci USA 73: 3584–3588

Schulz V P, Zakian V A, Ogburn C E et al 1996 Accelerated loss of telomeric repeats may not explain accelerated replicative decline of Werner syndrome cells. Hum Genet 97: 750–754

Shall S 1987 Mortalisation or reproductive sterility of animal cells in culture. In: Potten C S (ed) Perspectives on mammalian cell death. Oxford: OUP, 184–201

Sheshadri T, Campisi J 1990 Repression of c-fos and an altered genetic programme in senescent human fibroblasts. Science 247: 205–209

Sikora E, Kaminska B, Radziszewska E, Kaczmarek L 1992 Loss of transcription factor AP1 DNA binding activity during lymphocyte aging in vivo. FEBS Lett 312: 179–182

Silvestri G 1997 Age-related macular degeneration: genetics and implications for detection and treatment. Mol Med Today 3: 84–91.

Slagboom P E, Droog S, Boomsma D I 1994 Genetic determination of telomere size in humans – a twin study of 3 age-groups. Am J Hum Genet 55: 876–882

Smith J R, Whitney R G 1980 Interclonal variation in proliferative potential of human diploid fibroblasts: stochastic mechanism for cellular ageing. Science 207: 82–84

Smith S, de Lange T 1997 TRF1, a mammalian telomeric protein. Trends Genet 13: 21–26.

Solmi R, Tietz C, Zucchini C et al 1996 In vitro study of gingival fibroblasts from normal and inflamed tissue: age-related responsiveness. Mech Age Dev 92: 31–41

Stanulis-Praeger B M 1987 Cellular senescence revisited: a review. Mech Age Dev 38: 1–48

Stein G H, Dulic V 1995 Origins of G_1 arrest in senescent human fibroblasts. BioEssays 17: 537–543

Sugrue M M, Shin D Y, Lee S W, Aaronson S A 1997 Wild type p53 triggers a rapid senescence program in human tumor cells lacking functional p53. Proc Natl Acad Sci USA 94: 9648–9653

Technology Foresight Panel on Health and Life Sciences 1995 Progress through partnership. Tech Foresight 4: 20–22

Thomas E, Al-Baker E, Dropcova S et al 1997 Different kinetics of senescence in human fibroblasts and peritoneal mesothelial cells. Exp Cell Res 236: 355–358

Thweatt R, Lumpkin C K, Goldstein S 1992 A novel gene encoding a smooth-muscle protein is overexpressed in senescent human fibroblasts. Biochem Biophys Res Commun 187: 1–7

Van Hinsburgh V W M 1992 Arteriosclerosis: impairment of cellular interactions in the arterial wall. Ann NY Acad Sci 673: 321–330

van Steensel B, Smogorzewska A, de Lange T 1998 TRF2 protects human telomeres from end-to-end fusions. Cell 92: 401–413

Vazari H 1997 Critical telomere shortening regulated by the AT gene: a review. Biochemistry (Moscow) 62: 1306–1310

Vaziri H, Dragowska W, Allsopp R C et al 1994 Evidence for a mitotic clock in human hematopoietic stem cells: loss of telomeric DNA with age. Proc Natl Acad Sci USA 91: 9857–9860

Vaziri H, Schachter F, Uchida I et al 1993 Loss of telomeric DNA during aging of normal and trisomy-21 human-lymphocytes. Am J Hum Genet 52: 661–667

Vaziri H, West M D, Allsopp R C et al 1997 ATM-dependent telomere loss in ageing human diploid fibroblasts and DNA damage lead to the post-translational activation of p53 protein involving poly(ADP-ribose) polymerase. EMBO J 16: 6018–6033

Venable M E, Lee J Y, Smyth M J, Bielawska A, Obeid L M 1995 Role of ceramide in cell senescence. J Biol Chem 270: 30701–30708

Wang E 1987 Contact inhibition induced quiescent state is marked by intense nuclear expression of statin. J Cell Phys 133: 151–157

Wang S, Moerman E J, Jones R A, Thweatt R, Goldstein S 1996 Characterisation of IGFBP3, PAI-1 and SPARC expression in senescent fibroblasts. Mech Age Dev 92: 121–132

Watanabe Y, Lee S W, Detmar MAjioka I, Dvorak H F 1997 Vascular permeability factor vascular endothelial growth factor (VPF/VEGF) delays and induces escape from senescence in human dermal microvascular endothelial cells. Oncogene 14: 2025–2032

Wei X P, Ghosh S K, Taylor M E et al 1995 Viral dynamics in human-immunodeficiency-virus type-1 infection. Nature 373: 117–122

Weinrich S L, Pruzan R, Ma L B et al 1997 Reconstitution of human telomerase with the template RNA component hTR and the catalytic protein subunit hTRT. Nat Genet 17: 498–502

Weng N P, Granger L, Hodes R J 1997 Telomere lengthening and telomerase activation during human B cell differentiation. Proc Natl Acad Sci USA 94: 10827–10832

Weng N P, Levine B L, June C H et al 1995 Human naive and memory T-lymphocytes differ in telomeric length and replicative capacity. Proc Natl Acad Sci USA 92: 11091–11094

Weng N P, Palmer L D, Levine B L et al 1997 Tales of tails: regulation of telomere length and telomerase activity during lymphocyte development, differentiation, activation, and ageing. Immunol Rev 160: 43–54

West M D, Shay J W, Wright W E, Linskens M H K 1996 Altered expression of plasminogen activator and plasminogen activator inhibitor during cellular senescence. Exp Gerontol 31: 175-193

Wistrom C, Villeponteau B 1992 Cloning and expression of SAG: a novel marker of cellular senescence. Exp Cell Res 199: 355–362

Wolthers K C, Wisman G B A, Otto S A et al 1996 T-cell telomere length in HIV-1 infection – no evidence for increased CD4(+) T-cell turnover. Science 274: 1543–1547

Yasumoto S, Kunimura C, Kikuchi K et al 1996 Telomerase activity in normal human epithelial-cells. Oncogene 13: 433–439

Zeng G, McCue H, Mastrangelo L. Millis A J T 1996 Endogenous TGFβ activity is modified during cellular aging. Exp Cell Res 228: 271–276

Zeng G, Millis A J T 1996 Differential regulation of collagenase and stromelysin mRNA in late passage cultures of human fibroblasts. Exp Cell Res 222: 150–156

Simon S. Cross

Artificial neural networks in diagnostic pathology

Artificial neural networks were originally developed by psychologists who hoped that simulations of human cerebral function would allow the investigation of diseases such as schizophrenia. That expectation has been largely unrealised and artificial neural networks are used now as sophisticated statistical classifiers and image or signal processing devices. They have found widespread application reflected in the increase of the number of papers about them, from 84 in 1987 to 2974 in 1997, listed by the *Science Citation Index*. This chapter briefly reviews the principles of artificial neural networks and their usage and then critically assesses the published descriptions of their applications in pathology.

PARADIGMS OF MACHINE LEARNING

To understand the way in which artificial neural networks can be used as diagnostic aids in pathology, a brief overview of the different paradigms for machine learning is required. A simple problem will be used to make the differences between methodologies explicit. Figure 10.1 shows a diagram of a tennis court (without service or doubles lines). The court is equipped with pressure sensors beneath its surface so the position of a bouncing tennis ball will be recorded as x and y co-ordinates. The aim is to produce an automated line calling system that will indicate whether the bouncing ball is within, or outside, the limits of the court.

RULE-BASED SYSTEMS

In this simple example it is easy to generate a rule-based system that will work efficiently. The rules of tennis have been written by humans and are published

Dr Simon S. Cross, Department of Pathology, University of Sheffield Medical School, Beech Hill Road, Sheffield S10 2UL, UK

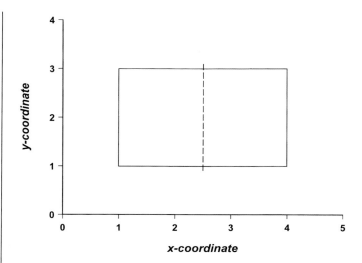

Fig. 10.1 Diagram of the boundaries of the 'tennis court' and their relation to the *x* and *y* co-ordinates. The 'net' is shown as a dotted line.

in explicit detail so it is easy to translate these into algorithms that can be interpreted by a computer. The co-ordinates of the court can be derived from Figure 10.1 and the following rules constructed:

If $1 \leq x \leq 4$ and $1 \leq y \leq 3$ then ball is IN   (1)

If $< x < 1$ or $x > 4$ then ball is OUT   (2)

If $y < 1$ or $y > 3$ then ball is OUT   (3)

which could be simplified to a single rule:

If $1 \leq x \leq 4$ and $1 \leq y \leq 3$ then ball is IN, else ball is OUT   (4)

SELF-LEARNING SYSTEMS

The self-learning paradigm makes no assumptions about the problem and requires no information apart from some input data with known outcomes. Figure 10.2 shows some data for the tennis court problem that could be used by a self-learning system. No information about the size or position of the court is given, but instead there is a set of points with the known outcome of whether each point is in or outside the court boundaries (points in court are circles, points outside court are triangles). These data could have been collected by recording the position of the bouncing ball using the pressure sensors and having a team of expert line judges calling each ball in or out. The data are presented to the self-learning system which uses it to construct a model of the problem. The system will have feedback mechanisms within it that will take the input data, make a prediction as to whether the ball is in or out, compare that prediction with the known outcome (the judgement of the expert line judges) of in or out and use a learning mechanism to adjust the model if the prediction is incorrect (Fig 10.3). After several cycles of prediction

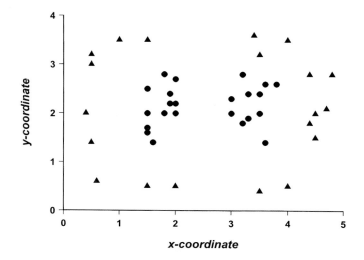

Fig. 10.2 A data set which could be used by a self-learning system to derive a model of the tennis court. The outcome of each point is shown by a circle (ball is IN) or a triangle (ball is OUT).

and adjustment of the model, the system will be able to correctly call the ball in or out for the points that it was given in the data set.

The model that the self-learning system has produced may not be explicit to a human user which is a problem with this technology. We are reluctant to believe the prediction of an opaque 'black box' system, and would prefer a system which also explained its decisions. In Figure 10.4, possible computed

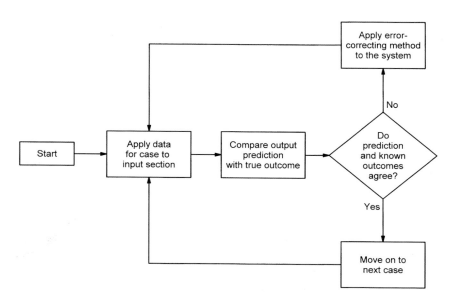

Fig. 10.3 A general algorithm used by self-learning systems. The differences between systems lie largely in the methods of error correction.

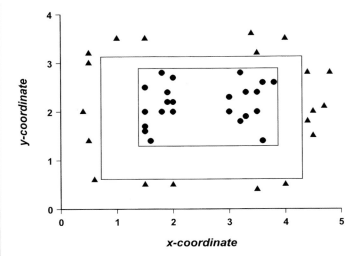

Fig. 10.4 Two models of the tennis court boundary that could be derived from the dataset given in Figure 10.2. Both models classify the points given correctly but neither corresponds with the known court boundaries shown in Figure 10.1.

models of the boundaries of the tennis court are shown, both of which would classify correctly the original dataset as being in or out, but neither of these models corresponds with the known boundaries shown in Figure 10.1. Why has this happened? The answer lies in the selection of the data used to train the self-learning system. The points shown in Figure 10.2 could have been obtained from observing two social tennis players warming up before a game, trying to hit the ball to each other to bounce midcourt; their skill deficiencies cause an occasional ball to fly far outside the court boundaries.

Figure 10.5 shows points that could have been obtained from two world class players during a series of sustained baseline rallies. Such players have the skill to hit the ball very close to the lines of the court and balls that are outside the boundaries are outside only by a small distance. If a self-learning system were to be supplied with these input data, the model of the court that would be derived would correspond closely with the actual boundaries of the court (Fig. 10.5). This illustrates the importance of using fully representative data when training and testing any system – especially those following a self-learning paradigm. It should be noted that the two social tennis players could supply data that would produce an accurate system but many more data points would have to be used to obtain a sample that would accurately map the boundaries of the court (Fig. 10.6).

In the tennis court example, the self-learning system is much more difficult and time-consuming to implement than the simple rule-based system because the problem has a known perfect model (the known boundaries of the court). In medicine, the converse is true in virtually all situations: there are input data with outcomes verified with a reasonable degree of certainty but no perfect model of the problem exists. It is in such situations that self-learning systems, as exemplified by artificial neural networks, have their greatest utility.

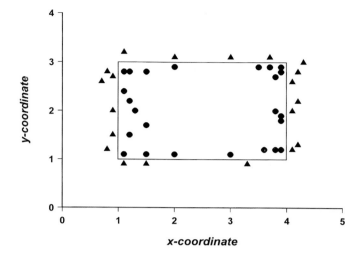

Fig. 10.5 A data set derived from highly skilled tennis players. The derived model (shown by the rectangle) must correspond closely with the known court boundaries if all the points are correctly classified.

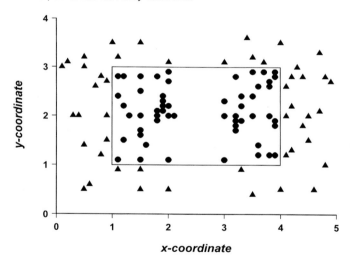

Fig. 10.6 The data set given in Figure 10.2 has been expanded with many more points from the relatively unskilled tennis players and the increased sample of points now gives a wide enough distribution to be able to derive an accurate model of the court boundaries (shown by the rectangle).

ARTIFICIAL NEURAL NETWORKS

WHAT IS AN ARTIFICIAL NEURAL NETWORK?

An artificial neural network is an emulation of a biological neural network that is implemented by a different substrate. Although artificial neural networks can be constructed as parallel circuits of discrete electronic components, such

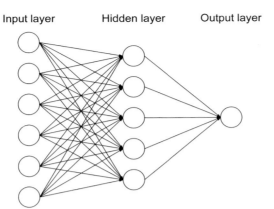

Input layer   Hidden layer   Output layer

Fig. 10.7 Schematic representation of the multilayer perceptron type of artificial neural network. The artificial neurones are shown as circles with each neurone in one layer connected to all the neurones in the next layer. The specific arrangement in this diagram would be described as a 6-5-1 architecture because of the number of neurones in each of the three layers.

circuits lack the flexibility required in developing self-learning systems. Most are created using software emulations running on standard serial computers. The means of implementation, however, does not affect the functional concept of such networks.

Figure 10.7 is a diagram of the most commonly used architecture of artificial neural network, the multilayer perceptron (Fausett 1994). The network is constructed of discrete artificial neurones (shown as circles) which are interconnected by routes that correspond to the axons in biological neurones. Like biological neurones, an artificial neurone summates the signal arriving from incoming connections. If this reaches a certain threshold, a signal is fired down the outgoing axons. The input data are presented to the layer of input neurones with one input neurone required for each item of input data (the tennis court problem would require two input neurones, one for the x co-ordinate and one for the y co-ordinate). The prediction of the neural network is given by the layer of output neurones which, for the tennis court problem, would be a single neurone with a threshold on its output above which the ball would be predicted as out, and below which the ball would be predicted as in. If an artificial neural network is constructed that consists solely of an input layer connected directly to an output neurone, then this network will function only as a linear regression classifier. If a hidden layer is interposed between input and output layers then the network will be able to perform more complex classification tasks.

A newly constructed artificial neural network will have random weighting applied to all the connections within the network and will give random predictions: in the tennis court problem, it would begin by calling 50% of balls in and 50% out. For the network to have any useful function it must be trained with input data which have a known outcome and the weights of the connections changed to give correct predictions by a feedback mechanism similar to the scheme given in Figure 10.3. The particular method of minimising errors will vary among different network architectures and it is important only that the general principle is understood. In multilayer perceptrons the most common method of learning is by back propagation in which the difference between the network's prediction and the true outcome is referred back through the network and minimised by changing the weight of connections (Fausett 1994).

The multilayer perceptron is only one type of neural network architecture and many other architectures have been described. Adaptive resonance theory neural network mapping (ARTMAP) is one that has attracted much attention. This system has a period of unsupervised learning which may reveal novel clustering of the data before they are linked with known outcome; explicit rules can be extracted from the trained network to give transparency to its internal workings (Carpenter et al 1991, Carpenter et al 1992, Carpenter & Tan 1993, Downs et al 1996). Other commonly used architectures include the radial basis function and Kohonen networks (Fausett 1994).

WHAT ARE THE THEORETICAL ADVANTAGES OF ARTIFICIAL NEURAL NETWORKS?

If artificial neural networks are to find widespread application in pathology, then there must a demonstrable advantage between these techniques and more conventional methods, such as multivariate linear or logistic regression. The main theoretical advantage is that they do not require any *a priori* model of the problem domain with associated judgements about the relevant importance of different input variables or their interaction. As most pathology problems do not have a clear-cut rule-based schema, in contrast to the tennis court problem, this advantage could be important. If we take the example of the distinction between chronic idiopathic inflammatory bowel disease and normality in endoscopic large bowel biopsies, we find that textbooks cite at least 30 microscopic features that are said to have discriminatory value. It is likely that the value of some of these features has been inflated by anecdote and single case reports, and that some features will represent extraneous data with no discriminatory value. In a system that requires some modelling of the problem before analysis, such as with most conventional statistical methods, relative values would have to be assigned to the different input variables that would influence the performance of the final system.

With an artificial neural network, each input variable is assigned small random weightings on the connections between the input neurone and the hidden layer neurones before training. During training, these weights are changed by the training algorithm to reflect the relative importance of each variable. If one input neurone represents a feature with no discriminatory value then the weight on the connections from that neurone will be reduced towards zero during training, effectively isolating it from making any contribution to the final prediction and so filtering useless data (acting as noise) from the system. Another stated advantage of artificial neural networks is a relative resistance to incomplete or partially erroneous input data that is important in the safety-critical medical environment. It should be pointed out that these theoretical advantages should not be accepted uncritically and in every circumstance in which an artificial neural network is used, a valid comparison should be made using more conventional statistical methods such as logistic regression.

HOW TO USE AN ARTIFICIAL NEURAL NETWORK

The popularity of neural network technology has led to the development of several user-friendly commercial packages which allow anyone with access to a reasonably fast and memory-rich computer (e.g. a Pentium-based PC with at least 16 MB of RAM) to run their own neural networks. These programs present a similar graphical interface to most common conventional statistical packages and are no more difficult to use.

The important aspects of developing a neural network system are the general principles of the training and testing cycle (Cross et al 1995). A data set with outcomes verified by a 'gold standard' method is required that is large enough to be split into three adequately sized subsets – an initial training set, a second training set for optimising the network, and an independent test set. The size of each set will vary with the number of different input and output variables, the number of neurones in hidden layers and the ranges that the variables have in the problem domain. A general rule of thumb is to have considerably more cases in each set than the total number of connections within the network. If a problem produced a network with 10 input neurones, one hidden layer of 5 neurones and a single output neurone, then at least 55 cases would be required in each set. If the number of cases is less than the total number of connections, then there is a high probability that each member of the training set can occupy a unique position in the multidimensional network, resulting in a network with 100% accuracy on the training set but poor generalisation and performance on test sets. This important feature is disregarded in most medical applications of artificial neural networks and results in an artificial reduction in the apparent performance of this technology.

APPLICATIONS IN CYTOPATHOLOGY

Although this account is primarily about the use of neural networks in histopathology, some mention should be made of the applications in cytopathology especially as this includes the only fully developed commercially available neural network system currently in use in pathology.

The problems of false negative smears in cervical cytology has been recognised since the start of this technique and there have been attempts from the 1940s onwards to produce automated systems for screening. With the advent of neural networks, a few systems have been developed which appear to offer a reasonable promise of automation, or least semi-automation, of the screening of cervical cytology. Foremost amongst these systems is PAPNET (Boon & Kok 1993, Koss et al 1994, Mango 1994, , Ouwerkerk et al 1994, Sherman et al 1994, Boon et al Beck S 1995): a commercially available system produced by Neuromedical Systems (New York, NY, USA). This system uses conventionally prepared specimens spread on a slide and stained by the Papanicolaou method. A slide is loaded into a scanning light microscope by a robot arm and examined at three magnifications with $\times 50$, $\times 200$ and $\times 400$

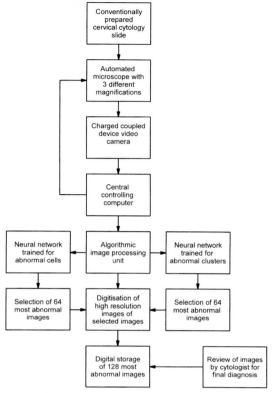

Fig. 10.8 Schematic diagram of the processes involved in the PAPNET system for screening cervical cytology smears.

objective lenses. At the lowest power, the machine maps the distribution of material on the slide. At medium power, some image-processing algorithms identify potentially abnormal cells. Digitised images of these are presented to two differently-trained multilayer perceptrons to produce a composite score of the object's resemblance to a training library of abnormal cells. A total of 128 fields, 64 from each network, of the objects that were rated as being most likely to be abnormal are digitised, at the highest magnification, and stored on tape together with their co-ordinates on the slide (Fig. 10.8). The final diagnosis is not made by the machine but by a human observer who looks at the digitised images of the cells rated as most abnormal and makes a final classification on the basis of the screen appearances and review down a light microscope. The machine attributes a numerical score to each cell and so it would be possible theoretically to set a suitable threshold and allow complete automation. This would subject the machine to much more stringent licensing procedures and the current system does have the advantage of human overseeing. As the problem of cervical cytology is not the interpretation of abnormal cells when detected but more the detection of these cells from a highly populous background of normal cells, then PAPNET represents a reasonable solution.

There have been a number of studies that have compared the performance of the PAPNET system with unassisted human screening. Some of these involved very small numbers of false negative smears and purported to show that the PAPNET system would have detected the abnormal cells which were initially missed (Boon & Kok 1993): the human interpreters of the PAPNET images do not appear to have been blind to the fact that these were false negative smears, which was likely to have biased the results. Much larger studies have been conducted which compare PAPNET screening with the results of human screening in retrospective studies. One of these studies (Ouwerkerk et al 1994) examined 1494 smears and found that there was a significantly increased rate of classification of smears as atypical (i.e. abnormal but less than mild dyskaryosis) rather than normal category when PAPNET was used. There was no statistically significant difference between PAPNET and unassisted cytologists for the detection of mild, moderate and severe dyskaryosis. The largest published study of PAPNET involved 42,134 smears screened by unassisted humans and 35,876 using PAPNET assistance (Boon et al 1995). The outcomes were validated by histological examination of tissue excised after abnormal smear reports but even with these large numbers there were only 24 cases of invasive carcinoma in the PAPNET group and 13 cases in the conventionally screened group.

Statistics were performed on the crude rate of abnormality detected in the two groups – the crude rates of diagnosis of carcinoma *in situ* and invasive carcinoma in the PAPNET-screened slides were significantly higher than those in the unassisted group. The balance of evidence suggests that the PAPNET system does improve performance in screening cervical smears and represents one of the few neural network systems that has made the transition from the development stage to a working production model that is used in everyday laboratory medicine practice. The PAPNET technology has also been applied to sputum (Hoda et al 1996), oesophageal (Morgenstern et al 1997), and urine (Hoda et al 1997) cytology. Other less developed systems using neural networks in cervical cytology have been described by Mehdi et al (1994) and Brouwer and Macauley (1995).

Breast cytodiagnosis is another area where neural network systems have been applied. Wolberg and Mangasarian have used a multilayer perceptron to diagnose breast cytology. The input data were nine defined human observations each rated on a scale of 1–10; e.g. for cellular dyshesion, clumps in which all marginal cells were adherent and not deformed were rated as 1 and those with little cohesion were rated as 10. All observations were made by a single experienced observer who was unaware of the outcome at the time of observation. The multilayer perceptron had nine input neurones, a single hidden layer of five neurones and a single output neurone for the dichotomous (benign/malignant) prediction. The network was trained on 420 cases and tested on a further 163. On the test set, the trained network produced only one false positive (a rate of 0.6%) and one false negative. One of the stated advantages of neural networks is their ability to produce classifiers with good generalisation and this is illustrated in this paper. In the 215 carcinomas in the study there were only two that shared the same scalar values for the nine input variables. Among the benign cases (total 368) there was more duplication; 175 cases had four or more identical input vectors, but there were still 146 with unique combinations of the scalar values. All but one of the cancers, and many of the benign cases, occurred as new combinations of scalar values for the nine input variables that were not encountered in the training set but were nonetheless classified correctly.

Downs and colleagues (Downs et al 1995a, Downs et al 1995b, Downs et al 1996) have reported similar studies on breast cytology using defined human observations but using the adaptive resonance theory mapping (ARTMAP) neural network architecture (Carpenter & Grossberg 1987a, Carpenter & Grossberg 1987b, Carpenter et al 1991, Carpenter et al 1992, Carpenter et al 1993). In their studies, there were 10 observations each coded in binary fashion: cellular dyshesion was coded as 0 if most epithelial cells were adhesive and 1 if most were dyshesive. These data are less information-rich than those used by Wolberg and Mangasarian (1993), but are more suitable for some biologically-dichotomous variables such as the presence or absence of intra-cytoplasmic lumina. The networks were trained on 313 cases and tested on a further 100.

ARTMAP networks cluster the input data in an unsupervised learning stage before these clusters are linked to the outcome (in this case a diagnosis of benignity or malignancy). The formation of the input clusters is dependent on the order in which the data are presented. Downs and colleagues exploited this property to produce multiple networks trained on different orders of the training data and then either selected the best performers or combined them into majority voting systems and finally into a cascaded voted system (Fig. 10.9). The cascaded voting system gives an indication of the confidence in the neural network prediction: if five networks optimised for sensitivity give a unanimous benign decision, then the prediction is highly likely to be correct, similarly for a unanimous malignant prediction from networks optimised for specificity. Using this system, 89% of cases were predicted by unanimous decisions of five networks pruned for either sensitivity or specificity (Fig. 10.9) and the accuracy for these cases was 100%. This left 11% of cases that were predicted by a majority decision of 5 networks optimised equally for sensitivity and specificity (i.e. overall accuracy) and these could have the Nottingham system of reporting suspicious cases applied to them with reports of 'suspicious, probably benign' and 'suspicious, probably malignant' according to the majority decision (Downs et al 1998). An advantage of the

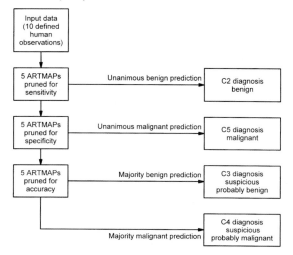

Fig. 10.9 The cascaded voting system of differently pruned ARTMAPs used by Downs and colleagues to make predictions on breast cytology specimens.

Artificial neural networks in diagnostic pathology

ARTMAP architecture is that explicit rules can be extracted from trained networks which give an indication of the decision-making process and help to overcome the user resistance to the impenetrable 'black box' technology (Hart & Wyatt 1990, Wyatt & Spiegelhalter 1991, Wyatt 1995). Downs et al (1966) extracted rules from their trained networks and compared them with canonical lists of diagnostic criteria in the published literature (Wells et al 1994). They found a close agreement with the exception of one feature, the presence or absence of foamy macrophages which, in the published literature, was said to favour a benign diagnosis but in the network rules, appeared with an equal frequency in benign and malignant tumours.

The same investigators have also published a study using image analysis parameters from fine needle aspirates of the breast to train a multilayer perceptron (Cross et al 1997). The measured variables included integrated optical density, fractal textural dimension, number of cellular objects, distance between cellular objects and derivatives (kurtosis and skewness) of these. The training set contained 200 cases and the test set 162 cases; the perceptron had a 15-12-1 architecture. The neural network produced a sensitivity of 83%, specificity of 85% and a positive predictive value of a malignant result of 85%. Logistic regression produced a virtually identical performance with no statistical difference. These performance values are well below what would be acceptable in a diagnostic situation but all the image analysis was performed automatically on a single low power field of view of each specimen. At this magnification, nuclear detail was not resolvable (a single nucleus would be represented as a single pixel) and most of the features cited as being important in the diagnosis of breast cytology are related to nuclear detail. It is thus possible that the reported system would give much better results of combined with an analysis of nuclear images.

Neural network systems have also been described in the cytodiagnosis of pleural and peritoneal effusions (Truong et al 1995), haemopoietic cells (Beksac et al 1997), oral epithelial lesions (Brickley et al 1996), thyroid lesions (Karakitsos et al 1996), gastric (Karakitsos et al 1996, Karakitsos et al 1997) and urothelial lesions (Hurst et al 1997).

APPLICATIONS IN HISTOPATHOLOGY

The main uses of artificial neural networks in histopathology have been as statistical classifiers on data generated by other analytical methods, but there are also reports where digitised images have been used as the input data for neural networks (Dytch & Wied 1990, Becker 1994, Cohen 1996).

HISTOLOGICAL DIAGNOSIS OF BREAST CARCINOMA

O'Leary et al (1992) have used data from image analysis of histological slides to train a neural network to distinguish between sclerosing adenosis and tubular carcinoma of the breast. They used an image analysis system to measure 18 morphological parameters and then used a modified Bonferroni analysis to select those features that were significant in discriminating between the two diagnoses. These two parameters (glandular surface density and the coefficient of variation of luminal form factor) were used as the input data to a multilayer perceptron with a single hidden layer of 4 neurones and one output neurone. The network was trained on 36 cases and tested on a separate set of 19 cases. It classified 33 out of 36 of the training cases correctly and all 19 in the test set. Comparison was not made with conventional statistical methods or human performance but the authors commented that they would have expected a pathologist reporting the 36 training cases to be able correctly to assign the test cases, and the 'gold standard' in this study was an expert human diagnosis. The preselection of input variables is worthy of comment, as one of the postulated advantages of neural networks is that irrelevant input data is ignored since the weighting on the routes from those input neurones will be adjusted during training to give no overall effect. In this study, the authors could have submitted all 18 measurements on each case to the network and it is possible that subtle interactions between these variables, not revealed by the Bonferroni analysis, could have acted to improve the performance. As the training set was small (36 cases), however, using 18 input variables would risk overtraining. Although the results of this study appear promising, they would need to be validated on much larger data sets and a problem with the overall system is that generation of the image analysis data is extremely time-consuming requiring tracing of glandular profiles with a light-pen after some image preprocessing and selection.

Fukushima et al (1997) have used neural networks in the histopathological diagnosis of intraductal proliferative breast lesions. The investigators measured 25 nuclear morphological features and 22 Markov textural parameters on 200 nuclei from each of 46 lesions that ranged from epithelial hyperplasia without atypia to the intraduct component adjacent to invasive carcinomas. The 'gold standard' in this study was the opinion of 2 experienced histopathologists. Various configurations of neural networks were trained using the data from two cases, which the authors selected as a 'typical' benign case and a 'typical' malignant case, and the networks were tested using the data from the other 44 cases. The parameters to be used as input data were selected by multiple regression analysis. The optimal network had 8 input neurones, a hidden layer of 20 neurones and 2 output neurones giving a total of 200 network connections. The overall agreement between the histopathologists' opinion and the neural network prediction was reported as 75% excluding the 13 cases that were classified as 'undetermined' by the histopathologists. The authors did not give a contingency table or parameters such as sensitivity and specificity. The main problems with this study are that only two cases were used to train the neural networks, that the optimal network had a hidden layer with many more neurones than the input and output layers, and that molecular biology has established that atypical ductal hyperplasia and intraduct carcinoma share similar genetic abnormalities, so that morphological distinction between them is likely to be a false arbitrary distinction.

AUTOMATED SEGMENTATION OF RENAL BIOPSIES

Serón et al (1996) have used a multilayer perceptron to segment automatically images from renal biopsies into tubules and interstitium (the ratio of these two areas correlates with renal function measured as the glomerular filtration rate). In digitised images, the authors applied a local granulometry method to each pixel to derive 8 numerical values which were input to the neural network, together with the grey-scale value of that pixel. The network had nine input neurones, two hidden layers of 10 and three neurones and a single output neurone. From images of eight biopsies, 160 pixels were selected randomly and the pixel visually classified as tubule or interstitium by a human observer. These values were used to train the network. The trained network was applied to all pixels in 202 images (a total of more than 13 million pixels) and the output (interstitium or tubule) was used to create a visual image and to calculate the area ratio of tubule to interstitium. The images produced had different qualitative appearances from a simple grey-scale thresholded image, but the correlation of both methods with the subject's glomerular filtration rate was the same ($r = 0.73$). The neural network method showed very close correlation with a manual point-counting method ($r = 0.92$), so it is possible that this could be implemented as an automated method of measuring these parameters.

HISTOLOGICAL DIAGNOSIS OF PARATHYROID LESIONS

Einstein et al (1994) have used quantitative measurements of nuclear diffuseness and nuclear profile area to train a multilayer perceptron to distinguish among normal parathyroid tissue, parathyroid adenoma and parathyroid carcinoma. They used a jack-knife ('leave one out') system of training and testing but had a very small study population of 16 cases (for a network with 50 weighted connections). The network classified 15 of the 16 cases correctly but clearly many more cases need to be examined to be able to evaluate the performance of this system.

HISTOLOGICAL DIAGNOSIS OF HEPATOCELLULAR CARCINOMA

Erler et al (1994) have used measurements from an image analysis system to train a neural network to discriminate between well-differentiated hepatocellular carcinoma and dysplastic hepatocytes. An image analysis system was used to measure 35 nuclear morphometric and densitometric parameters of 100 nuclei from each of 90 cases (56 hepatocellular carcinomas, 34 normal or dysplastic). Stepwise discriminant analysis was used to identify the parameters which gave the lowest classification error rates and these were used as input data. The selected morphometric variables were area, skewness of area, length of major axis, nuclear roundness factor and circularity factor. The network was a multilayer perceptron with an architecture of five input neurones, a single hidden layer of five neurones and one output neurone which was trained with 45 cases and then tested with a further 45. On the test set, the neural network gave a positive predictive value of 100% and a negative predictive value of 85% that compared favourably with 86% and 81%, respectively, for linear discriminant analysis and 86% and 77% for quadratic discriminant analysis. The criticisms that can be made of this study are similar to those of the breast carcinoma study reviewed above (O'Leary et al 1992), in that the image analysis process is too time-consuming to be used in routine practice and that the validation of the outcome (by expert human diagnosis) is open to some doubt, as the difficulties in this diagnostic area were identified as the motivation for the study.

HISTOLOGICAL GRADING OF ASTROCYTOMAS

The histological grading of astrocytomas is important for the selection of appropriate therapy, disease prognosis and a standardisation of disease for comparison of trials of different treatments. Studies using the World Health Organization (WHO) classification have shown a large amount of inter- and intra-observer variation is assigning tumours to one of the four grades, especially in the two intermediate grades. Kolles et al (1995) have developed an automated image analysis grading system based on neural networks. From previous studies, they selected four morphometric parameters – the relative nuclear area of all cells per field of vision, the relative volume weighted mean nuclear volumes of proliferating (proliferating cellular nuclear antigen, MIB1, positive) nuclei and the mean value and variation coefficient of the secant lengths of the minimal spanning trees per field of vision. They used these parameters on a set of 68 tumours and applied cluster analysis to derive their own quantitative system of grading astrocytomas into three grades. They then used neural networks (multilayer perceptrons with a 4-30-10-3 neurone/layer architecture) and discriminant analysis on training and testing sets to classify the tumours using their own unique grading system. The neural networks showed a 60% accuracy of assigning tumours to the WHO grades (as subjectively assessed by a neuropathologist) and a 99% accuracy of assigning tumours to the authors' cluster analysis-derived grades. By comparison, discriminant analysis gave overall accuracies of 62% and 92%, respectively. The main defect of this study is that the authors derived their own grading system by cluster analysis which the neural network could reproduce very well which shows only that neural networks are efficient at approximating the technique of cluster analysis which the authors used. In a follow-up study, Kolles et al (1996) used a number of different neural networks on a data set similar to the first study

HISTOLOGICAL GRADING OF PROSTATE CANCER

Stotzka et al (1995) have published a comprehensive study of a sophisticated image analysis-based system of grading prostatic carcinomas. The basic data structure used in the study was a 64×64 binary pixel array representing the spatial position of the nuclei in an area of prostatic carcinoma. When viewed alongside the photographic image of the same area, this array is a great simplification of the original image that would be viewed down the microscope by a histopathologist but it still contains 4096 items of information that require an immense amount of computation if input into a neural network in its raw unprocessed form. In one part of this paper, the investigators reduced the size of the binary pixel array to 45×45 and presented this to a multilayer perceptron with 2025 input neurones, a single hidden layer of 35 neurones and one output neurone. Training of this network required 3 weeks of computing time on a Sun SPARC workstation.

The authors used a conventional statistical method (quadratic Bayes classifiers) to classify the images into classes corresponding to moderate or poor differentiation, with all the usual caveats for such dichotomous divisions of biological continuums. Using this classification, the trained network classified the training set with an accuracy of 82%, 65% for the test set. The authors then developed an interesting hybrid system, where a partially trained multilayer perceptron was used to preprocess the binary image before presentation of outputs from the hidden layer of neurones to a set of statistical classifiers (Fig. 10.10). This system produced an accuracy of classification of 96% on a training set and 77% on a test set but this was an improvement of only 2% on the test set performance when compared with a more conventional statistical method (Bayes classifier). This well-written paper contains much useful discussion for any investigators contemplating using image analysis systems and neural networks as classifiers.

PREDICTION OF STAGING IN TUMOURS

Staging provides the most important prognostic information for most tumours, but the surgery required to sample lymph nodes for staging often has significant morbidity – axillary sampling in breast carcinoma is a common example. If the stage, particularly the lymph node status, could be predicted accurately from data from the primary tumour, then such sampling procedures would be unnecessary. Naguib and colleagues (Naguib et al 1996, Naguib et al 1997) used neural networks to predict the axillary node status in patients with

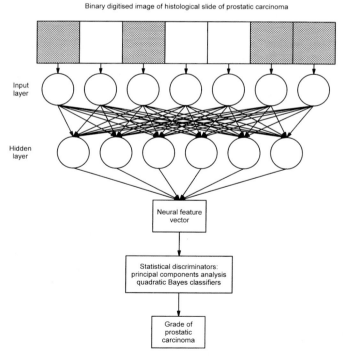

Binary digitised image of histological slide of prostatic carcinoma

Input layer

Hidden layer

Neural feature vector

Statistical discriminators: principal components analysis quadratic Bayes classifiers

Grade of prostatic carcinoma

Fig. 10.10 Schematic diagram of the hybrid neural network/statistical discriminators system used by Stotzka et al (1995) to grade prostatic carcinoma.

breast carcinoma. They studied histological grade, tumour size, oestrogen and progesterone receptor status, p53, nm23 and RB1-3 protein product expression as input data with 50 training cases and 31 test cases. The optimal combination of input variables and network structure gave an overall accuracy of 84% but the sensitivity of prediction of nodal metastases was only 73% which is unacceptably low for clinical practice. Moul and colleagues (Moul 1995, Moul et al 1995) used histological features of testicular teratomas to predict the stage of the tumour at presentation; the seven histological features used included vascular invasion in the primary tumour and percentage of tumour composed of embryonal carcinoma component. Stage was predicted with an accuracy of 92% using custom-developed neural networks and 80% accuracy using commercially available neural network software.

CONCLUSIONS

Histopathology is almost entirely based on subjective human interpretation of visual images. The dominant role of human interpretation is explained by the complexity of the images seen down the microscope and the very efficient processing of this information by the human brain. A single binary image at a resolution of 256×256 pixels contains over 65,000 bits of information, which places an enormous computational burden on an artificial neural network implemented on a digital computer if this is presented as raw input data, but which is a very crude representation of a microscopic image. Images at a resolution of 1024×1024 pixels and 64,000 colours are closer to the appearances seen down the microscope but still have far less resolution: finer detail, which may be important diagnostically, is not visible. Evolution has produced *Homo sapiens* with high resolution vision and a large biological neural network to interpret those data; artificial neural networks are unlikely to compete with this in the immediate future even with the accelerated evolutionary forces that exist *in silico*. However, this review has shown that neural networks can compete with human performance in areas where constant vigilance or objective weighting of multiple probabilities are required. The only commercially available neural network system, PAPNET, uses a hybrid of neural networks to perform the vigilance task and human observers to make the final diagnosis and this may be the way forward for other neural network systems in histopathology.

References

Becker R L 1994 Computer-assisted image classification: use of neural networks in anatomic pathology. Cancer Lett 77: 111–117

Beksac M, Beksac M S, Tipi V B, Duru H A, Karakas M U, Cakar A N 1997 An artificial intelligent diagnostic system on differential recognition of hematopoietic cells from microscopic images. Cytometry 30: 145–150

Boon M E, Kok L P 1993 Neural network processing can provide means to catch errors that slip through human screening of pap smears. Diagn Cytopathol 9: 411–416

Boon M E, Kok L P, Beck S 1995 Histologic validation of neural network-assisted cervical screening: comparison with the conventional procedure. Cell Vision 1: 23–27

Brickley M R, Cowpe J G, Shepherd J P 1996 Performance of a computer simulated neural network trained to categorise normal, premalignant and malignant oral smears. J Oral Pathol Med 25: 424–428

Brouwer R K, MacAuley C 1995 Classifying cervical cells using a recurrent neural network by building basins of attraction. Anal Quant Cytol Histol; 17: 197-203.

Carpenter G A, Grossberg S 1987a A massively parallel architecture for a self-organizing neural pattern recognition machine. Computer Vision, Graphics Image Processing 37: 54–115

Carpenter G A, Grossberg S 1987b Discovering order in chaos: stable self-organization of neural recognition codes. Ann N Y Acad Sci 504: 33–51

Carpenter G A, Grossberg S, Markuzon S, Reynolds J H, Rosen D B 1992 Fuzzy ARTMAP: a neural network architecture for incremental supervised learning of analog multidimensional maps. IEEE Trans Neural Networks 3: 698–712

Carpenter G A, Grossberg S, Reynolds J H 1991 ARTMAP: supervised real-time learning and classification of non-stationary data by a self-organizing neural network. Neural Networks 4: 565–588

Carpenter G A, Tan A-H 1993 Rule extraction, fuzzy ARTMAP, and medical databases. Proc World Congress Neural Networks 1: 501–506

Cohen C 1996 Image cytometric analysis in pathology. Hum Pathol 27: 482–493

Cross S S, Bury J P, Stephenson T J, Harrison R F 1997 Image analysis of low magnification images of fine needle aspirates of the breast produces useful discrimination between benign and malignant cases. Cytopathology 8: 265–273

Cross S S, Harrison R F, Kennedy R L 1995 Introduction to neural networks. Lancet 346 : 1075–1079

Downs J, Harrison R F, Cross S S 1995a A neural network decision-support tool for the diagnosis of breast cancer. In: Hallam J (ed) Hybrid problems, hybrid solutions. Amsterdam: IOS Press, 51–60

Downs J, Harrison R F, Cross S S 1995b: Evaluating a neural network decision-support tool for the diagnosis of breast cancer. In: Barahona P, Stefanelli M, Wyatt J (eds) Artificial intelligence in medicine – lecture notes in artificial intelligence. Berlin: Springer, 239–250

Downs J, Harrison R F, Cross S S 1998 A decision support tool for the diagnosis of breast cancer based upon fuzzy ARTMAP. Neural Comput Applications 7: 147–165

Downs J, Harrison R F, Kennedy R L, Cross S S 1996 Application of the fuzzy ARTMAP neural network model to medical pattern classification tasks. Artif Intell Med 8: 403–428

Dytch H E, Wied G L 1990 Artificial neural networks and their use in quantitative pathology. Anal Quant Cytol Histol 6: 379–393

Einstein A J, Barba J, Unger P D, Gil J 1994 Nuclear diffuseness as a measure of texture: definition and application to the computer-assisted diagnosis of parathyroid adenoma and carcinoma. J Microsc 176: 158–166

Erler B S, Hsu L, Truong H M et al 1994 Image analysis and diagnostic classification of hepatocellular carcinoma using neural networks and multivariate discriminant functions. Lab Invest 71: 446–451

Fausett L 1994 Fundamentals of neural networks: architectures, algorithms and applications. Englewood Cliffs, NJ: Prentice-Hall

Fukushima N, Shinbata H, Hasebe T, Yokose T, Sato A, Mukai K 1997 Application of image analysis and neural networks to the pathology diagnosis of intraductal proliferative lesions of the breast. Jpn J Cancer Res 88: 328–333

Hart A, Wyatt J 1990 Evaluating black-boxes as medical decision aids: issues arising from a study of neural networks. Med Inf (Lond) 15: 229–236

Hoda R S, Saccomanno G, Schreiber K, Decker D, Koss L G 1996 Automated sputum screening with PAPNET system – a study of 122 cases. Hum Pathol 27: 656–659

Hoda R S, Tahirkheli N, Koss L G 1997 PAPNET screening of voided urine sediments: a study of 100 cases. Lab Invest 76: 186

Hurst R E, Bonner R B, Ashenayi K, Veltri R W, Hemstreet G P 1997 Neural net-based identification of cells expressing the p300 tumor-related antigen using fluorescence image analysis. Cytometry 27: 36–42

Karakitsos P, Cochand-Priollet B, Guillausseau P J, Pouliakis A 1996 Potential of the back propagation neural network in the morphologic examination of thyroid lesions. Anal Quant Cytol Histol 18: 494–500

Karakitsos P, Stergiou E B, Pouliakis A et al 1996 Potential of the back propagation neural network in the discrimination of benign from malignant gastric cells. Anal Quant Cytol Histol 18: 245–250

Karakitsos P, Stergiou E B, Pouliakis A et al 1997 Comparative study of artificial neural networks in the discrimination between benign from malignant gastric cells. Anal Quant Cytol Histol 19: 145–152

Kolles H, von Wangenheim A, Rahmel J, Niedermayer I, Feiden W 1996 Data-driven approaches to decision making in automated tumor grading. An example of astrocytoma grading. Anal Quant Cytol Histol 18: 298–304

Kolles H, von Wangenheim A, Vince G H, Niedermayer I, Feiden W 1995 Automated grading of astrocytomas based on histomorphometric analysis of Ki-67 and Feulgen stained paraffin sections. Classification results of neuronal networks and discriminant analysis. Anal Cell Pathol 8: 101–116

Koss L G, Lin E, Schreiber K, Elgert P, Mango L 1994 Evaluation of the PAPNET cytologic screening system for quality control of cervical smears. Am J Clin Pathol 101: 220–229

Mango L J 1994 Computer-assisted cervical cancer screening using neural networks. Cancer Lett 77: 155–162

Mehdi B, Stacey D, Harauz G 1994 A hierarchical neural network assembly for classification of cervical cells in automated screening. Anal Cell Pathol 7: 171–180

Morgenstern N, Tahirkheli N, Schreiber K, Koss L G 1997 Evaluation of esophageal cytology with an interactive neural net based automated scanning system (PAPNET). Lab Invest 76: 198J, Harrison R F, Kennedy R L, Cross S S

Moul J W 1995 Proper staging techniques in testicular cancer patients. Tech Urol 1: 126–132

Moul J W, Snow P B, Fernandez E B, Maher P D, Sesterhenn I A 1995 Neural network analysis of quantitative histological factors to predict pathological stage in clinical stage I nonseminomatous testicular cancer. J Urol 153: 1674–1677.

Naguib R N, Adams A E, Horne C H, Angus B, Sherbet G V, Lennard T W 1996 The detection of nodal metastasis in breast cancer using neural network techniques. Physiol Meas 17: 297–303

Naguib R N, Adams A E, Horne CH et al 1997 Prediction of nodal metastasis and prognosis in breast cancer: a neural model. Anticancer Res 17: 2735–2741

O'Leary T J, Mikel U V, Becker R L 1992 Computer-assisted image interpretation: use of a neural network to differentiate tubular carcinoma from sclerosing adenosis. Mod Pathol 5: 402–405

Ouwerkerk E, Boon M E, Beck S 1994 Computer-assisted primary screening of cervical smears using the PAPNET method: comparison with conventional screening and evaluation of the role of the cytologist. Cytopathology 5: 211–218

Serón D, Moreso F, Gratin C et al 1996 Automated classification of renal interstitium and tubules by local texture analysis and a neural network. Anal Quant Cytol Histol 18: 410–419

Sherman M E, Mango L J, Kelly D et al 1994 PAPNET analysis of reportedly negative smears preceding the diagnosis of a high-grade squamous intraepithelial lesion or carcinoma. Mod Pathol 7: 578–581

Stotzka R, Manner R, Bartels P H, Thompson D 1995 A hybrid neural and statistical classifier system for histopathologic grading of prostatic lesions. Anal Quant Cytol Histol 17: 204–218

Truong H, Morimoto R, Walts A E, Erler B, Marchevsky A 1995 Neural networks as an aid in the diagnosis of lymphocyte-rich effusions. Anal Quant Cytol Histol 17: 48–54

Wells C A, Ellis I O, Zakhour H D, Wilson A R 1994 Guidelines for cytology procedures and reporting on fine needle aspirates of the breast. Cytopathology 5: 316–334

Wolberg W H, Mangasarian O L 1993 Computer-designed expert systems for breast cytology diagnosis. Anal Quant Cytol Histol 15: 67–74.

Wyatt J 1995 Nervous about artificial neural networks. Lancet 346: 1175–1177

Wyatt J, Spiegelhalter D 1991 Field trials of medical decision-aids: potential problems and solutions. Proceedings of the 15th Symposium on Computer Applications in Medical Care 1991; 3–7

F. Joel W-M. Leong   Andrew K. Graham
Thomas Gahm   James O'D. McGee

CHAPTER 11

Telepathology: clinical utility and methodology

Most histopathologists are aware of the ability to transmit textual, numerical, macroscopic and microscopic images via telecommunication technologies, though the majority have yet to see it work in practice. Telepathology and medical telematics, however, have progressed beyond the experimental stage and advances in computer image processing, the development of the Internet and telecommunications technology have evolved so that telepathology is now used in many institutions.

Telepathology is the acquisition of histological and or macroscopic images for transmission along telecommunication pathways for diagnosis, consultation or continuing medical education. In brief, a telepathology system comprises a conventional microscope; a method of image capture, commonly a camera mounted on a light microscope; telecommunications link between sending and receiving sites; and a workstation at the receiving site with a high-quality monitor to view the images (Fig. 11.1). There may also be mechanical hardware to allow the receiving pathologist to control the microscope from a distance and view the entire slide in 'real-time'. The images are viewed on a computer screen, rather than through microscope oculars.

Telemicroscopy, in its current form, falls short of what pathologists are used to seeing through their conventional microscopes. Despite this, recent work suggests that, in most cases, an accurate diagnosis can still be made (Eide & Nordrum 1992, Wold & Weiland 1992, Ito et al 1994, Olsson & Busch 1995, Weinberg et al 1996, Eusebi et al 1997, Weinstein & Epstein 1997, Weinstein et al 1997). The authors experience in this area is that image quality is such that

Dr F. Joel W-M. Leong, Nuffield Department of Pathology and Bacteriology, University of Oxford, John Radcliffe Hospital, Academic Block, Level 4, Headington, Oxford OX3 9DU, UK
Dr Andrew K. Graham, Nuffield Department of Pathology and Bacteriology, University of Oxford, John Radcliffe Hospital, Academic Block, Level 4, Headington, Oxford OX3 9DU, UK
Dr Thomas Gahm, Autocyte Inc., Burlington, NC 27215, USA
Prof. James O'D. McGee, Nuffield Department of Pathology and Bacteriology, University of Oxford, John Radcliffe Hospital, Academic Block, Level 4, Headington, Oxford OX3 9DU, UK

diagnosis is unduly difficult and cannot be made with the same level of confidence as with conventional microscopy.

We describe the recent advances in this field and discuss the exponential growth and popularity of the Internet and how various spin-off technologies in image delivery may be utilised. This chapter is presented in two parts: the first describes and delineates the clinical utility of telepathology, and to a lesser extent telecytopathology; the second describes the technological background on which future developments in telepathology will evolve.

CLINICAL UTILITY OF TELEPATHOLOGY

HISTORY

The initial impetus in the development of telepathology was the provision of the best possible diagnostic opinion to all patients irrespective of location and socio-economic circumstances. Telepathology has its origins in telemedicine, a generic term encompassing the use of visual telecommunications in health care. Radiology was one of the earliest medical specialties to use this as early as 1959 when Albert Jutra used co-axial cable to transmit videotaped telefluoroscopy examinations between two hospitals in Montreal, some 5 miles apart (Weinstein et al 1987). Pathologists employed the technology somewhat later, probably because image resolution was not of a sufficient standard; a histological image is exponentially more complex than a black-and-white radiological image and colour television was not then mass-produced. One of the earliest instances of telepathology took place in Boston in 1968 when a microwave-based telecommunications system was established, linking Massachusetts General Hospital with a medical station at Logan Airport, outside downtown Boston (Bird 1975). Live black-and-white images of histological sections and stained blood smears were transmitted from a clinic at the airport to the hospital. The video quality was equivalent to the then current US commercial television (300–330 lines). A technician at the airport was directed by the pathologist at the hospital and also provided information on stain colours as requested. The aim of this experiment, organised by Dr K.T. Bird, a Harvard physician, was to demonstrate the feasibility of remote physical diagnosis, telestethoscopy, teleauscultation, teledermatology, speech pathology and even telepsychiatry (Weinstein et al 1989). Interestingly, even at this embryonic stage of development, Prof. Scully made the correct diagnosis on all microscopic images (Saunders J, personal communication).

In 1974, satellite communication was used to transmit histological images and clinical data from a 17-year-old male on a hospital ship moored near Brazil to a hospital in Washington DC (Riggs et al 1974). The system provided the equivalent of two telephone lines, one of which was used for voice communication, the other to transmit images of tissue sections, blood and bone marrow smears from a microscope video camera. In addition, teletype provided textual data communications while facsimiles of drawing and diagrams were sent at a rate of one page every 6 minutes. An electrocardiogram transmission unit and electronic stethoscope relayed ECGs and heart sounds. While the patient was not actually visualised, the data provided allowed a team of specialist consultants to diagnose

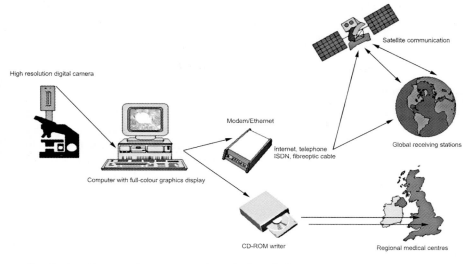

Fig. 11.1 A diagramatic representation of telepathology.

'mediastinal lymphosarcoma with leukemic transformation', initiate chemotherapy and irradiation to the mediastinum, and even transmit a relevant journal article to the ship. During follow-up under similar circumstances 35 days later, a chest radiograph showed a reduction in tumour size.

Telepathology became a newsworthy item on 20 August, 1986 with a public demonstration of a satellite-linked colour-video dynamic telepathology system between Fort William Beaumont Army Medical Center in El Paso, Texas and Washington DC (Colburn 1986). In Texas, a frozen section slide of breast tissue was placed on the stage of a custom-designed, Olympus Vanox motorised microscope equipped with a video camera. The full-colour image was transmitted via the SBS-3 COMSAT satellite (Communications Satellite Corp, Washington DC) to Washington DC where a pathologist seated at a prototype workstation (Corabi International Telemetrics, Rockville, MD) was able to control stage movements, magnification, focus and illumination while viewing a real-time image at 525 lines of resolution. A second monitor displayed other parameters such as location of the image in relation to the whole slide, co-ordinates, and stage speed. Two-way audio communication was also available. The exercise was a success, though the *Washington Post* afforded it only page seven newsworthiness.

Since then, work by independent groups in Europe (Kayser et al 1991, Nordrum et al 1991, Kayser & Drlicek 1992, Martin et al 1992, Schwartzmann 1992, Kayser et al 1993, Martin et al 1995, Nordrum & Eide 1995, Olsson et al 1995), the USA (Wold & Weiland 1992, Weinstein et al 1995, Halliday et al 1997) and Japan (Shimosato et al 1992, Ito et al 1994, footnote [a]) have each made significant contributions to the development and assessment of the clinical utility of telepathology equipment.

---

[a] http://telepath.med.cornell.edu/pathmaker.html

TYPES OF TELEPATHOLOGY

Telepathology or telemicroscopy has developed along two lines designated 'static telepathology' and 'robotic interactive pathology' (RITPath). The former is also referred to as 'store-and-forward' or passive telepathology.

Static imaging

The static or 'store-and-forward' approach to telepathology is cheap, simple and needs only a standard telephone line or Internet connection (Eusebi et al 1997). By definition, the images are static – there is no facility for recipient control. In practice, only a limited number of images are captured for each case, varying between 1–40 (Eusebi et al 1997, Halliday et al 1997) with the average number varying between 4.9 (Halliday et al 1997) and 6.3 (Eusebi et al 1997). To the pathologist trained in the doctrine that one must view the entire slide in order to make a confident diagnosis, this method would appear suboptimal, and many initially find it quite disconcerting. And yet, international static telepathology consulting services do exist (Eusebi et al 1997, Halliday et al 1997).

The major disadvantage is, of course, sampling error, though interpretation and video image quality have also been cited as problems (Weinberg et al 1996). Sampling error has been well-demonstrated in various studies (Eide & Nordrum 1992, Ito et al 1994, Halliday et al 1997, Weinstein et al 1997). Attempts to overcome this have included use of a trained pathologist to select the images (Halliday et al 1997, Weinstein et al 1997); however, few pathologists are completely happy to relinquish control to another person. Halliday et al (1997) pointed out that referring pathologists would tend to select images that supported their own diagnosis and that ambiguous fields were often ignored. The limited number of images could under-represent the complexity of the case and lead to a false sense of security as to the ease of the diagnosis. Sampling error or bias remains a serious flaw as the pathologist being consulted cannot identify significant regions of the slide while scanning at low-power.

Assessing the accuracy of telepathology is difficult. Involving multiple pathologists is the best option as the results from a single pathologist is influenced by the skill and experience in viewing static images. Eusebi et al (1997) used the Pathmaker image acquisition software (footnote [b]) to package 36 diagnostically difficult cases from a quality assurance program over the course of a year. Images included immunohistochemistry and were digitised at $640 \times 480 \times 24$ bit colour resolution before being sent as E-mail attachment to Dr Juan Rosai, in the Memorial Sloan-Kettering Center, New York. Of the 36 cases, 35 were also sent for final diagnosis as actual histological slides and/or further stains. Dr Rosai deferred a telepathology diagnosis in 8 cases. In 3 of these cases, his final diagnosis concurred with the referring pathologists. While a telepathology diagnosis was provided in only 77% of the cases (27/35) the concordance with the final diagnosis in those 77% was 100%. It is difficult to ascertain whether this is due to the accuracy of the technique or the skill of the histopathologist. Anecdotal evidence would suggest the latter.

Shimosato et al (1992) reported a diagnostic accuracy of 88.1% also based upon the performance of one pathologist. Weinberg et al (1996) used four patho-

[b] (http://telepath.med.cornell.edu/pathmaker.html)

logists at the Brigham and Women's Hospital in Boston, showing them 50 static images selected from cases on CD-ROM and comparing their diagnoses with the conventional light microscopy diagnoses they gave at a later date. The overall diagnostic accuracy was 88.5%, but marked interobserver variability was noted.

Weinstein et al (1997) examined the diagnostic accuracy of static imaging telepathology in assessing archival frozen sections of 46 skin excisions showing a spectrum of benign ($n = 9$) and malignant ($n = 37$) lesions. Using a single pathologist, they found 100% concordance in discriminating benign from malignant lesions, with minor discrepancies relating to precise characterisation of the lesion (actinic keratosis versus irritated seborrhoeic keratosis, basal cell carcinoma versus squamous cell carcinoma). Where errors occurred in determining clearance at the margin, they were attributed to field selection error. The images were stored at 1024 × 768 × 24-bit colour with no complaints about image quality.

Results from the Arizona-International Telemedicine Network (AITN) (Halliday et al 1997) showed an 88.2% concordance (127/144) between tele-pathology and glass slide diagnosis on a variety of referred cases, with 96.5% concordance (139/144) for clinically important diagnoses. They divided the reasons for discordance into three categories – field selection, diagnostic interpretation, and video image quality. Diagnostic interpretation was the most commonly cited reason, with field selection second. Poor image quality was not a problem at a resolution of 1024 × 768 × 24-bit colour and 6.5:1 JPEG compression. Comments were made on a possible reluctance by the telepathologist to overturn the provisional diagnosis provided by the referring pathologist based upon a small set of images.

Weinstein and Epstein (1997) conducted an analysis of the diagnostic accuracy of a static telepathology system in the interpretation of prostatic needle biopsies. They examined 200 needle biopsies of prostate divided into two groups and cited accuracy of up to 99%. However, no mention was made of image resolution, colour depth or the colour depth of the computer monitor used for viewing. Average image size was 300 Kb using JPEG compression (incorrectly referred to as a lossless algorithm) which would correspond to a 1024 × 768 image using moderate compression.

These studies have provided us with an indication of the skill of several individual pathologists in interpreting 'bitmapped' histological images. It is difficult to make comparisons between studies, however, due to the lack of standardisation in hardware, image resolution, storage format and colour-depth. This, combined with the narrow range of pathologists and wide range of cases, is a limitation preventing the extrapolation of results. The future of this technique may lie in education and external quality assessment rather than as a diagnostic tool.

Robotic interactive telepathology (RITPath)

RITPath systems allow the receiving pathologist to control the movement of the slide on the stage and to see the image in 'real-time' on a high-resolution monitor. Synonyms used for this modality include dynamic telepathology, active telepathology and real-time telepathology.

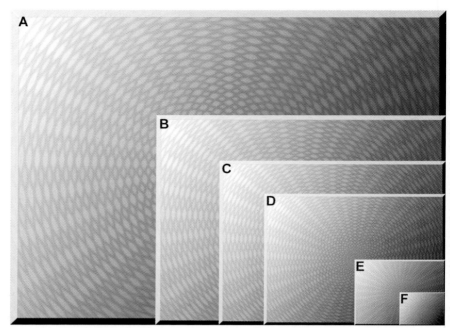

Fig. 11.2 A graphical representation of image resolutions and resultant file sizes (see Table 11.1 for details).

The limiting factor in RITPath is transmission time; an understanding of the various types of telecommunications protocols is essential for assessing the appropriateness of a dynamic system.

Norwegian geography necessitated development by the Norwegian health care system in 1991 of one of the earliest working European frozen section telepathology services. This was established between the University Hospital of Tromsø, Tromsø and an outlying hospital, Kirkenes Hospital, 420 km to the north-east (Nordrum et al 1995). Supported by a Norwegian Telecom network with a 2 Mb/s capacity, both dynamic or static resolution images could be transmitted. In 1991, the average time taken for assessment of a frozen section was 15 min, but it ranged from 5–30 min. An image resolution of 256 × 286 pixels appears quite small by present standards (Fig. 11.2, Table 11.1). Magni - fication shifts are performed manually by the local technician, although there are plans to automate this. Recently, two additional diagnostic centres hasve been established in Oslo and Trondheim.

The HISTKOM RITPath system (footnote [c]) is a joint project of the Institut für Physikalische Elektronik of the University of Stuttgart and Deutsche Telekom. The prototype has been tested in our department under simulated line speeds. It consists essentially of a robotic Zeiss microscope with a triple charge-coupled device sensor (CCD) Sony video camera transmitting images to a remote station. At this station, the user is able to control all the functions of the

[c] (http://www.uni-stuttgart.de/UNIuser/ipe/res/ip/histkome.html)

Table 11.1 Image resolutions, resultant file sizes and current popular usage (refer to Fig. 11.2 for graphical comparison)

Key	Image dimen. (pixels)	Size using 24-bit colour	Size in grey scale or 8-bit colour (256 shades/colours)	Current usage
F	160 × 120	57 KB	19 KB	♦ Video conferencing
E	320 × 240	225 KB	75 KB	♦ High-quality video conferencing ♦ Approximate resolution using Apollo/Corabi telepathology system in dynamic mode (actual resolution 352 × 288) ♦ Early digital snapshot cameras ♦ Personal digital assistants, high-end electronic diaries
D	640 × 480	900 KB	300 KB	♦ High-end personal digital assistants ♦ Outdated computer systems with 14 inch monitors ♦ Entry-level digital snapshot cameras ♦ Home digital video (DV) cameras ♦ Most microscope cameras used by pathology departments for clinical presentations
C	800 × 600	1.37 MB	469 KB	♦ Budget-priced computer systems ♦ Mid-range digital snapshot cameras ♦ Approximate resolution of HISTKOM dynamic telepathology system resolution (actual resolution 768 × 576)
B	1024 × 768	2.25 MB	768 KB	♦ Entry-level office workstations (requires 2 Mb graphics RAM and 15 inch flat screen monitor for best viewing) ♦ Upper-range digital snapshot cameras
A	1536 × 1152	5.06 MB	1.69 MB	♦ Minimum resolution for desktop publishing, computer graphics editing, computer-aided design (requires > 19 inch monitor) ♦ Static image resolution using Apollo/Corabi telepathology system
	2048 × 1536	9.00 MB	3.00 MB	
	3072 × 2304	20.3 MB	6.75 MB	♦ Upper limit of Jenoptik ProgRes 3012 ultra high resolution digital camera

Key: KB, kilobytes; MB, megabytes (1024 KB = 1 MB); Dimen. = Dimensions.

microscope, including the scanning stage, magnification and light intensity. Manual focussing may also be used in preference to the autofocus. Designed to be used with low-bandwidth networks, e.g. Integrated Services Digital Network (ISDN), compression algorithms are employed to minimise the data transmitted. Transmission along multiple ISDN channels is also possible. The system also conforms to Transmission Control Protocol/Internet Protocol (TCP/IP), the *de facto* standard for data transmission over networks to ensure compatibility with current network systems. The remote station is designed for ease of use with two monitors, one displaying the current position relative to the whole slide, the other providing the current view at $768 \times 576 \times 24$-bit colour (*see* Table 11.1, Fig. 11.2 for a comparison with other systems). Stage movement is controlled with a joystick, with optional mouse control. The images are transmitted in compressed JPEG format (see below for an explanation of image compression formats), encoded 'on-the-fly' via a hardware JPEG board. The software at the receiving station 'stitches' the images together, thus simulating a moving image. The degree of JPEG compression employed is proportional to the speed of movement, with the image quality improving when the slide is at rest. Images and position on the slide can be marked and saved. Response time is sufficient to review a slide in under 10 min, though in preliminary studies, experienced users have been able to reduce this to less than 3 min.

Two field trials were conducted in 1997 using this system (Schmid et al 1996). A prototype was tested in Stuttgart in a double blind study involving three pathologists, 118 lung frozen sections and a single ISDN connection providing a 64 Kb/s transmission rate. Overall accuracy of telepathology diagnosis was 73.1% compared with 89.8% using conventional light microscopy. Transmission time was unsatisfactory. A second field trial was conducted in the University of Tübingen, using two pathologists, 139 frozen sections of lung and eight times the bandwidth (8×64 Kb/s). The two pathologists averaged 105 s and 124 s per case, respectively, compared with 24 s using conventional light microscopy. Concordance with conventional light microscopy was 92.8% and 94.2%, respectively. There were no complaints about image quality.

The Apollo Image Management System/Corabi® Dynamic Module (IMS/CDM™) is based around the Corabi DX 1000, the result of a corporately-financed joint US-Japanese venture. It was first used in 1986 and since then has been tested in several American universities (Weinstein 1991). Apollo Software, a corporation in Maryland, has licensed a telepathology system patented by Prof. R.S. Weinstein and Corabi International Telemetric, Inc. and coupled it with its own image management software and teleconferencing facilities. The system provides remote stage movement, focus, light intensity and magnification, as well as the ability to view a gross image of the slide with the relative position of the current objective over the specimen. It also has the capability of functioning as a fully bi-directional telepathology system. This system differs from the Histkom system in that it is a hybrid system capable of both static telepathology, at resolutions up to $1520 \times 1144 \times 24$-bit colour, and dynamic images at $352 \times 288 \times 24$-bit colour via video codec over a T-1 line. One disadvantage of using video conferencing technology is susceptibility of the system to blurring or interruptions in image display. The use of a T-1 line greatly improves transmission speeds compared with ISDN (Table 11.2).

This system is used in the Veterans Affairs Hospitals in Milwaukee, Wisconsin and Iron Mountain, Michigan. Dunn et al (1997) reported that they achieved an overall concordance with consensus 'truth' diagnoses of 97.5% based upon a test set of 100 consecutive routine surgical pathology cases. The quality of the video images was cited as the reason for diagnostic error in two cases. The rest were attributed to diagnostic difficulty. The time spent on each slide varied between 2.8–4.7 min.

Table 11.2 Comparison of telecommunication line speeds

Device/ protocol	Speed	Speed relative to telephone service	Approximate time to transmit *Encyclopedia Britannica*
SINCGARS (tactical radio)	16 Kb/s	1/3	2.5 days
Digital telephone (DS-0)	56 Kb/s	1	18 h
ISDN	64/128 Kb/s	2	8 h
Broadband ISDN	1.5 Mb/s	30	40 min
Fractionated T-1	multiple (n) of 56 Kb/s	1n	
Standard leased line (DS-1/T-1)	1.5 Mb/s	30	38 min
Ethernet	10 Mb/s	180	6 min
High capacity leased line (DS-3/T-3)	44.7 Mb/s	800	1.5 min
SONET/ATM (STS-1/OC-1)	52 Mb/s	900	60 s
Fast ethernet (100Base-T)	100 Mb/s	1800	30 s
SONET/ATM (STS-3/OC-3)	155 Mb/s	2700	20 s
SONET/ATM (STS-12/OC-12)	622 Mb/s	11,000	6 s
Gigabit ethernet	1 Gb/s	17,900	< 4 s
SONET/ATM (STS-48/OC-48)	2.5 Gb/s	45,000	< 2 s
SONET/ATM (STS-192/OC-192)	10 Gb/s	190,000	< 0.5 s

Key: ATM, asynchronous transfer mode; Gb/s, gigabits (1000,000 kilobits) per second; ISDN - integrated services digital network; Kb/s, kilobits per second (8 bits = 1 byte); Mb/s, megabits (1000 kilobits) per second; SINCGARS, single channel ground and airborne radio; SONET, synchronous optical network, a protocol for transmission along fibre-optic cables.

OTHER SIGNIFICANT AREAS OF DEVELOPMENT

Internet

The World Wide Web was invented by Tim Berners-Lee in 1990 while working for the European Laboratory for Particle Physics (CERN) in Geneva. In 1993, the first graphical Web browser, Mosaic, was released by the National Center for Supercomputing Applications (NCSA). The exponential growth of the Internet can be attributed to the popularity of this graphical, animated, interactive interface. In the long-term, developers would like the Internet to become as ubiquitous and as simple to use as the television set and such enticing terms as 'WebTV' and 'Digital TV' have already appeared in the popular press. In the short-term, however, full-motion Internet video and video-conferencing is erratic and possible only with software technologies that circumvent the immediate problems of narrow bandwidth and network congestion.

The advantage of using the Internet for telepathology is cost and availability. Sending static images as E-mail attachments is not only easy for most people, it costs nothing to send. The Internet, however, is too slow and unreliable for satisfactory dynamic telepathology. Another consideration is the issue of security, which has yet to be adequately addressed. Encryption techniques of varying levels do exist, but a discussion of what is a satisfactory level of encryption goes beyond the scope of this review. Nonetheless, there are several examples of novel approaches to Internet telepathology and as advances in video-conferencing and presentation of graphical images takes place, telepathology can only benefit.

Wolf et al (1998) have used the cross-platform Java programming language to allow 'net-surfers' to control an automated microscope through a web browser. They cite the considerably lower cost of the telemicroscopy server software compared with remote station hardware as being an important advantage. Small images (360 × 270) are viewed within a Java-compliant browser, such as a recent version of Netscape Navigator or Microsoft Internet Explorer, with the option to capture larger ones (720 × 540) for closer inspection. The user has control of the stage movement, objectives and focus. The site is open to the public and, presumably, if there is more than one person viewing the site, there may be a fight for control.

Web-based remote control is not an original idea, the UK Leica site (footnote [d]) showcases a primitive slide viewer, and there are many sites which offer controllable robotic arms or real-time views from a user-controllable camera, often pointed into a street scene or room. However, this is the first time someone has attempted to match the features offered by a dedicated dynamic telepathology system. In real-terms it is not practical: response times are slow, and transmission via the Internet lacks the reliability of a dedicated line.

The exact number of Internet host sites (sites which form part of the Internet) is difficult to estimate. Anecdotal figures place it in the range of 29 million. In 1989, this figure was around 100,000. In 1996 it was 12.8 million (footnote [e]). The actual number of Internet users is far greater. The problem of Internet bandwidth was addressed by the US President Bill Clinton, in his 1998 State of the Union Address where he advocated US Congressional support for a Federal organisation, the Next Generation Internet (NGI) initiative. This initiative began under the Clinton administration in 1996 with three goals. First, to connect universities and national laboratories with high-speed networks, the majority operating at 100 times current Internet speeds, with a selected few operating at 1000 times normal. Second, to promote experimentation within research networks of networking technologies, such as high-quality video-conferencing, thus accelerating the introduction of new commercial services. Third, to demonstrate new applications that utilise this higher-speed and meet 'national goals and missions'.

The third goal involves development of applications in the areas of health care, national security, distance education, energy and biomedical research, manufacturing and environmental monitoring. Telemedicine represents a major investment within the health care component. In addition to video-conferencing and secure, reliable remote use of scientific facilities, other avenues of development include virtual reality environments with real-time interaction, creation of virtual supercomputers from multiple networked workstations, and centralised databases capable of handling terabytes (a trillion bytes) of

[d] http://www.leica.co.uk
[e] http://info.isoc.org:80/guest/zakon/Internet/History/HIT.html

data daily. With US government funding and access to the resources of other government agencies, such as the National Institutes of Health, Department of Defense, Department of Energy and National Aeronautical and Space Agency, this initiative will be a major influence on the course of Internet development and telepathology, at least within the US.

A less-powerful organisation, Internet2 or I2, is a non-Federal collaboration of over 100 universities, predominantly in the US. It too has a primary goal of developing the next generation of computer network applications particularly in the area of multimedia broadband networking and also collaborates with various government organisations within the NGI. Unlike the NGI initiative, however, the I2 agenda is focused towards facilitating the research and education agendas of the universities with the aim of ensuring new developments benefit all computer networks, not just those deemed suitable by the US government. Membership to the I2 is open to all universities and non-profit organisations involved in Internet development.

Slide digitisation

Digitisation is the conversion of an analogue source into a digital format that can be stored by a computer and recreated at a later date. The difficulty with doing this to a histological image is that the amount of digitisable data is a function of both the magnification and the image resolution. A single slide could potentially generate terabytes of data, an amount incompatible with current storage capacities. There are currently no studies that have reported on the minimum acceptable amount of data to make a diagnosis: this is not surprising, as the pathology community is still struggling with minimum criteria for such analogue functions as macroscopic specimen sampling. With respect to single images, past studies have shown that pathologists do not complain of poor image quality at resolutions above or equal to $1024 \times 768 \times 24$-bit colour (Halliday et al 1997, Weinstein et al 1997); however, small sample size precludes final judgement.

APPLICATIONS

Removal of the spatial constraint of physical proximity is the motivation behind telepathology development. Often, a remote-site cannot support a full-time pathologist due to lack of interest or economics, yet frozen section consultation or semi-urgent surgical pathology consultation may be needed. In countries such as Australia, pathologists are reluctant to work in the more isolated country areas. At least for frozen section work, telepathology offers a feasible solution to this problem. In this area, serious errors vary between 0–5% (Weinstein & Epstein 1997) with sampling and lack of adequate communication being major causes for error in static systems.

Even where a pathologist is on-site for consultation, the need often arises to consult a colleague or someone with more experience. Telepathology can satisfy this desire without the delays associated with the postal service.

External quality assessment and teaching

External quality assessment programs (EQA) can benefit from the convenience in mass delivery that static telepathology offers. Rather than cut multiple sections for distribution via mail, selective images for each case can be sent via E-mail, and these cases may now also include cytology specimens without fear of irreparable damage or loss. Participants have the added benefit of being able to keep the case images for review at a later date. Educational cases can easily be distributed to trainees throughout the country. Time zone differences notwithstanding, the potential exists for conferences to be hosted in cyberspace, with a slide being demonstrated to an international audience, each remaining in their home countries.

Image libraries, databases, archiving

Pathologists are fortunate that they are not dependent only upon clinical experience and patient contact to broaden their knowledge. Slide sections may be kept in archive for retrospective studies or self-education long after the patient has left hospital. Stained sections will, however, fade with time and paraffin blocks are finite in the number of sections they can yield. Image storage in digital form offers a longer lifespan, in addition to rapid recall and infinite reproduction.

There are several Internet sites which already offer image databases. Unfortunately, it is difficult to find high-resolution images and network congestion makes downloading the images time consuming. Hopefully, with improvements to the Internet, centralised image repositories may become a viable alternative to looking through a colleague's slide collection.

INTERNATIONAL CONSORTIA

Individuals and government agencies in several countries have recognised the need for international collaboration in telemedicine in general. The Atlantic Rim network was established to encourage interchange of ideas and information among Europe, the US and South America. The more specific brief was to encourage the exchange of protocols and expertise on both sides of the Atlantic and establish a strategically-significant network for use in medical consultation and education. The first scientific meeting was held in Boston in 1997 and was attended by academics, major telecommunications companies, major commercial organisations, and the military. It is planned to repeat such a meeting, probably in Europe, in 1999.

The International Consortium on Internet Telepathology (ICIT) was formed by a group of pathologists from Japan, the UK and US at a meeting in Washington DC in 1996. The aims were to exchange images between the Armed Forces Institute of Pathology (AFIP), the National Cancer Centre in Tokyo, and the University of Oxford. These images were transmitted at various levels of resolution and by at least two forms of telecommunication, namely telephone lines and the Internet.

The European Pathology Assisted by Telematics for Health (Europath) project is a consortium of engineers, computer experts, biologists and pathologists. The aims of Europath are: to establish guidelines for usage of static telepathology systems; to evolve a robotic interactive telepathology system; to enable fluid interoperability between static and robotic systems; and to establish pathology databases for use in oncology research within the European Union and elsewhere. Europath is sponsored by the European Union.

TECHNICAL ASPECTS OF TELEPATHOLOGY

IMAGE ACQUISITION

The scope of this article does not allow for detailed discussion of the various image types nor the principles of digital image manipulation. This has been previously discussed by other authors (Weinberg & Doolittle 1996, Furness 1997).

Early studies in telepathology were concerned with establishing whether video images displayed on a cathode ray tube (CRT) screen were of sufficient quality for microscopic diagnosis (Bloom et al 1987, Weinstein et al 1987, Weinstein et al 1992). The standard of even domestic television screens has improved much since then and 19-inch flatscreen computer monitors with resolutions up to 1600×1200 pixels are now available. The next problem is the best technique of image 'capture' or conversion of an image into a digital form. This technique needs to be rapid and result in an image which is of adequate size to satisfy a pathologist without being so large that it becomes impractical to transmit.

Digitised images can be divided into vector images and bitmaps – a pathologist need only be concerned with the latter. These are images represented digitally by a two-dimensional array of dots. Resolution refers to the number of dots. The cathode ray tube produces colour by combining red, green and blue at different intensities. The physiology of colour interpretation is very complex (Stiles 1964, Wald 1964). The human eye has difficulty appreciating more than 16.8 million colours (2^8 shades of red $\times$ 2^8 shades of green $\times 2^8$ shades of blue) or 256 shades of grey. When an image is viewed from a palette of 16.8 million colours, it is referred to as a true-colour or 24-bit colour image. When the colour palette has only 256 colours, it is referred to as an 8-bit image. Greyscale images are also 8-bit images as they use greys from a palette of 256 shades. Consequently, half-tone radiological images can be digitised at a considerably smaller size than histological images. Table 11.2 shows file sizes according to image dimensions and colour depth. Greyscale refers to images in shades of grey.

Work by Doolittle et al (1997) suggested that 8-bit colour may be sufficient for histological image assessment; however, the methodology behind that study has been questioned and 24-bit colour appears to be a *de facto* standard. Some scanners and graphics cards are now offering 32-bit colour but this has not yet been adopted for mainstream use.

Image acquisition may occur in a variety of ways. Most commonly, a camera is mounted on the top of a microscope and the image viewed in a small preview window within a computer software package. The user then 'captures' the desired fields. Both the video camera, the digital snapshot camera and optical scanner utilise a solid-state CCD sensor, to receive and convert images to an electronic form. A CCD contains a series of tiny, light-sensitive photosites capable of producing varying amounts of charge in response to the amount of light they receive. CCDs are usually arranged as either a line of cells or a rectangular array of cells. Sensors employing video technology have rectangular pixels, while sensors with square pixels were created specifically for use on computers. The performance of a CCD is often measured by its output resolution, a function of the number of photosites on the CCDs surface.

Most CCD video cameras have colour capability which, in a single chip system, is accomplished by striping columns of cells in alternating red, green, and blue filters. All pixels, taken in order, are used for luminance. Every third pixel represents one of the three colours. The colour quality of the single chip cameras is limited by the fact that the luminance signal is sequential rather than a true monochrome signal, and that any single colour has only one-third of the luminance resolution. A more subtle problem is that any one primary colour is not sensed over the entire surface of the CCD. The effect is similar to looking through a vertical venetian blind and becomes noticeable when the subject has vertical bands of colour.

Three chip cameras solve these problems with three identical CCDs (each handling one of the primary colours – red, green or blue) and a prism block incorporating dichroic filters that improve colour and sensitivity. Since each CCD produces only one colour, all components of the signal are at full system resolution. The penalty is cost, size, and weight.

CCDs are not digital devices as light is continuously variable in colour and intensity and the output from a CCD is an analogue voltage, not a discrete number. When we refer to a digital camera we are considering a device in which the analogue CCD output is immediately converted to digital. All subsequent processing of the signal is done digitally. As processing of the raw signal from a CCD comprises most of the work of a video camera, doing this digitally results in substantially better picture quality.

Something that is not often realised by those who have not used image capture systems is not only is the field rectangular, the field area is considerably less than the view through the microscope oculars. It is possible to increase this area with optical adaptors between the camera and the microscope; however, the only reliable way to increase the area captured is to increase the size of the CCD.

The output from a digital video camera may be either converted back to an analogue signal for viewing on an analogue television monitor, for teaching or demonstration, or sent unchanged to a computer with appropriate hardware and software for recording.

Originally intended for presentations, lower-priced analogue cameras combine all the visual information into a single video signal (composite video). This can result in inferior colour and spatial resolution. Video-capture units ('image-grabbers') will accept input from any analogue source such as a digital video camera with analogue output, standard home video camera, or even video cassette player and 'capture' images at resolutions of up to 1500×1125 pixels through a technique based upon oversampling the analogue signal. In reality, though, the quality of the images are at their best at 640×480 resolution.

One complementary method of image acquisition is to 'scan in' an entire glass slide using a digital scanner for 35 mm slides or negative strip film. We use a Polaroid SprintScan 35 and there are comparable models produced by other photographic companies. Maximum resolution is 2700 dots per inch (dpi) with 24-bit colour which produces an uncompressed file in the region of 30 megabytes size. This is a complementary rather than alternative technique because the image is only a low-power view without the aid of lens magnification. In theory, a resolution of 2700 dpi defines each dot at 9.4 µm, though in practice this is far larger. Even in optimum conditions, this figure is insufficient to show nuclear detail. If this resolution could be trebled and magnification aided with lenses, then it could become independently useful.

It may also be necessary to improve the image brightness, contrast or colour or even crop or annotate the image. This may be done using any one of a number of commercially available graphics software such as Adobe Photoshop, or with less expensive products such as Paintshop Pro. Use of graphics software also allows the possibility of digital magnification.

STORAGE

For short-term storage, the hard-drive offers the fastest access and greatest convenience. Those using SCSI (small computer system interface) architecture remain the fastest. SCSI has the advantage of being capable of handling multiple devices such as extra hard drives, scanners, CD-ROMs, simultaneously along a single interface. Several generations of SCSI protocols exist. SCSI-3 or SCSI UltraWide offers 40 megabytes per second (MB/s) data transfers across a 16-bit bus (the connection between the interface card and the motherboard).

Unfortunately for most PC users, SCSI has never been offered as a standard interface, with the less-expensive IDE (integrated drive electronics) hard-drives being commonplace. Like SCSI, it too has undergone improvements and the current protocol, Ultra-ATA (AT attachment), is capable of up to 33 MB/s data transfers.

Size and speed of the hard-drive is also an issue, as operating systems such as Windows 95, Windows NT, or Mac OS will use the hard-drive as a temporary holding area when system requirements exceed random access memory (RAM). Even with 64 MB of RAM, this will occur frequently when manipulating high-resolution digital images.

IMAGE COMPRESSION

In the past, some authors have stressed the importance of storing images in a form than does not compromise image quality. Indeed, those involved in computer graphic design realise the importance of working on an image in its optimum form before finally employing a compression algorithm to reduce it to a more practical size. This, however, is impractical for transmission of images as Table 11.1 demonstrates.

A severe hindrance to the wider use and effectiveness of telepathology is a lack of international standards for communication protocols, image resolution and compression. At present, those institutions using telepathology do so within a limited network, often not exceeding three institutions. It is possible to send static images as an E-mail attachment and institutions such as the Armed Forces Institute of Pathology will accept consults in this form; however, they provide no strict recommendations with respect to image size, type or degree of compression.

Radiologists were faced with a similar problem well over a decade ago. The American College of Radiology, in association with the National Electrical

Manufacturers Association addressed this lack of interoperability between different institutions by developing the Digital Imaging and Communications in Medicine Standard (DICOM(SM)) standard in 1984. DICOM is now in its third major revision and provides standardised formats for image capture and storage coupled with definitions and protocols for communication for radiological equipment and images (footnote [f]).

The DICOM(SM) standard is internationally recognised for medical imaging and has been adopted by the European standards body, Comité European de Normalisation (CEN TC 251) for use within the European Standard MEDICOM (SM). The Japanese Industrial Association of Radiation Apparatus has done the same. The College of American Pathologists (footnote [g]) is defining standards for telepathology and a current draft standard (DICOM Supplement 15 Visible light image for endoscopy, microscopy and photography) (DICOM 1997) is available via the Internet (footnote [h]).

A discussion of the more popular image formats follows. There are many more then those listed here, but lack of widespread appeal precludes their use from mainstream technologies. They can be divided into two broad categories – 'lossy' algorithms that discard 'unnecessary' data in the course of compression and 'lossless' algorithms that preserve data at the expense of compressed image size. Repeated editing and saving of an image using a lossy technique will result in image degradation. This is not an important issue if no further editing is performed, as is the case with telepathology.

JPEG

The Joint Photographics Experts Group (JPEG) established the JPEG standard for the purpose of storing high-resolution photographic images (Leger et al 1991). It is accredited as an industry standard by the International Standards Organisation, has universal multi-platform support on web browsers and graphics editing software and is the dominant format for still-image compression. Using a lossy compression technique known as discrete cosine transformation, it offers configurable compression ratios up to 20:1.

Work by Doolittle et al (1997) on 8-bit versus 24-bit colour images overlooked the use of compression techniques. Although their images were stored in tagged image file format TIFF format, which offers up to 10 different kinds of compression algorithms, no reference was made to which, if any, were utilised. For a JPEG compression algorithm, the difference in file size between an 8-bit and 24-bit colour image is almost negligible. As this compression method discards data in the process, excessive compression leads to false colour and blockiness which is noticeable in areas of high contrast.

Graphics interchange format (GIF)

The GIF format was introduced by the US online service provider, Compuserve, and is popular in web page design. Unisys now holds the patents to several aspects of the algorithm. The GIF 89a format features background transparency

[f] http://ftp.nema.org/medical/temp/broch95.htm
[g] http://www.cap.org
[h] http://idt.net/~dclunie/dicom-status/status.html

and animation, neither of which is of immediate value in the field of telepathology. Its utilisation of the lossless Lempel-Ziv-Welch (LZW) compression algorithms makes it suitable for images that have high-contrast, e.g. line drawings; however, support only for 8-bit colour prevents it from being a satisfactory format for histological images. Recently, the Unisys company, which owns patents to several key components within the LZW algorithm, has begun to charge a licensing fee for any commercial company wishing to write applications that use GIF compression. This has effectively ceased all further development in this area by third-party software companies and prompted development to focus on the superior portable network graphics (PNG) format. Those looking for a lossless form of compression should consider PNG.

Portable network graphics (PNG)

The PNG format has been approved as a standard by the World Wide Web consortium (footnote [i]) to replace the GIF format for use in web pages. This is a superior lossless compression format which supports 24-bit colour. With planned support within both Netscape Navigator and Microsoft Internet Explorer, it may provide a possible solution for those seeking uncompromised image storage.

Flashpix

This recent format developed by a consortium called the Digital Imaging Group has the advantage of multilayering of image resolutions. This may have application in image digitisation though it has yet to gain widespread acceptance.

Wavelet (WSQ)

Wavelet scalar quantitisation is a technology originally developed at the Los Alamos National Laboratory for the US Federal Bureau of Investigation as a method of storing and transmitting fingerprint data. It is a lossy compression technique that will most likely supersede JPEG due to its better compression ratios and preservation of image detail. There are multiple vendors offering wavelet compression software but, unfortunately, no industry standard or compatibility among different companies. Without a recognised standard, images saved using one type of wavelet compression will be able to be viewed only by those with similar software. Many companies circumvent this problem by offering file viewers as free software and also offering 'plug-ins' – program code which integrates with a web browser (Netscape Navigator, Microsoft Internet Explorer) and allows viewing of these images when they appear on a web page. This, however, does not allow image manipulation except with graphics software offered by the same company. Influential software companies such have Adobe (manufacturers of the industry-standard graphics software, Photoshop) have stated that they will not support wavelet

---

compression until a standard has been determined. Until a particular format is recognised by a major software company or the ISO, it would be unwise to store images solely with this method.

Tagged image file format (TIFF)

TIFF is a heterogeneous group of image formats, varying from greyscale images to 24-bit colour bitmaps which may optionally employ the lossless LZW compression algorithm used by the GIF format. It is difficult to find software which supports all possible TIFF formats. There are advocates of TIFF who argue that preservation of data is of medicolegal significance. Use of TIFF images is perhaps more relevant when repeated graphical editing will take place and the ultimate output is paper rather than computer monitor, e.g. desktop publishing, graphic design.

Fractals

In 1975, mathematician Benoit Mandelbrot coined the term 'fractal' to describe shapes that were 'self-similar' that is, they looked the same at different magnifications. He found that by using relatively simple mathematical equations, it was possible to create complex structures, often resembling those seen in nature. The aim of fractal compression is to do the reverse – to find a small finite set of mathematical equations that describe an image. In so doing, some data are discarded from the original image. It is a technique that is more effective the larger the image. Fractal compression appears ideally suited to real-world image compression, due to the inherent fractal nature of many natural images (e.g. histological sections). This has proved not to be the case for several reasons. There is no universal standard, the compression scheme is not documented in the public domain, and the source code is not widely available for development. More importantly, software compression times are very long, unless hardware assisted.

NETWORKING AND LINE SPEEDS

Robotic telepathology is so dependent on telecommunication transmission speed that some basic knowledge of telecommunications protocols and line speeds is important. As it becomes more prevalent, a knowledge of networking will be necessary to structure the most cost-efficient way of communicating between local and remote stations. Table 11.2 offers a comparison of different telecommunication line speeds.

Plain old telephone service (POTS)

This is the cheapest but slowest method of data transmission and is impractical for dynamic telepathology. Under optimum circumstances the maximum speed of this analogue service between two 33.3 Kb/s modems is 4.2 KB/s (33000 bits / 8 = 4200 bytes). 56 Kb/s modems (V.90) have now been standarized and are widely available; however, to attain such speeds requires a digital connection at the other end, such as is currently offered by many commercial Internet service providers. Even then, the maximum download speed in the US is limited to 53 Kb/s. Uploading does not exceed 33.3 Kb/s. The maximum speed attainable between two 56 Kb/s modems is still 33.3 Kb/s.

Integrated services digital network (ISDN)

ISDN is an international communications standard for sending voice, video and data over digital phone lines at speeds up to 64 Kb/s. ISDN basically is offered in two packages:

Basic rate interface ISDN (BRI-ISDN) is defined as two circuit-switched bearer (B) channels of 64 Kb/s each and one packet-switched delta (D) control channel of 16 Kb/s. The usable bandwidth of BRI-ISDN is 128 Kb/s.

Primary rate interface ISDN (PRI-ISDN) is defined in the US to match the bandwidth of the T-1 definition. It combines 23 B channels and 1 D channel to a total bandwidth of 1.544 Mb/s. In Europe, it matches the bandwidth of the existing E-1/CEPT definition of 2.048 Mb/s (30 B + 1 D). It is common for two ISDN lines to be employed, allowing for simultaneous voice and data or pure data transmission at 128 Kb/s. Requiring special metal wiring, early ISDN uses baseband transmission, in which one wire carries one signal at a time. A recent technology, broadband ISDN (B-ISDN), uses broadband transmission, in which a single wire may carry multiple signals simultaneously. Requiring fibre-optic cables, this offers speeds of up to 1.5 Mb/s, roughly 23 times the capacity of ISDN.

Asynchronous transfer mode (ATM)

ATM is a network technology that overlaps with B-ISDN and is capable of speeds from 25–622 Mb/s. B-ISDN employs the ATM protocol within one of its several 'layers'. Suitable for both local and wide area networks it transmits data in packets of fixed size at variable speeds determined by the nature of the data and the type of service subscribed to by the user. It is however, extremely expensive and currently limited in its use.

T-1/T-3

A T-1 carrier (also referred to as DS-1 line) is a dedicated phone connection supporting data transmission rates of up to 1.544 Mb/s. It actually consists of 24 individual channels, each supporting 64 Kb/s. A T-3 carrier (or DS-3 line) consists of 672 channels and can provide speeds of around 44.736 Mb/s. The Internet is based upon a T-3 carrier. Even a T-1 carrier does not come cheaply and telephone companies will often offer fractional T-1 access in multiples of 56 Kb/s.

Cable modems/Digital subscriber lines

These technologies are already in the United State and are a superior alternative to ISDN. Cable modems use a computer network interface card and operate via cable television. Working speeds are very much manufactuirer and service provider specific. Realistic figure vary between 3–10 Mb/.s for downloading and 200 Kb/s – 2Mb/.s uploading.

xDSL refers collectively to all types of digital subscriber lines, a transmission protocol which utilises unused frequencies in normal copper telephone wires. The two main categories are Asymmetric DSL (ADSL) and Symmetric DSL (SDSL). xDSL offers up to 32 Mb/.s for downstream traffic, and from 32 Kb/s to over 1 Mb/s for upstream traffic. The International Telecommunication Union recently approved the G.992.2 (*G.lite*) protocol which provides upstream access of up to 512 Kb/s and downloads of up to 1.5 Mb/s. It is imagined that installation of a G.992.2 modem will be as easy as installing a V.90 modem.

Unfortunately, availability of these services within Britain will be most likely be determined by economics and profitability from the telecommunications corporation point of view, the same companies which have an investment in ISDN.

COMPUTER NETWORKS

Computer networking is a key tool used by companies and institutions worldwide. A local area network (LAN) is a high-speed communications system designed to link computers and data-processing devices together within a small geographic area such as a department, or single-floor of a building. Users may then share resources such as printers or other CD-ROM drives. Multiple LANs may be linked together over a distance to form a wide area network (WAN), the means by which most robotic telepathology systems will communicate.

LANs were traditionally designed for 'bursty' or 'transaction-orientated' data with all devices connected to a common, dedicated, private medium. Data within a LAN is broken up into 'packets' and transmitted along the network until it reaches the intended recipient. Contrary to connection-oriented techniques like the common telephone service, where a busy signal is returned if a connection is already established between two parties and somebody tries to use the same circuit, LANs simply slow down as the traffic increases, without returning a busy signal. This presents a severe problem for voice and online image transmission, resulting in stilted speech and motion.

The bandwidth of different LAN technologies ranges from the low-speed token ring (4 Mb/s) through ethernet (10 Mb/s) and high-speed token ring (16 Mb/s) to the high-end fibre distributed data interface (FDDI) technology with typical bandwidth values around 100 Mb/s. Depending on the bandwidth, still image transmission, robotic telepathology, video-conferencing and even multiples of these applications are possible (Fig. 11.3).

Wide area network (WAN) services can be broken up into two broad categories: access and transport. Contrary to LANs, the networks normally do not belong to the network user but are operated by inter-exchange carriers such as telephone companies. To create a WAN between two LANs, each must have a connection to their inter-exchange carrier. These access channels can be dedicated digital circuits with a high bandwidth. The advantage of getting a high data throughput has to be weighed against the disadvantage of excluding all 'external' participants who do not have the same dedicated access connections. Use of switched access services eliminates this problem. Instead

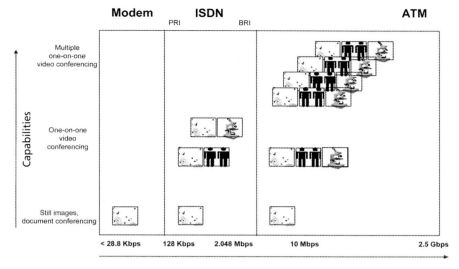

Fig. 11.3 Capabilities of different WAN technologies.

of dedicated circuits, the services of a local exchange carrier are used to connect the user to whatever inter-exchange carrier he chooses.

The telephone network is probably the best known example of a WAN. In the US, it is based on the North American digital hierarchy that defines packages of different bandwidth. DS-0 characterizes the lowest available bandwidth of 64 Kb/s. This number is derived from converting the traditional analogue 4 kHz voice channel to digital using pulse code modulation. The next step in the hierarchy is DS-1, also called T-1 (already discussed), combining the bandwidth of 24 DS-0 channels to a total of 1.544 Mb/s using time division multiplexing. Further steps up are DS-2, which combines 4 T-1 channels to a total of 6.312 Mb/s and DS-3 which has the capacity of 28 T-1 channels (44.736 Mb/s).

Although the 'transport part' of the US telephone network is completely digital, the local access to the inter-exchange carrier often for historical reasons is still analogue. In such a situation, digital data created by a computer have first to be converted to analogue via a high-speed modem before they are sent through the analogue channel to the inter-exchange carrier, where they are reconverted to digital. Use of ISDN has superseded this.

THE FUTURE

Telepathology in its current form is far from being an alternative to conventional reporting, but it offers a new approach to diagnostic services. After tissue processing and staining, everything seen by microscopy is an artefact, and the art of histopathology has evolved around the interpretation of these. Telepathology brings with it a new set of artefacts which, for many, is quite disconcerting.

We would like to think that progress in the digitisation of histological images will continue until the quality equals that which is seen through the standard microscope and this will be true up to a point. However, what is more likely and perhaps more feasible, is that pathologists' skill in interpreting digitised images will improve until it matches their skill with conventional images.

References

Bird K 1975 Telemedicine concept and practice. In: Bashshur E, Armstrong P, Yussel Z (eds) Telemedicine: explorations in the use of telecommunications in health care. Springfield, IL, USA: Charles C Thomas, 89–112

Bloom K J, Rozek L S, Weinstein R S 1987 ROC curve analysis of super high resolution video for histopathology. SPIE Proceedings Visual Communications Image Processing II 845: 408–412

Colburn D 1986 The next best thing to being there. And now, diagnosis by satellite. Washington Post, August 27: 7

DICOM 1997 Digital Imaging and Communications in Medicine. NEMA PS 3 Supplement 15: Visible light image for endoscopy, microscopy and photography. Rosslyn, VA: The National Electrical Manufacturers Association

Doolittle M H, Doolittle K W, Winkelman Z, Weinberg D S 1997 Colour images in telepathology: how many colors do we need? Hum Pathol 28: 36–41

Dunn B E, Almagro U A, Choi H et al 1997 Dynamic robotic telepathology: Department of Veterans Affairs feasibility study. Hum Pathol 28: 8–12

Eide T J, Nordrum I 1992 Frozen section service via the telenetwork in Northern Norway. Zentralbl Pathol 138: 409–412

Eusebi V, Foschini L, Erde S, Rosai J 1997 Transcontinental consults in surgical pathology via the internet. Hum Pathol 28: 13–16

Furness P N 1997 The use of digital images in pathology. J Pathol 183: 253–263

Halliday B E, Bhattacharyya A K, Graham A R et al 1997 Diagnostic accuracy of an international static-imaging telepathology consultation service. Hum Pathol 28: 17–21

http://www.nema.org/medical/dicom.htm

http://idt.net/~dclunie/dicom-status/status.html

http://info.isoc.org/guest/zakon/Internet/History/HIT.html

http://telepath.med.cornell.edu/pathmaker.html

http://www.cap.org

http://www.leica.co.uk

http://www.uni-stuttgart.de/UNIuser/ipe/res/ip/histkome.html

http://www.w3.org

Ito H, Hironobu A, Kiyomi T et al 1994 Telepathology is available for transplant-pathology: experience in Japan. Mod Pathol 7: 801–805

Kayser K, Drlicek M 1992 Visual telecommunication for expert consultation of intraoperative sections. Zentralbl Pathol 138: 395–398

Kayser K, Drlicek M, Rahn W 1993 Aids of telepathology in intraoperative histomorphological tumour diagnosis and classification. In Vivo 7: 395–398

Kayser K, Oberholzer M, Weiss G et al 1991 Long distance image transfer: first results of its use in histopathological diagnosis. Acta Pathol Microbiol Immunol Scand 99: 808–814

Leger A, Omachi T, Wallace G K 1991 JPEG still picture compression algorithm. Optic Eng 30: 947–954

Martin E, Dusserre P, Fages A et al 1992 Telepathology: a new tool for pathology? Presentation of a French national network. Zentralbl Pathol 138: 413–417

Martin E, Dusserre P, Got C L et al 1995 Telepathology in France: justifications and developments. Arch Anal Cytol Pathol 43: 191–195

Nordrum I, Eide T J 1995 Remote frozen section service in Norway. Arch Anat Cytol Pathol 43: 253–256

Nordrum I, Engum B, Rinde E et al 1991 Remote frozen section service: A telepathology project to northern Norway. Hum Pathol 22: 514–518

Olsson S, Busch C 1995 A national telepathology trial in Sweden: feasibility and assessment. Arch Anat Cytol Pathol 43: 234–241

Riggs R S, Purtillo D T, Connor D H 1974 Medical consultation via telecommunications. JAMA 228: 600–602

Schmid J, Schwarzmann P, Binder B, Burkat J, Klose R 1996 Field test to evaluate telepathology with remote driven microscopy – Project HISTKOM. Cell Vision 3; 479–481

Schwartzmann P 1992 Telemicroscopy: design considerations for a key tool in telepathology. Zentralbl Pathol 138: 183–187

Shimosato Y, Yagi Y, Yamagishi K et al 1992 Experience and present status of telepathology in the National Cancer Center Hospital, Tokyo. Zentralbl Pathol 138: 413–417

Stiles W S 1964 Foveal threshold sensitivity on fields of different colors. Science 145: 1016–1017

Wald G 1964 The receptors of colour vision. Science 145: 1007–1016

Weinberg D S, Allaert F-A, Dusserre P et al 1996 Telepathology diagnosis by means of still digital images: an international validation study. Hum Pathol 27: 111–118

Weinberg D, Doolittle M 1996 Image management in pathology. Am J Clin Pathol 105 (Suppl 1): S54–S59

Weinstein L J, Epstein J I, Edlow D, Westra W H 1997 Static image analysis of skin specimens: the application of telepathology to frozen section evaluation. Hum Pathol 28: 30–35

Weinstein M H, Epstein J I 1997 Telepathology diagnosis of prostate needle biopsies. Hum Pathol 28: 22–29

Weinstein R S 1991 Telepathology comes of age in Norway (editorial). Hum Pathol 22: 511–513

Weinstein R S, Bhattacharyya A, Halliday B E et al 1995 Pathology consultation services via the Arizona-International Telemedicine Network. Arch Anat Cytol Pathol 43: 219–226

Weinstein R S, Bloom K J, Rozek L S 1987 Telepathology and the networking of pathology diagnostic services. Arch Pathol Lab Med 111: 646–652

Weinstein R S, Bloom K J, Rozek L S 1989 Telepathology. Long distance diagnosis. Am J Clin Pathol 91 (Suppl 1): S39–S42

Weinstein R S, Bloom R J, Krupinski E A et al 1992 Human performance studies of the video microscopic component of a dynamic telepathology system. Zentralblat Pathol 138: 399–401

Wold L E, Weiland L H 1992 Telepathology at the Mayo. Clin Lab Manage Rev 1: 174–175

Wolf G, Petersen D, Dietel M, Petersen I 1998 Telemicroscopy via the internet. Nature 391: 613–614

Jem Rashbass

Internet resources in histopathology

During the last decade, advances in molecular biology have revolutionised the science and practice of histopathology; in the next 10 years, we are likely to experience as great a change, if not greater, due to the exploitation of advances in information technology. The development of shared communication standards and advances in software design, and the timeliness of several aspects of communication technology have culminated in the arrival of the information age (Coiera 1996). Global networks such as the Internet have the potential to provide access to information resources on computers anywhere in the world. Diverse areas of pathology, whether basic research, routine diagnosis, training or teaching, will all be affected as these facilities become more readily available and achieve a wider degree of acceptance among the profession.

I shall focus first on the technological changes that have been necessary to produce the infrastructure for these international networks. Then, rather than catalogue and compare the range of resources available, I have chosen to look at how these facilities might be used in three separate areas of histopathology: first as part of an integrated pathologist's workstation (Aller 1997) used alongside the microscope for reporting routine histopathology; second the use of Internet-based information resources in the context of teaching and training; finally, the use of algorithms and programs on super-computers on the Internet and World Wide Web for disease modelling and research. The use of the Internet as an infrastructure for telepathology has become increasingly important and is covered elsewhere in this book.

BASIC ADVANCES IN TECHNOLOGY

The Internet is a worldwide network of smaller networks of computers that share a common communication protocol called TCP/IP (transmission control

Dr Jem Rashbass, Clinical and Biomedical Computing Unit, Cambridge Clinical School, Box 11, Addenbrooke's Hospital, Box 111, Hills Road, Cambridge CB2 2QQ, UK

Table 12.1 Summary of the principal changes in technology and information standards required for the development of the WWW

1. A worldwide network of computers called the Internet exists sharing a communication protocol called TCP/IP
2a. A set of document encoding standards have been adopted that allow information in a wide variety of formats to be accessed and interpreted
2b. Hypertext links allow access to information stored anywhere on a computer on the WWW
3. Browser software has been developed that allows information to be interpreted on the user's machine
4. Information entered through a browser on a local computer can be transferred over the Internet for processing on remote computers

protocol/Internet protocol). The basic specifications of TCP/IP arose from ARPAnet, an American defence department network that was developed towards the end of the 1960s at the height of the cold war. TCP/IP was designed to ensure that data could be sent between military sites by a variety of different networks, irrespective of the type of wiring. Each piece of information sent on the network from one site to another is broken down into small discrete packets each of which is electronically tagged with its origin and destination. Each packet is then routed by hardware on the network to its destination using the fastest path possible. If one route becomes blocked or broken during transmission, the subsequent packets are automatically redirected by the hardware routers along another path in an attempt to reach their target. Only when packets reach their destination are they re-assembled. Advantages of the specifications of this communication protocol are that the transfer of information is essentially independent of the type of network wires linking the two computers and that a permanent, fixed link between computers is unnecessary. The simplicity of the protocol also makes it compatible with many computer types and essentially independent of the operating system.

TCP/IP as a communication protocol that allowed information to be sent on networks from one computer to another has been around since the late 1960s, but there was no agreed format for encoding the information by the transmitting computer so that it could be interpreted when it arrived at its destination (Coiera 1997). The situation was analogous to having decided that one should use the Roman alphabet to transmit a document, but not which European language it should be written in. To resolve this problem, scientists led by Tim Berners-Lee working at CERN, the high energy physics research laboratories in Switzerland, produced a series of standards to permit documents to be shared on the Internet between research groups.

1. *Hypertext mark-up language (HTML)* defined a standard by which to incorporate text, images, sound and video (multimedia) into a document. Documents could contain links to other documents within them so called 'hypertext' links.

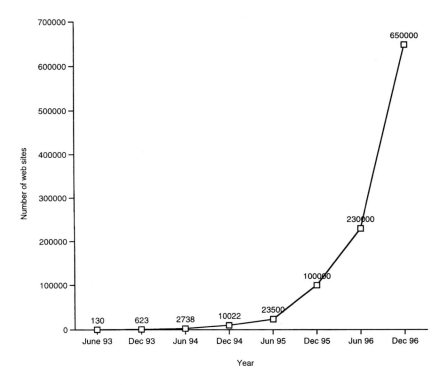

Fig. 12.1 Number of sites on the WWW (data from Matthew Gray of the Massachussets Institute of Technology).

2. The *uniform resource locator* (URL) specified the standard way of formatting a hypertext link which made it capable of encoding the address of any document on the Internet.

3. *Hypertext transfer protocol (http)* defined a method by which information could be transferred between computers and determined how the document should be displayed on the screen when it arrived.

The combination of the network wires with the communication protocol TCP/IP comprise the Internet: the standards defined at CERN by Berners-Lee for sharing information on the Internet form the basis of the World Wide Web (WWW). The standards for the Web have been rapidly adopted (see Table 12.1, Fig. 12.1). Programs have been developed that permit computers to supply information (servers) to users equipped with software (browsers) on their machines capable of interpreting the hypertext links and multimedia resources that any server on WWW produces. The basic standards of HTML coding have been maintained and greatly enhanced by adding new technologies.

INTERNET, INTRANETS AND EXTRANETS

The increased use of the Internet that occurred with the development of the WWW rapidly resulted in network congestion. In addition, information

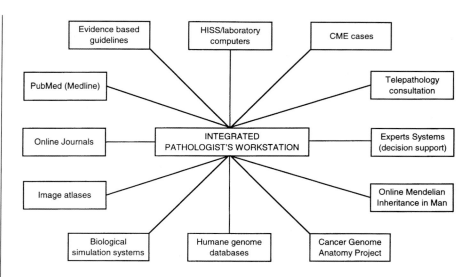

Fig. 12.2 A schematic diagram illustrating the range of Internet-based resources that could be accessed on an integrated pathologist's workstation.

transferred on the Internet could be easily read by anyone connected to the network and data was neither secure nor confidential. To address these problems, secure gateways or firewalls have been developed that allow networks within organisations to be connected to the Internet. All network traffic through the firewall is monitored and access can be restricted. This separate internal network is an *intranet*. Intranets use all the technologies of the Internet but are either completely separate or connected to it through a firewall.

Data encryption methods have been developed that permit information to be encoded so that it is not easily read on the open networks that make up the Internet (Makris et al 1997). These methods of encryption allow two networks, each protected by its own firewall, to be linked using the global network of the Internet. The data transferred between the two is encoded so that others cannot read it. Such a system, an *extranet*, permits international organisations to use otherwise insecure international networks to join separate sites together and share data confidentially.

INTERNET RESOURCES FOR THE PATHOLOGISTS WORKSTATION

During the next few years, hospital laboratories will make greater use of Internet technologies, including intranets and extranets, to access their local systems (Berrios et al 1995, Lowe et al 1996). With this will come the potential for the seamless integration of web-based resources accessible through secure gateways that are beyond the confines of a hospital's information system (Fig. 12.2). Aller (1997), writing on the design of an integrated pathologist's workstation, notes that after the local laboratory and hospital information systems, the WWW provides access to the third most valuable information resource for the diagnostic pathologist. An indication of the variety, integration and depth of these resources is given below; the extensive use of the Internet as a medium for telepathology (Mun et al 1995, Della Mea et al 1996, Balis 1997) is covered elsewhere (*see* Chapter 11).

INTEGRATED BIOMEDICAL DATABASES

With the rapid increase in biomedical knowledge, new tools have been developed which allow close integration of separate databases of biological information. The greatest impetus for this has come from the human genome project and related studies on the molecular biology and genetics of disease. To deal with this information deluge, the National Center for Biotechnology Information, part of the National Library of Medicine in the US, has developed an integrated, WWW-based information system. This project combines the Medline reference databases (as PubMed) with the DNA and protein sequence databases (Benson et al 1998), which are in turn linked to chromosome maps within the human genome mutation database and the electronic online version of Victor McCusick's genetic disease database, On-line Mendelian Inheritance in Man. In addition, a new project, the Cancer Genome Anatomy Project aims to link histopathological features of individual malignancies with specific molecular mutations in the tumours. Each of these resources provides valuable, up-to-date information of use to the diagnostic histopathologist.

PUBMED

The data within PubMed are drawn from Medline dating back to the 1966 database and contain the whole of the Medline citation with abstracts from more than 3800 biomedical journals and over 8.6 million records. Each reference before entry into Medline is manually coded with keywords using Medical Subject Headings (MeSH), which results in a delay of 1–6 months before a reference enters the formal Medline or PubMed databases. Medline is updated weekly but, in addition, a new pre-Medline database has been added within PubMed which is updated daily and contains references prior to the formal Medline entry which has the MeSH headings. This pre-Medline project and PubMed itself is a collaboration between the National Library of Medicine and publishers of biomedical literature who submit data to the pre-Medline database electronically. Hypertext links are available from the PubMed references to such full text journal articles that are made available on-line by the publishers themselves. The relationship between the National Library of Medicine and the publishers is symbiotic. The publishers may use the PubMed citation number in the electronic resources for their journals while the National Library of Medicine provides a hypertext link to the full text on-line version of the published article. Access to most full text journals is not free and users pay either a standard subscription to the journal or are charged on a pay-per-view basis.

The distribution and development of full text electronic journals has been relatively slow. The publishers have clearly been anxious about the potential loss of revenue and have been slow to embrace the new technology. Recent evidence, however, suggests that paper subscriptions can increase as a result of the introduction of an on-line version. Academic-based companies such as the High-wire press that was formed out of work conducted in Stanford University's medical library have developed techniques for converting full text journals from their paper format into electronic versions. To date, they have 27 projects, including journals such as *Science* and *Blood*, but by the middle of 1998 will have added another 70 journals, including the *British Medical Journal* (Delamothe 1997).

ON-LINE MENDELIAN INHERITANCE IN MAN (OMIM)

OMIM (Brandt 1993, McKusick & Amberger 1993, Rashbass 1995) is the electronic version of Victor McCusick's database of genetic diseases with more than 8000 entries. Twelve subject editors are responsible for the individual areas of the database and information is updated daily. Before June 1994, each new entry was given a 6 digit number (the MIM number) where mode of inheritance was coded by the first digit (1 = autosomal dominant; 2 = autosomal recessive; 3 = X-linked; 4 = Y-linked; and 5 = mitochondrial). Since June 1994, all new entries are given sequential MIM numbers from 600000. Within each database entry are fields for the disease title, allelic variants, references and clinical synopsis. The title can be marked by an asterisk (*) if the entry has been confirmed as a unique Mendelian locus or by a hash (#) if the entry is a general phenotypic description. There is in-depth information on the clinical manifestations and the relevant pathology, and each entry is linked by hypertext to PubMed, DNA sequence and protein databases.

The histopathological manifestations of uncommon genetic diseases can be found by searching the OMIM database, providing the pathologist with access to information and references that may be extremely difficult to find in all but the largest of specialised textbooks.

HUMAN GENOME MUTATION DATABASE (HGMD)

Illustrating the global nature of the Internet and WWW, the HGMD (Cooper et al 1998, Krawczak & Cooper 1997), though linked to OMIM and PubMed from the National Library of Medicine, is maintained in Cardiff, UK. The HGMD collects published information on details of mutations associated with specific inherited diseases to identify the mutations and their pathological significance. It aims to provide information for researchers and diagnosticians involved in molecular medicine. The use of such molecular databases in diagnostic histopathology is likely to increase as pathologists increasingly correlate molecular abnormalities with the morphological features seen on routine microscopy. The ability to analyse specific mutations by the polymerase chain reaction on wax-embedded tissue places diagnostic histopathology in the front line of work to correlate microscopic phenotype with genotype.

CANCER GENOME ANATOMY PROJECT

The main focus of the human genome project has been the identification of the molecular basis of inherited diseases. Somatic mutations that occur as part of malignant transformation of cells are specifically excluded from both the

HGMD and OMIM databases except where they are part of an inherited predisposition to malignancy. The aim of the CGAP from the National Cancer Institute is to address this deficiency and to provide a comprehensive genetic profile of normal cells and those at all stages of cancer development (Kuska 1996, O'Brien 1997). The aim is to identify specific and sensitive molecular markers of neoplasia by studying the molecular differences between tumours, even when those tumours appear similar histopathologically. The project is at an early stage and the first phase is the development of a tumour gene index for all genes expressed in breast, prostate, lung, colon and ovarian cancers. Microdissection techniques are being used to isolate areas of tumours believed to be most informative and therefore most likely to produce cDNA libraries that best represent the diversity of transcripts expressed in these tumours. The work is closely correlated with the morphology of individual tumours.

The CGAP has the potential to provide valuable information for diagnostic pathologists. Internet access to the CGAP databases provides images of the morphological features of individual tumours and the molecular alterations common to that tumour type. Pathological diagnoses of solid tumours in the early years of the next millennium will no doubt proceed along a similar route to the cytogenetic analysis in correlations that are now routine in haemato-pathology.

ONLINE IMAGE ATLASES

High quality images can be distributed relatively easily over the WWW and have the potential to provide a valuable reference resource for the diagnostic pathologist (Lowe et al 1996, Rashbass & Vawer 1996, Della Mea et al 1997, Eusebi et al 1997, Flandrin 1997, Horn et al 1997). The cost of storage and production of each image is small, so that, in contrast to conventional printing in books, many different views of one entity can be provided. The technical aspects and the strengths and weaknesses of image capture, digitisation and storage have been extensively reviewed (Balis 1997, Balis 1997, Furness 1997). Issues of copyright, validation and authentication applies to images in the same way as other Internet based resources (see below) and is one of the most significant problem facing the development of this new technology. Nevertheless, as a diagnostic support in histopathology extensive, well catalogued image archives will be invaluable.

CONTINUING MEDICAL EDUCATION VIA THE INTERNET

Continuing medical education over the WWW has been hailed as an efficient means of delivering CME to the community at large (Kruper et al 1994, Bouffard 1996, Frisby 1996, McEnery et al 1996, Shortliffe et al 1996, Horn et al 1997, Richardson & Norris 1997), but formal studies of its effectiveness are sparse and much of the evidence of is anecdotal. Web technology lends itself to the cost effective distribution of CME material which can be combined images, text, sound and video (Horn et al 1997, Rashbass 1998). Case histories, clinical summaries, laboratory investigations and micrographs can all be accessed and made available from a variety of different servers. Pathologists can access the information at leisure any time of the day and the cost of

Table 12.2 Strengths and weaknesses of the use of the WWW to distribute and access information

Advantages	Disadvantages
An extensive amount of information	Information may not be reviewed or verified
Combines text, images sound and video	It can be difficult to know the original source or publisher
Access is relatively easy	The large amount and poor quality of much of the information can make finding specific resources difficult and time consuming
Information is easily updated and corrected if necessary	Out of date information may never be removed
Can be accessed by hundreds of users simultaneously	Copyright controls are unclear
Not restricted to a single make of computer	Internet access is not encouraged in the NHS. Sophisticated security systems are essential to protect HISS systems
Resources anywhere on the Internet can easily be linked together and, therefore, one is not limited to in-house facilities	Can be very wasteful of time and in some cases even addictive
Information is cheap and easy to produce – few production or distribution overheads	
Allows users to exploit the power of remote computers to perform complex tasks	

accommodation and travel to meetings is reduced. Answers to CME questions can be submitted electronically and marked anonymously by the computer, significantly reducing the administrative burden of the system and removing the sense of judgement associated with peer assessment. Computer systems can also be used to monitor the amount of time each participant spends on individual CME exercises and there is the potential for individual resources to be linked together (for example to PubMed references). Inevitably, the knowledge that a pathologist visited a Web site to complete a CME exercise is no guarantee that any benefit was actually achieved (Wyatt 1997), but the same could be said of those who attend meetings but doze during the presentations!

CME over the Internet is not without its problems (Table 12.2). Connections can be difficult or slow when standard telephone lines are used and those cases with a significant image content can be an inefficient use of time if each image takes several minutes to download. In histopathology, selected digital images are no replacement for formal evaluation of microscope slides and electronic CME should not be seen as a replacement for slide clubs. The recent development of a Web accessible microscope where the stage and objectives can all be controlled through a web browser may well revolutionise teaching and CME (Burton & Farkas 1998, Wolf et al 1998).

The quality of digital images can be highly variable. In radiology, where digital image transfer is now commonplace, there is much discussion of the effects that 'lossy' compression techniques (extracting data from the original image to reduce the file size) may have on the diagnostic quality of the images. This problem is, in general, not seen in histopathology where the combination of tissue architecture with the ability to increase resolution by changing microscope objectives can provide more information. However, if digital images are to be used in cytopathology, 'lossy' compression of images may affect the resolution and lose details in features such as nuclear chromatin.

Technological problems that arise in electronic systems are relatively easy to overcome when compared with the administrative and practical aspects involved in the introduction of new teaching methods (Wyatt 1996, Impicciatore et al 1997, Wyatt 1997). Friedman has listed 10 reasons why the WWW may fail to change education and many of these focus on the difficulties that medical schools face when trying to introduce and evaluate new electronic resources in the curriculum (Friedman 1996). As with many technological advances they are often, of necessity, enthusiast lead and evaluation is performed by groups committed to the system who are likely to be much more tolerant of faults than the final users. Considerable care must be taken when designing Internet-based CME systems to produce well structured questionnaires for feedback and to evaluate usage statistics intelligently. Rigorous and specific methods of evaluation designed for information technology and informatics need to be applied to ensure that the appropriate variables are measured (Friedman & Wyatt 1997). There is a danger as Wyatt has noted (Wyatt 1996) that we are led by technology push rather than clinical pull.

VALIDATION OF INFORMATION ON THE INTERNET

Anyone with Internet access can easily publish information on the WWW. As a result, the amount of information is vast, most of it is not peer reviewed and it can be difficult or even impossible to check the origin of the information. In addition, hypertext technology allows the user to move from one Web site to another and for the unwary to drift into uncharted territories at the fringes of the Internet (Weisbord et al 1997). There have been several studies on the evaluation and validation of Web resources, the results of which confirm the anxieties that many have that misleading information of dubious value is easily found (Bower 1996, Impicciatore et al 1997, Wyatt 1997). The problem of validating published works is nothing new. Even in the sixteenth century, pamphlets produced by Martin Luther in Wittenbourg in Saxony were reprinted and distributed by sympathetic printers elsewhere in Europe and had a considerable influence on public opinion. The Web only represents the latest technology for publishing and distribution of information and, as such, will require a range of new guidelines and standards that go beyond simply the assessment of the content by which to judge Web sites. Methods that have been applied to other electronic distribution systems such as electronic textbooks, telemedicine and decision support systems will need to be adapted so that they can be applied to the Internet (Friedman & Wyatt 1997).

Traditional medical training teaches aspects of critical appraisal of information from published journals and textbooks. The speed of the arrival of the information age has left much of the medical profession unprepared and untrained in the formal aspects of information evaluation from Web sites. New methods of evaluation of electronic resources are an essential new generic skill which should underpin electronic methods of CME. These need to be acquired by ward clinicians, not just pathologists, as the advances in information technology provide ever increasing amounts of information in relatively easily accessible ways.

EXPERIMENTAL SYSTEMS IN HISTOPATHOLOGY ACCESSIBLE OVER THE INTERNET

The Internet is valued as a vast information storage and retrieval system – essentially a global electronic library. However, this use obscures the much smaller, but intellectually more challenging, use of the network, where the Internet provides access to computer applications of considerable complexity available on remote supercomputers. Some of these systems we take for granted: for example, the search engine AltaVista™ is provided free to the Internet community by Compaq. This supercomputer program has the ability to search databases of millions of Web pages within milliseconds and also to translate retrieved links from one European language to another on-the-fly. In molecular biology, largely as a result of the discipline Bioinformatics, computational resources are widely available over the Internet. These provide the bench scientist with a range of tools, such as access to complex sequence alignment algorithms and secondary structure prediction models that are now routine tools in the molecular and cell biology laboratory (Benson et al 1998).

The last few years have begun to see the development of cellular modelling systems directly applicable to the histopathologist. Amongst these are cybermouse, cybermensch (Sieburg 1994, Sieburg & Clay 1991) and the Biological Toolbox (Rashbass 1996, Vawer & Rashbass 1997) (see below). These are based upon mathematical models of disease mechanism which have been adapted for use by biologists as *in silico* experimental systems. As our understanding of basic disease mechanisms grows and we accumulate more pieces of data of how cellular pathways interact, it becomes increasingly difficult to predict how these systems combine to produce the overall cellular environment. One traditional approach to these problems has been to model or describe each step in the system mathematically and then combine the equations to test the simulation (Hills 1993). This approach is particularly valuable where the data are largely quantitative or where two disparate hypothesis need to be distinguished. However, in many of the analyses the results are presented as complex differential equations which are difficult for the biologist without extensive mathematical knowledge to interpret or are difficult to compare with data derived directly from laboratory experiments. In some cases, visual displays of cellular behaviour have been introduced and these provide a simulacrum of the biological behaviour (Stekel et al 1995, Rashbass et al 1996). Many of these are highly stylised and produce only a snapshot of the process. Furthermore, they do not provide the experimental biologist who does not have extensive computer programming experience with the tools necessary to perturb or alter the system and therefore perform the *in silico* experiments.

With the arrival of improved computer communication and Web browser interfaces, Internet-based, accessible cellular environments designed specifically for biologists with little specialist computer expertise have been developed. Hans Sieburg from UCSD has developed the cybermouse and cybermensch as part of the virtual Wet lab (Sieburg 1994, Sieburg 1996). This system is designed to allow biologists to manipulate a virtual immune system and to study the spread of HIV infection in immunocompromised Hu-SCID mice. A new programming language called SLANG (Simulator LANGuage) written specifically for biologists has been developed in which each cell type can be allocated rules of how the cells interact with other cells of the immune system and whether the interactions produce cell proliferation or cell death (Sieburg & Clay 1991). The model has proved valuable and provided interesting insights into how CD4 cells respond to different viral strains of HIV and gave information on the rates of cell turnover that occur following HIV infection (Sieburg et al 1993).

More complex models of pathological processes are beginning to emerge, for example the Biological Toolbox (Rashbass 1996, Vawer & Rashbass 1997). This is an entirely Web-based experimental system developed to provide a simulation environment for biological experiments. Each cellular resource (division, differentiation, release or response to a morphogen or cytokine) can be defined and cells distributed in the spatial array in the model using a Web-based form. The model will then calculate cell growth, differentiation and movement as the system develops over a period of time and 'grows' through a series of biological cycles. The growth cycles are then combined in a short video sequence showing the cellular movement, growth and differentiation; these movies can be viewed over the Internet by the experimental biologist. In addition, the system can be perturbed by the introduction of somatic mutations that alter the properties of individual cells during the differentiation process and the effects of this visualised. The program provides a computer simulation environment that biologists can access at the laboratory bench and run in parallel with wet experiments. The power of the system comes from its flexibility and though, of necessity it is only an approximation to the biological system, it permits complex hypotheses to be tested in parallel with the wet experimental system.

Inevitably, computational models are limited by a lack of our understanding of the underlying biology and the need to introduce approximations into the mathematical analyses. Most simulations with only a few exceptions are based on two dimensional cellular interactions. Although they may appear removed from true biology it is perhaps of value to remember that many cell biological analyses take place in immortalised cell lines containing numerous uncharacterised molecular defects where the experimental perturbation involves the transfection of virally driven, non-physiological quantities of biologically active compounds. The *in silico* environment is in its infancy, but is one of the few methods with the potential to permit the simulation of complex biological pathways that are beginning to dominate our understanding of cell biology.

FUTURE DEVELOPMENTS

On average, the power of a computer doubles every 18 months, while the cost halves (Moore's Law) and new advances in technology occur all the time.

Pathology is one of the most IT intensive environments in the medical field with a long history of the use of computers to store and administer data. The introduction of the shared communication standards discussed in this chapter are likely to see the breakdown of barriers that, to date, have made most laboratory computer systems unable to share information. With this will come a greater emphasis on distributed information, with repositories of images, references and guidelines all provided from centrally managed national and international computers. Disciplines such as evidence based pathology (Fleming 1996) are beginning to emerge, and this will inevitably draw on Internet technologies to make the latest, best practice available to the pathologist in the reporting room. Access to decision support systems such as those developed by Diamond and co-workers (Diamond et al 1994a, 1994b) in haematopathology will begin to appear on the Internet, and will be come an integral part of the pathologists workstation. Telepathology (Della Mea et al 1997b), with the ability to discuss cases in real-time online with international experts will become common practice.

These advances are not without their problems; careful evaluation, validation of information and the cost-benefits will need to be addressed before they are widely implemented. Nevertheless, these changes in information technology are already affecting our everyday life and have the potential to revolutionise the practice of many aspects of histopathology.

References

Aller R D 1997 The pathologist's workstation. Clin Lab Med 17: 201–228

Balis U J 1997 Imaging input technology. Clin Lab Med 17: 151–174

Balis U J 1997 Optical considerations in digital imaging. Clin Lab Med 17: 189–200

Balis U J 1997 Telemedicine and telepathology. Clin Lab Med 17: 245–261

Benson D A, Boguski M S, Lipman D J et al 1998 GenBank. Nucleic Acids Res 26: 1–7

Berrios D C, Dreyer J, Newman T et al 1995 Design of a hypertext clinical laboratory testing database and implementation of a World Wide Web test information service. Am J Clin Pathol 104: 327

Bouffard K 1996 CME today looks to the future. Mich Med 95: 26–30

Bower H 1996 Internet sees growth of unverified health claims [news]. BMJ 313: 381

Brandt K A 1993 The GDB Human Genome Data Base: a source of integrated genetic mapping and disease data. Bull Med Libr Assoc 81: 285–292

Burton K, Farkas D L 1998 Telemicroscopy. Net progress Nature 391: 540–541

Coiera E 1996 The Internet's challenge to health care provision. BMJ 312: 3–4

Coiera E 1997 Guide to medical informatics, the Internet and telemedicine. In: London: Chapman and Hall, 376

Cooper D N, Ball E V, Krawczak M 1998 The human gene mutation database. Nucleic Acids Res 26: 285–287

Delamothe T 1997 Developing www.bmj.com. BMJ 315: 1558

Della Mea V, Puglisi F, Forti S et al 1996 Telepathology through the Internet. J Telemed Telecare 2: 24–26

Della Mea V, Puglisi F, Forti S et al 1997 Expert pathology consultation through the Internet: melanoma versus benign melanocytic tumours. J Telemed Telecare 3: 17–19

Diamond L W, Mishka V G, Seal A H et al 1994a A clinical database as a component of a diagnostic hematology workstation. Proc Annu Symp Comput Appl Med Care 298–302

Diamond L W, Nguyen D T, Andreeff M et al 1994b A knowledge-based system for the interpretation of flow cytometry data in leukemias and lymphomas. Cytometry 17: 266–273

Eusebi V, Foschini L, Erde S et al 1997 Transcontinental consults in surgical pathology via the Internet. Hum Pathol 28: 13–16

Flandrin G 1997 Image bank, diagnostic codification and telediagnosis in hematology. Leuk Lymphoma 25: 97–104

Fleming K A 1996 Evidence-based pathology [editorial]. J Pathol 179: 127–128

Friedman C P 1996 Top ten reasons the World Wide Web may fail to change medical education. Acad Med 71: 979–981

Friedman C P, Wyatt J C 1997 Evaluation methods in medical informatics. In: Orthner H F (ed) Computers in medicine. New York: Springer, 311

Frisby A J 1996 The Internet and medical education. Del Med J 68: 602–605

Furness P N 1997 The use of digital images in pathology. J Pathol 183: 253–263

Hills W D 1993 Why physicists like models and why biologists should. Curr Biol 3: 79–81

Horn K D, Sholevhar D, Nine J et al 1997 Continuing medical education on the World Wide Web (WWW). Interactive pathology case studies on the Internet. Arch Pathol Lab Med 121: 641–645

Impicciatore P, Pandolfini C, Casella N et al 1997 Reliability of health information for the public on the World Wide Web: systematic survey of advice on managing fever in children at home [see comments]. BMJ 314: 1875–1879

Krawczak M, Cooper D N 1997 The human gene mutation database. Trends Genet 13: 121–122

Kruper J A, Lavenant M G, Maskay M H et al 1994 Building Internet accessible medical education software using the World Wide Web. Proc Annu Symp Comput Appl Med Care 32–36

Kuska B 1996 Cancer genome anatomy project set for take-off [news]. J Natl Cancer Inst 88: 1801–1803

Lowe H J, Antipov I, Walker W K et al 1996 WebReport: a World Wide Web based clinical multimedia reporting system Proc AMIA Annu Fall Symp 314–318

Makris L, Argiriou N, Strintzis M G 1997 Network and data security design for telemedicine applications. Med Inf (Lond) 22: 133–142

McEnery K W, Roth S M, Walkup R V 1996 Radiology CME on the Web using secure document transfer and internationally distributed image servers. Proc AMIA Annu Fall Symp 37–40

McKusick V A, Amberger J S 1993 The morbid anatomy of the human genome: chromosomal location of mutations causing disease. J Med Genet 30: 1–26

Mun S K, Elsayed A M, Tohme W G et al 1995 Teleradiology/telepathology requirements and implementation. J Med Syst 19: 153–164

O'Brien C 1997 Cancer genome anatomy project launched [news]. Mol Med Today 3: 94

Rashbass J 1995 Online Mendelian inheritance in man. Trends Genet 11: 291–292

Rashbass J 1996 Modelling tissues on the computer. Trends Cell Biol 6: 280–281

Rashbass J 1998 Why use the Internet to teach pathology? J Clin Pathol 51: 179–182

Rashbass J, Stekel D, Williams E D 1996 The use of a computer model to simulate epithelial pathologies. J Pathol 179: 333–339

Rashbass J, Vawer A 1996 A networked computer program for managing a national external quality assurance scheme in cytopathology. Cytopathology 7: 377–385

Richardson M L, Norris T E 1997 On-line delivery of continuing medical education over the World-Wide Web: an on-line needs assessment. Am J Roentgenol 168: 1161–1164

Shortliffe E H, Barnett G O, Cimino J J et al 1996 Collaborative medical informatics research using the Internet and the World Wide Web. Proc AMIA Annu Fall Symp 125–129

Sieburg H B 1994 Methods in the Virtual Wetlab I: rule-based reasoning driven by nearest-neighbor lattice dynamics. Artif Intell Med 6: 301–319

Sieburg H B 1996 *In silico* environments augment clinical trials. IEEE Eng Med Biol 47–59

Sieburg H B, Baray C, Kunzelman K S 1993 Testing HIV molecular biology in *in silico* physiologies ISMB 1: 354–361

Sieburg H B, Clay O K 1991 The Cellular Device Machine Development system for modelling biology on the computer. Complex Systems 5: 575–601

Stekel D, Rashbass J, Williams E D 1995 A computer graphic simulation of squamous epithelium. J Theor Biol 175: 283–293

Vawer A, Rashbass J 1997 The biological toolbox: a computer program for simulating basic biological and pathological processes. Comput Methods Programs Biomed 52: 203–211

Weisbord S D, Soule J B, Kimmel P L 1997 Poison on line – acute renal failure caused by oil of wormwood purchased through the Internet. N Engl J Med 337: 825–827

Wolf G, Petersen D, Dietel M et al 1998 Telemicroscopy via the Internet. Nature 391: 613–614

Wyatt J C 1996 Commentary: telemedicine trials – clinical pull or technology push. BMJ 313: 1380–1381

Wyatt J C 1997 Commentary: measuring quality and impact of the World Wide Web. BMJ 314: 1879–1881

Index